DATE DUE			
GAYLORD			PRINTED IN U.S.A.

D1505549

Complementary and Integrative Medicine in Pain Management

Complementary and Integrative Medicine in Pain Management

Michael I. Weintraub, MD, FACP, FAAN

Ravinder Mamtani, MBBS, MD, FACPM

Marc S. Micozzi, MD, PhD

Editors

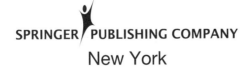

SPRINGER PUBLISHING COMPANY
New York

Springer Publishing Company, LLC
11 West 42nd Street
New York, NY 10036
www.springerpub.com

Acquisitions Editor: Sheri W. Sussman
Production Editor: Julia Rosen
Cover design: Joanne E. Honigman
Composition: Apex Publishing, LLC

08 09 10 11/ 5 4 3 2 1

Library of Congress Cataloging-in-Publication Data

Complementary and integrative medicine in pain management / Michael I. Weintraub, Ravinder Mamtani, Marc S. Micozzi, editors.
    p. ; cm.
Includes bibliographical references and index.
ISBN 978-0-8261-2874-4 (alk. paper)
1. Pain—Alternative treatment. I. Weintraub, Michael I. II. Mamtani, Ravinder. III. Micozzi, Marc S., 1953–
[DNLM: 1. Pain—therapy. 2. Complementary Therapies. WL 704 C7367 2008]

RB127.C643 2008
616'.047—dc22   2007051943

Printed in the United States of America by Book-Mart Press.

Dedicated to Anita, Jeffrey, and Lisa, my central energy source.

—Michael I. Weintraub

To Mother Teresa, with whom I had the distinct pleasure of working in Albania in 1991. From her I learnt the value of focusing on the patient as a whole with the symptoms, rather than on the symptoms alone that the patient has.

To my esteemed colleague and my mentor, late Joseph A. Cimino, MD, who continued to encourage and support me in my endeavors aimed at promoting health, and alleviating human pain and suffering.

To my wife, Jaishree, and my children Raashi and Ronac, who have always believed in my work, and continue to remain a constant source of inspiration in furthering my goals of empowering people with information that would enable them to make informed choices concerning health.

—Ravinder Mamtani, MD

Contents

PART II. MANUAL AND HAND-MEDIATED MODALITIES

PART III. ASIAN MEDICAL THERAPIES

PART IV. HERBAL MEDICINE, PLANT-BASED THERAPIES AND HOMEOPATHY

Editors

Michael I. Weintraub, MD, FACP, FAAN, is a neurologist and pain medicine specialist and a leading proponent of complementary and alternative medicine (CAM). He served as the first Director of American Academy of Neurology Course on Alternative Medicine in 1999 and 2000. He has performed original and pioneering research with laser biostimulation in carpal tunnel syndrome and magnetic biostimulation using both static and time-varying magnetic fields to reduce neuropathic pain in diabetic peripheral neuropathy and carpal tunnel syndrome. He has published over 200 articles in leading peer-reviewed journals, provided chapters for several textbooks, written three books, and edited several books.

He has received many awards including being the recipient in 1991–1992 of American Journal of Pain Management Award for Outstanding Contribution to the Interdisciplinary Pain Management Literature with paper "Litigation-Chronic pain syndrome: a distinct entity. Analysis of 210 cases." He has been named in "Best Doctors in New York" (*New York Magazine*) 4 years in a row voted by his peers.

Dr. Weintraub attended medical school at State University of New York (SUNY) at Buffalo and completed his neurology training at Yale University School of Medicine. He has held faculty positions at SUNY–Buffalo, Yale, Boston University, Albert Einstein College of Medicine as well as his current faculty appointments as Clinical Professor of Neurology and Medicine at New York Medical College, and also Adjunct Clinical Professor of Neurology at Mt. Sinai School of Medicine.

Ravinder Mamtani, MBBS, MD, FACPM, is a preventive and occupational medicine specialist. He was a Professor of Clinical Community and Preventive Medicine, and Associate Professor of Clinical Medicine at New York Medical College, and the Section Chief of Complementary Medicine at the Westchester Medical Center, New York. Effective December 2007 he assumed a senior faculty position at Weill Cornell Medical College and has been seconded to its medical school facility in

Qatar. Dr. Mamtani is a keen teacher, educator and takes pride in his clinical and research accomplishments.

Dr. Mamtani earned his medical degree from University of Delhi, India, and received his postgraduate training in United Kingdom and at New York Medical College/Our Lady of Mercy Medical Center. He is a Diplomate of the American Board of Preventive Medicine in the specialties of general preventive medicine and public health, and occupational medicine. Well-known for his evidence-based approach to medicine, he sees patients/persons with an interest in preventive and integrative approaches. His clinical interests include lifestyle medicine, and management of patients with chronic pain, women's health issues, stress-related conditions, cancer, and other chronic health problems.

Marc S. Micozzi, MD, PhD, is a physician–anthropologist who has worked to create science-based tools for the health professions to be better informed and productively participate in the new fields of CAM and integrative medicine. He was the founding editor-in-chief of the first U.S. journal in CAM, *Journal of Complementary and Alternative Medicine: Research on Paradigm, Practice, and Policy* (1994). He organized and edited the first U.S. textbook, *Fundamentals of Complementary & Alternative Medicine* (1996), now entering a fourth edition (2008). He served as series editor for *Medical Guides to Complementary and Alternative Medicine* with 20 titles in print on a broad range of therapies and therapeutic systems within the scope of CAM. In 1999, he edited *Current Complementary Therapies,* focusing on contemporary innovations and controversies, and *Physician's Guide to Complementary and Alternative Medicine.*

He organized and chaired six national continuing education conferences on the theory, science, and practice of CAM during 1991 to 2001, cochaired with former Surgeon General C. Everett Koop and Dr. Dean Ornish. In 2002, he founded the Policy Institute for Integrative Medicine in Washington, DC to educate policy makers, the health professions, and the general public about needs and opportunities for integrative medicine. From 2003 to 2005, he accepted an interim appointment as executive director of the Center for Integrative Medicine at Thomas Jefferson University in Philadelphia. He is presently an adjunct professor at the University of Pennsylvania in Philadelphia, and at Georgetown University School of Medicine in Washington, DC, and teaches at Drexel University in Philadelphia, Johns Hopkins University in Baltimore, University of California at Irvine and at San Diego, and George Washington University in Washington, DC.

Contributors

Donna Alderman, DO
Hemwall Family Medical Centers
Glendale, CA

Donald Bisson, RRPr
Ontario College of Reflexology
New Liskeard, Ontario, Canada

Elaine Calenda, AOS, NCTMB
Boulder College of Massage
Therapy
Boulder, Colorado

Peggy Codding, Ph.D, MT-BC
Berklee College of Music
Boston, MA

Michael Cohen, JD, MBA
Harvard School of Public Health
Boston, MA

Arthur Fass, MD, FACP, FACC
Phelps Memorial Hospital
Sleepy Hollow, NY

Mark Friedman, DDS
New York Medical College
Valhalla, NY

William H. Frishman, MD
New York Medical College
Valhalla, NY

**Suzanne Hanser, EdD, BMus,
MMus**
Berklee College of Music
Boston, MA

Alan R. Hirsch, MD
Smell & Taste Treatment and
Research Foundation
Chicago, IL

Eric Leskowitz, MD
Spaulding Rehabilitation Hospital
Harvard Medical School
Boston, MA

Angele McGrady, PhD
The University of Toledo
Toledo, OH

Terry Oleson, PhD
California Graduate Institute
Los Angeles, CA

Daniel Redwood, DC
Cleveland Chiropractic College
Overland Park, KS

Amy Tyberg, MD
New York Medical College
Westchester Medical Center
Valhalla, NY

Sharon Weinstein, MD
Huntsman Cancer Institute
University of Utah
Salt Lake City, UT

**Ronald Whitmont, MD, DABIM,
DABHM**
Private Practice
Rhinebeck, NY

Preface

Complementary and alternative medicine (CAM) approaches are currently riding the crest of public enthusiasm. The medical and scientific community, however, remain relatively skeptical and are basically unfamiliar with the specific applications, background history, and specific clinical studies. The pharmacological approach to treatment of various medical conditions is often limited, associated with side effects and high costs. Thus individuals tend to search for another approach that can relieve their pain and suffering.

Specifically, pain syndromes are multifactorial and the role of the psyche is paramount. The goal of this text is to de-mystify the many types of CAM so that physicians can appreciate a potential role in helping patients in a safe and cost-effective manner. We have asked our many expert contributors to provide evidence-based approaches to specific clinical pain syndromes and conditions and a wide range of related neurological conditions. The book is organized according to therapeutic modalities and is divided into four broad sections. The first section relates to modalities that are considered to operate in the realm of mind-body and bioenergetic mechanisms. The second section discusses manual and hand-mediated modalities. The third section addresses alternative medical therapies from Asian healing traditions. The fourth section focuses on the use of herbal remedies, their essential oils, and homeopathy. We also include innovative therapies from within western biomedicine as well as some general, ethical and medical-legal considerations.

We wish to thank our many contributors who have provided their expertise and experience toward making this a clinically useful textbook.

We also want to thank our publisher, Springer Publishing, for all their support and specifically Sheri Sussman and Alana Stein.

Michael I. Weintraub, MD
Briarcliff, NY

Ravinder Mamtani, MD
Valhalla, NY

Marc S. Micozzi, MD, PhD
Bethesda, MD

Introduction

Pain is a commonly reported symptom. Patients with chronic pain and other neurological conditions feel helpless and frustrated. The events and stories surrounding their suffering are innumerable and continue to pose challenges for all those concerned with human welfare and health.

Science and medicine have made remarkable progress in many realms. Mortality rates have declined, and people are living longer. This outcome has resulted in changes in disease patterns and patient priorities. Chronic diseases such as arthritis, musculoskeletal pain, mental health problems and neurological conditions such as Alzheimer's and stroke are becoming more common. Those who suffer continue to live and look for ways and means to alleviate their pain and agony.

The modern medicine of today views the human body as a biomedical machine which can be analyzed, and when needed repaired, altered or modified structurally. Surgery remains an efficacious and effective treatment for many trauma situations. The skill of doctors treating acute emergency illnesses remains high. However, the current, high-technology based health care system is not without its limitations and problems.

While the modern health care system is effective in managing infectious diseases, traumatic injuries, and other acute problems, it is limited in helping those with chronic diseases, the causes of which are related to a number of factors. Modern chronic pain treatments such as surgical interventions and pain medications are inadequate for most and, in many instances, are not safe. Those using pain and other medications remain at risk for developing serious side effects.

Therefore, approaches which encourage patients to participate in programs that integrate conventional and complementary/alternative medicine (CAM) treatments are gaining popularity worldwide. Such approaches are producing positive scientific results, as well as forming the basis of a refreshing and a novel integrative method of treatment and healing.

Evidence from scientific studies is beginning to emerge, documenting both usefulness and limitations/risks associated with various treatments. There is sufficient evidence, for example, to support the use of (a) acupuncture for chronic low back pain and dental pain, (b) hypnosis for pain and anxiety; and (c) mind-body techniques such as meditation, yoga, and biofeedback for chronic pain. Medical doctors who utilize these therapies in their practice report benefits both for their patients and themselves. There are some CAM therapies, however, that have yet to show a benefit or might even present an unjustifiable risk to patients. Examples of those therapies include coffee enemas, Laetrile, ozone therapy, megadoses of vitamins and shark cartilage. Use of these unproven or disproven therapies may also result in loss of valuable time and the opportunity to receive potentially beneficial therapies. This book omits these unproven approaches and focuses on those that have proven benefits.

Fostering and nurturing an evidence-based integrative approach that combines both modern medicine and efficacious CAM will not only promote health but also improve the quality of life for patients with chronic pain and other neurological conditions.

PART I

Mind-Body and Bioenergetic Modalities

Social and Cultural Perspectives on Complementary/ Alternative Medicine in Pain

Marc S. Micozzi

Pain and headache (head pain) are perhaps the two most common functional disorders of the human condition, experienced by virtually everyone on an acute basis, and by many on a chronic, episodic, or recurring basis. Much of the effort in human healing traditions throughout history has been directed at analgesia—the alleviation of pain—through discovery and development of materia medica (opiates, salicylates, etc.), manipulation (e.g., bone setting, chiropractic, traditional osteopathy, physical therapy), manual therapies and massage, yoga, acupuncture, and mind-body approaches, all of which are topics in this book. Energy healing represents a new frontier with ancient roots.

In the history of American medicine, alleviation of pain, together with prevention of death, was one of the two central tenants of rational medicine. Rational medicine in clinical practice was a conscious result of the eighteenth-century Scottish Enlightenment (as manifested by the social philosopher, Adam Smith, in economics, for example). It was brought to the then American Colonies by Drs. Morgan and Hutchinson from the University of Edinburgh to the College of Philadelphia (now the University of Pennsylvania), where they established the first school of medicine in what was to become the United States by charter from Colonial Governor Thomas Penn in 1765. The rest is history.

3

Today, pain is understood as a dynamic condition, not a static pathologic state or lesion. And while curing or removing a painful lesion may eliminate the pain (with the curious exception of phantom pain such as the phantom limb syndrome of amputees), pain exists in many other contexts where there is no lesion to cure or remove. Therefore, the assessment and management of pain, whether alternative or mainstream, must lie in the interaction between mind and body, healer and patient, patient and therapy.

Pain is a subjective complaint, and therefore its improvement is also subjective, yet associated with very high levels of patient satisfaction. That mind-body approaches are proving so successful in the management of pain is another sign that the Cartesian separation of mind and body has been an artificial accommodation to once-limited philosophical and naturalistic understandings of health and healing. This outdated separation in western biomedicine (which is not a factor in Asian medical traditions, for example), perhaps even influences how we are conditioned to experience and express pain itself. In traditional societies in Africa, and elsewhere, psychic pain is often somatized to a specific area of the body and presents as pain in a particular organ rather than as a general mental state.

If the entire body acts beyond the brain-body barrier as the organ of consciousness through the movements of "molecules of emotion" (as postulated by Candace Pert and others), mind-body distinctions begin to lose their meaning. A "gut feeling" is really being felt in the gut. And some of the diffuse pain associated with chronic fatigue syndrome and fibromyalgia, for example, may ultimately be a conditioned response emanating from elsewhere.

The successful alleviation of pain and treatment of other neurological conditions can no longer be considered alternative vs. mainstream—what works should simply be considered good medicine.

CHAPTER 1

Biofeedback

Angele McGrady

Biofeedback (BF) is a mind-body therapy based on operant learning theory. The fundamental principle of BF is that a patient receives information about a specific physiological parameter and with practice, learns to control that aspect of the physiological responses to stress. BF requires monitoring and displaying accurate and meaningful information from a body site in an easily recognizable form. Correct responses are reinforced by sound or visual feedback, facilitating learning. With the guidance of a mental health provider and assuming regular practice of BF, the person can repeatedly and reliably control one or more physiological responses. For example, muscle tension is measured with surface sensors from the forehead; the output is converted to a visual or auditory signal that is made available to the patient, such as a sound that fluctuates depending on the level of tension. Knowing which muscles are tense or relaxed allows the person to learn to self-regulate the physiological process. Undesirable internal states are associated with increased levels of sound or light, and reinforcement is provided for desired responses, such as relaxed muscles.[1] There are three broad categories of BF treatment: stress reduction in which lower arousal is reinforced; muscle retraining, in conditions where muscle tone is lower than desired; and brain wave training, for disorders in which EEG patterns are associated with specific problems of attention and concentration.

MODALITIES AND DEVICES

Electromyograph (EMG), thermal, skin conductance, blood pressure (BP), brain wave, and heart rate are the most common types of feedback. The EMG measures levels of skeletal muscle contraction, and the raw signal is converted usually to an auditory signal. For disorders in which excess muscle tension and over-arousal are associated with symptoms and lowered responsiveness is the goal, surface monitoring (SEMG) is most appropriate. However, when the objective is to increase motor unit potentials, needle technique is often used. Thermal biofeedback (TBF) provides information about the temperature of the skin, which is correlated with blood flow in the small arterioles underlying the area where the sensor is placed; the most common placement is on the palmer surface of the index or middle finger of either hand, with occasional placement on the underside of the toes. Skin conductance feedback monitors the activity of the sweat glands directly beneath the sensors. Brain wave (electroencephalogram, or EEG) feedback, also called neurofeedback involves monitoring brain wave activity of certain areas of the brain underlying the electrodes. Heart rate and BP feedback provide information about dysregulation of the cardiovascular system.[2] A newer form of BF is heart rate variability, which facilitates patient learning to control the oscillation (variability) of heart rate.[3] Lower heart rate variability has been linked to medical illness, particularly cardiovascular disease. No matter the specific type of BF, all applications share these factors: an instrument is utilized; the person receives information; correct responses are reinforced; and repetition is necessary for success.

MULTICOMPONENT TREATMENT

BF is often coupled with symptom monitoring, relaxation therapy (RT), patient education, psychotherapy, and medical pharmacotherapy. When the primary objective of treatment is lower arousal, relaxation is an integral part of therapy. Relaxation is of two basic types: active or passive. Active relaxation is defined as producing lower arousal by voluntarily tensing and releasing tension from specific muscle groups and learning to differentiate between tension and relaxation. The goal is to be able to consciously lower tension.[4] Passive relaxation consists of deep breathing or using words, phrases, or imagery. For example, autogenic relaxation uses specific phrases dealing with sensations of heaviness in the muscles and warmth in the hands.[5] The key to effective relaxation is repetition of phrases or behavior (such as breathing) on a daily basis until a reliable relaxation response can be produced quickly when needed.[6] Home practice of relaxation with or without portable feedback devices is critical to learning and long-term maintenance of newly acquired skills. Generalization of the relaxation response to conditions of daily living allows the patient to use relaxation to counter the effects of stressful situations. The experience of decreasing the severity of a stress response or blocking the response with relaxation rather than relying solely on medication increases patients' confidence in their ability to use the technique.[7] Because different relaxation techniques have specific effects, the provider guides the patient to learn to differentiate among multiple maladaptive psychophysiological responses and to match each signal to a strategy: breathing, passive or active relaxation, or imagery.[8]

Patients are asked to record symptoms and these data are reviewed with the provider at each session. Reliable symptom monitoring prior to, during, and following treatment is necessary to first establish the baseline, then monitor the progress of treatment, and finally determine outcome. Symptom monitoring informs treatment and serves as a source of reinforcement of progress. A pretreatment baseline can be easily established if the patient tracks frequency, duration and severity of symptoms, and use of medication prior to the initiation of BF. The length of the baseline and post treatment is determined by the frequency of the symptom. In addition, the patient becomes fully engaged in the therapeutic process when the occasion of the symptom and the patient's attempts to manage the symptom are discussed.

Patient education provides easy-to-understand explanations of the rationale for BF based on physiological principles. The use of SEMG feedback for disorders of excess muscle tension and tension-type headaches is logical and quickly grasped; the relationship between a high-pitched or high-frequency sound and high tension is intuitively obvious. Other symptom-feedback pairs are less so, necessitating greater efforts to make the required tasks comprehensible to patients. For example, a patient with migraine who is going to learn to warm her hands with TBF might be told the following: "When you are in a stressful situation, your body gets ready to react. This reaction includes tensing your muscles, increasing your pulse rate, and sending blood to your muscles. Thus blood is diverted away from nonessential tissues, like your digestive system and your hands and feet. When there is less warm blood in your fingers, they get cold. With feedback, you will learn to warm your hands consciously. This is part of learning how to decrease excessive responses to stress, which seem to be related to your headaches." Regarding EEG feedback, the explanation for its effects may be as follows: "Certain brain wave patterns are associated with sleep, others with attention and good concentration, and still others with lack of attention or daydreaming. You will be able to learn to generate brain waves that are associated with good concentration and paying attention, instead of being distracted or unfocused."

Psychotherapy is combined with BF for patients who have comorbid conditions such as mood or anxiety disorders. For example, patients with episodic headache may also have generalized anxiety disorder or adjustment disorder with anxiety. Clinical depression is often prominent in patients with chronic headaches or other pain syndromes. A recent study of prevalence of depression and chronic headache showed that in women, chronic severe headache and disability were associated with depression in women. A neuron-psycho-chemical association that supports both pain and negative emotional states was suggested.[9] Cognitive-behavioral therapy (CBT) is a type of psychotherapy commonly used in conjunction with BF in anxiety and mood disorders. CBT explores negative and irrational thoughts that are contributing to mood symptoms and teaches the patient to counter these thoughts with more realistic approaches to situations. Therefore, the therapy emphasizes generating more positive thinking patterns and acquiring effective coping skills.[10,11]

It is best but not always possible for the same practitioner to provide both psychotherapy and BF. When a clinical psychologist, clinical counselor, social worker, or psychiatric nurse is also trained in BF, single sessions can integrate psychotherapy, hypnosis, or imagery with BF. For example, the patient might spend the first 30 minutes of a 50-minute session engaged in psychotherapy, and the last 20 minutes practicing BF. On the other hand, the session might consist of 20 minutes of guided imagery-assisted BF to create an atmosphere of trust between patient and practitioner followed by 30 minutes of psychotherapy. The stages of change model may be useful to assess how willing the person is to change,[12] and an experienced therapist is equipped to manage the lack of motivation evidenced by patients in the precontemplation stage or the uncertainty of the contemplation stage.

TREATMENT PROTOCOLS

The number and structure of sessions should be matched to the patient's condition(s) and the severity of the disorders for which treatment is sought. Three basic formats are used in the lower arousal applications of BF: standard, brief, and psychotherapy based. After the clinical interview, and before beginning any BF treatment, a psychophysiological assessment is carried out. This profile consists of measuring muscle tension, skin temperature, heart rate, heart rate variability, and skin conductance under various conditions. First, the patient is asked to sit quietly with eyes closed and then with eyes open. Then, stressful mental imagery or mental arithmetic is used to determine which physiological system responds most acutely. Finally, the patient is then asked to attempt to relax in any familiar way. Information collected during the last phase of the assessment suggests the extent of past experience that the patient brings to the therapeutic setting.[13]

The standard format of BF therapy consists of 8 to 12, 50-minute sessions of BF, RT, and stress management-oriented counseling.[14,15] The limited contact protocol includes 3 to 4 sessions of BF and emphasizes home practice of relaxation. This is appropriate for patients who are highly motivated, can follow directions, and have no more than mild psychopathology.[16] An intensive BF treatment protocol is one in which BF and RT are used as adjuncts to psychotherapy, as is common in treating patients with chronic pain.[17] This format is recommended for patients who have long-standing moderate or severe symptoms, who are poorly motivated, whose lives are focused on pain, or who need in-depth psychotherapy to explore emotional conflicts or interpersonal difficulties. New treatment paradigms continue to emerge. Telemedicine can be considered when the clients are separated from the BF clinic by large distances. In a multi-case report, BF was provided through long distance video conferencing with moderate additional expense but successful pain reduction in migraine.[18] A more intriguing suggestion is that of deCharms et al to provide information from real time functional MRI of the rostral anterior cingulate cortex, the area thought to be involved in pain perception.[19]

It is important to note that BF and RT are not contraindicated in patients who are also medically managed by physicians. In fact, if pain or disability is severe, the BF practitioner may request that the patient return to the physician for medication to facilitate the relaxation process. As symptoms improve, the need for some types of medicine, particularly analgesics or antianxiety agents, may decrease. When log sheets indicate steadily decreasing symptoms that required medication, the patient is encouraged to talk to the physician about lessening the dosage of drugs. The joint management of patients by physicians and BF practitioners is more the norm than the exception.

Headache

This section addresses BF treatment of tension-type and migraine headache with briefer discussions of application of BF to posttraumatic headache and medication overuse headache. A typical 8- to 12-session treatment protocol for tension-type headache includes the following: SEMG BF with sensors placed on the forehead or back of the neck, active and then passive RT, home practice of relaxation, daily symptom logging, and psychotherapy or stress management as appropriate. Patients are trained to decrease tension levels and to produce a general relaxation response. Because surface sensors placed on the forehead detect a wide range of muscular activity, responding to grimacing, frowning, and teeth clenching helps patients to regulate muscle tension and decrease pain.[17] The relaxation process is then generalized to stressful situations where patients feel their muscles tensing or notice the early signs of headache. A typical 8- to 12-session treatment protocol for tension-type headache includes the following: EMG BF with sensors placed on the forehead or back of the neck, active and then passive RT, home practice of relaxation, daily symptom logging, and psychotherapy or stress management as appropriate. Patients are trained to decrease tension levels and to produce a general relaxation response.

The literature on BF in tension type headache supports the effectiveness of EMG BF combined with RT. An excellent review of 30 years of research on behavioral therapy of recurrent headaches summarizes the experimental literature on BF.[20] In tension-type headache, EMG BF combined with relaxation was superior to wait list control, relaxation alone, and amitriptyline. Two earlier reviews investigated the efficacy of BF through an extensive literature review and analysis by a panel of experts.[21,22] In the case of chronic pain, there was strong evidence to support relaxation techniques and hypnosis, and moderately strong evidence for BF and CBT. BF worked best with tension-type headaches.[21] A meta-analysis of 78 publications that included 2,866 participants found that EMG BF alone or combined with RT was superior to no treatment and to pseudo-placebo therapy in tension-type headache.[22]

The most common treatment model for nonpharmacological therapy of migraine headache is TBF accompanied by RT. The treatment regimen used in the author's clinic for patients with migraine consists of four sessions of EMG BF and six to eight sessions of TBF combined with passive relaxation, home practice of relaxation, symptom logging, and stress management or psychotherapy as appropriate.[23] Rigorous evaluation criteria have been used to evaluate controlled studies of psychosocial interventions in migraine. Conclusions were that "thermal biofeedback plus relaxation . . . qualifies as an efficacious treatment for migraine headaches."[24] BF has also been compared with medical therapy in migraine.[25] Abortive ergotamine tartrate was associated with a 30% decrease in headache index in the first month of treatment and an additional 11% decrease later. TBF resulted in an early reduction of 25% and an additional 26% at post-treatment. Seventy-eight percent of the BF group and 40% of the medication group decreased analgesic use by a minimum of 50%.[26] In a meta-analysis involving 2,445 patients with migraine, BF was found to be equivalent to propranolol; both resulted in a 43% improvement in headaches according to patients' diaries. Placebo yielded a 14% improvement, and monitoring alone produced no changes.[27] For migraine headache, temperature BG and relaxation was comparable to propranolol, superior to wait list control or placebo medication and not as effective as flunarizine.[20] Vasudeva et al compared the results of BF in migraineurs with and without aura.[28] Although MA demonstrated the more typical patterns of cerebral blood flow, both groups responded equally well to improvement not related to presence of aura or to differences in CBF.[23] Long-term maintenance of headache improvement mediated by BF and RT therapy is good if patients are able to generalize the relaxation response to stressful situations and continue to use the adaptive coping techniques learned during therapy.[29]

Posttraumatic headache and high medication consumption headache are two problems that pose special therapy challenges for practitioners of BF. Forty subjects with posttraumatic head pain were treated with EMG BF, TBF, and RT. Of the subjects, 53% reported at least moderate improvement in the number of headaches, and 80% found that the therapy increased their ability to relax and cope with the pain. In general, chronicity of posttraumatic pain predicts a poorer response for improvement in therapeutic paradigms dominated by BF.[30] Another challenging population of headache patients is the group who use high doses of multiple classes of medication. Withdrawal of medication, which can be accomplished, although with difficulty, on an outpatient basis, should precede treatment in this group. In a small study of 10 patients, progressive relaxation and BF were found to be helpful in 6 of the 10 patients who were treated. Pain levels and medication use were reduced. However, the involvement of the therapist who provided the CBT was critically important to success.[31]

Grazzi et al tested the effects of BF in a groups of patients with transformed migraine who overused analgesics.[32] The protocol called for inpatient setting with either a complicated pharmacology management program or with the addition of BF with relaxation. The combined group showed fewer headache days and fewer patients relapsed than the group with medicine alone. Although trends were observed earlier, significant group differences were founds only at 36 months, which emphasizes the difficulty in obtaining successful outcome in this patient group.

Children and the elderly are also appropriate candidates for BF therapy. Although the widespread belief that children acquire BF skills much faster than adults is not supported by statistical analysis of outcome data, children's success rate are higher than adults, perhaps because most children do not present with the depressive features so common in adults who struggle with daily pain.[33] Younger patients are often intrigued by the BF equipment, are comfortable with video game type technology, and adapt to the treatment setting quite easily. Holyrod and Drew provided a relaxation CD for children with headaches to use at home and obtained a successful outcome.[34] Both standard and minimal contact models of treatment have been tested and found to be effective in childhood migraine and tension headache.[35-38] Trautman et al conducted a meta-analysis of 23 studies comprising 935 children and adolescents with recurrent headache in which relaxation, biofeedback, CBT, or combined treatments were tested.[39] The success rate of 70% in the treated subjects was significantly better than the 30% of controls who were successful. Elderly persons often require additional sessions and learning may be somewhat slower. Nonetheless, EMG BF has been found to help decrease total headache activity and increase headache-free days in elderly persons.[40]

Musculoskeletal Pain

Patients with chronic pain often report a myriad of psychological and physical symptoms. In addition to pain, patients suffer from sleep disturbance, vague sensations of discomfort, anxiety, and depression. Therefore, successful treatment must comprise interventions for each dysfunction of mind and body. For example, treating patients with chronic low back pain requires a multimodal approach that combines BF with other modalities such as physical therapy, exercise, correction of gait and posture, and CBT.

Although BF will not be the sole therapy, BF is useful in training general relaxation and in correcting specific muscle tension problems. Fifty-seven patients with chronic back pain were provided with EMG BF from the site of the pain and were taught tension-reduction exercises. The EMG BF group did better than either the CBT group or the patients who continued medical treatment alone. At 6- and 24-month follow-up in the BF group, there were significant reductions in pain severity and fewer visits to the health care system.[17] It is important to monitor tension when the patient is in postures other than reclining in a chair because muscles automatically relax if the head is supported by a head rest. Poor posture, bracing, insomnia, and depression are often contributory or perpetuating factors in the long-term pain patient. So EMG BF is provided to the patient while he or she is in the sitting and standing positions. In addition, CBT may be necessary to modify maladaptive thoughts and behaviors as with other chronic pain conditions.[41] In this population, follow-up sessions are strongly recommended because continued relaxation practice is a key component in maintaining improvement. Relapse can occur after patients have learned the basic skills, particularly if lifestyle and posture have not changed.[42]

Similarly to the findings in the headache literature, age past 60 years does not contraindicate BF treatment of patients with chronic pain.[43] Review of mind-body therapies for older adults with pain from osteoarthritis showed that older and younger adults did equally well on achieving the criterion of 50% reduction in symptoms after BF; there was moderate evidence to support progressive muscle relaxation and guided imagery.[44] A 12- to 16-session EMG BF and RT protocol integrated within a multidisciplinary pain program was used to treat an elderly group of patients with cervical pain. The older adults did as well as the younger adults in acquiring self-regulation skills and achieving reduction of pain.[45] A Cochrane review summarized the effectiveness of behavioral therapies in chronic back pain and concluded that mind-body therapies have a moderate positive effect on pain compared with usual medical care or controls (effect size .62).[46]

Fibromyalgia is a complex psychophysiolgical disorder that is manifested by muscle pain, tender points, and sleep disturbance; many sufferers also report headache, fatigue, memory problems, anxiety, and depression. Environmental conditions such as changes in weather and noise level that interrupts sleep are often reported to exacerbate the pain and discomfort. This chronic illness is severely distressing; and physical symptoms are intensified by chronic stress. The person who is already anxious is more aware of body pain and then becomes more anxious when feeling pain.[47]

Management of fibromyalgia syndrome is guided by an evidenced based step wise treatment plan.[48] Mention that chronic pain changes the brain action potential summation of pain stimuli. CBT decrease severity and improve function. Step 1 is diagnosis, then beginning low dose tricyclic antidepressant and CBT. The cognitive component is of major importance, since more intense pain due to mood state may be misinterpreted as worsening of the syndrome. There is strong evidence for efficacy of CBT and moderately strong evidence for the efficacy of BF in fibromyalgia. According to Astin, mind-body therapy in fibromy-algia was effective in increasing self efficacy but not specifically pain.[49] A program of 6 weeks of symptom monitoring followed by 12 sessions of EMG BF was associated with a reduction in pain intensity. The num-ber of doctor and hospital visits was another factor contributing to the reduction of pain.[50] Change in perception of pain from an experimental thermal pain stimulus was reported in normal subjects and in eight pain patients after training with feedback from the rostral anterior cingulate cortex. A protocol of 3 training days, 1–5 runs of 13 minutes each was associated with decreases in the intensity of pain in the patients.[19]

In therapy of temporomandibular disorders, Sherman and Turk recommend that the psychological-behavioral approaches be used with the medical-dental treatments at the time of the initiation of care and not as a last resort.[51] Supporting this contention is the observation that tension levels may not be significantly higher in patients compared to nonpain controls, so factors besides actual muscle tension must be considered in treatment.[52] Positive outcomes in pain reduction were found in almost twice the number of patients treated with SEMG BF compared to no treatment.[53] The incorporation of four sessions of CBT (including progressive relaxation, diaphragmatic breathing, and home practice) into usual care improves pain and decreases the extent of interference with normal activity. The review by Crider et al concludes that surface EMG with adjunctive CBT is efficacious in temporomandibular disorders.[54]

Once again, therapy of chronic neck pain must comprise patient education, relaxation, BF, and CBT. Patients receive explanations of the transmission of the pain signal, increase awareness of and reduce the bracing response, and learn the muscular relaxation response. CBT is used to decrease the habitual negative cognitions that impact the pain experience, including the concept of maladaptive muscle contractions.[55] In a 3-year follow-up of workers with neck or back pain who were on sick leave, the workers who were treated with CBT including relaxation and imagery demonstrated increased scores on the SF-36 (a quality of life inventory that assesses the interference of physical and emotional symptoms on function); more employees returned to work in comparison to the usual care group.[56] The cost effectiveness parameter was significant only for the women in the study. Although not specifically BF because a monitoring instrument was not used, a unique educational feedback intervention was tested in 126 patients with uncomplicated cervical strain who presented to their local emergency room. The experimental group watched a 12-minute video that consisted of education about muscle strain, psychological factors that may affect pain perception and demonstration of deep breathing. All variables assessed (verbal pain rating, ER visits, taking narcotics, and number of urgent care visits) were significantly lower than patients receiving usual care.[57]

Osteoarthritis (OA) and rheumatoid arthritis (RA) are two disorders that differ biologically but share the pain disability associated with pain and emotional distress. Dixon et al grouped data from patients with either OA or RA in a meta-analysis to investigate the effects of psychosocial interventions.[58] A compilation of 23 CBT studies and 5 stress management studies resulted in significantly lower pain post treatment and improved coping compared to control conditions in both RA and OA. Grouping data from patients with both forms of arthritis makes more sense if the primary outcome variables are nonbiological but rather reported pain and psychosocial factors that affect pain. Similarly to other pain conditions, older adults with arthritis pain do as well as younger adults; a review of mind-body therapies for older adults supported the application of BF, guided imagery, and progressive relaxation.[44]

ANXIETY AND MOOD DISORDERS

Anxiety and mood disorders are common psychiatric conditions as well as frequent companions to medical complaints, such as chronic pain. Anxiety disorder may present as cognitive symptoms such as fear of losing control, dying, or going crazy, or as somatic symptoms such as racing heart, sweating, or shortness of breath. Sub-clinical anxiety syndromes often cause sufficient distress and functional impairment to merit therapy.[11] Appropriate candidates for BF include patients with psychiatric illnesses who can learn to modify specific physiological or psychological responses associated with their disorder.[59] In one study of school-age children, teachers identified 150 students as "anxious," although the children were not diagnosed with a specific disorder by a mental health provider. Twelve sessions (six SEMG and six TBF) were provided during a 6-week period. Significant reductions in situational and trait anxiety were reported.[60]

Learning facial relaxation with BF promotes lower central and autonomic nervous system activity and can be effective in managing both the somatic and cognitive components of anxiety.[61] Generalized anxiety disorder was treated in 38 diagnosed adults and in an additional 7 subjects with sub-clinical symptoms. Fifteen sessions of EEG feedback resulted in decreased self-reported and observer-rated anxiety and in improved quality of life.[62] The effects of eight sessions of frontal EMG BF or EEG feedback to increase or to decrease alpha wave activity, or pseudo-meditation control, were compared using a standardized self report inventory. All treated subjects reported significantly decreased anxiety symptoms, which were maintained at 6-weeks follow-up. The authors suggest that in anxiety, the effects of BF may be nonspecific.[63]

With phobic patients, RT is integral to systematic desensitization therapy; gradual exposure to the phobic stimulus is combined with guided relaxation. Psychophysiological approaches including BF and RT are suggested as a first step in management, to be followed by medication if necessary. BF can shorten the time required to learn relaxation under conditions of exposure to the phobic stimulus.[64] Syncope (discussed in more depth in the subsequent section) can also be symptomatic of simple phobia. For example, the sight of blood or injury can result in loss of consciousness in susceptible individuals. In a single case study, EMG and TBF were combined with systematic desensitization to treat an individual with long-standing blood injury phobia. With therapy, the individual learned to identify presyncopal cues and used BF and RT to block syncope when confronted with the phobic stimulus.[65] Neurofeedback has also been used to treat anxiety disorders, particularly generalized anxiety and phobias.[66] Combined with EMG feedback, alpha enhancement training produced a decrease in anxiety scores beyond the placebo effects. According to APA criteria, neurofeedback is categorized as probably efficacious for anxiety.[66] It should be mentioned that working with patients with PTSD, another of the anxiety disorders will always require therapy beyond BF and relaxation. Because some of the causes of chronic pain are events, like motor vehicle accidents or serious work injury, patients should be evaluated for the presence of posttraumatic stress disorder before BF is initiated.[67]

BF has not traditionally been recommended for patients with major depressive disorder or dysthymia. Although there are no contraindications or reports of worsening of depression after BF, the stress management applications presuppose a higher level of sympathetic autonomic arousal, which has not been a characteristic of depression. However, depressed chronic pain patients' sense of helplessness regarding their pain and the limitations induced by pain is a common observation. Because BF is based on the principle of patients' gaining a sense of control over their maladaptive physiology, the experience of success can be translated into a sense of self efficacy. During the course of therapy, the major nonspecific effect of BF, that is, developing the sense of control over physiological responses to stress can facilitate learning of pain control.[68] In summary, assessment of mood is recommended as part of the evaluation for BF for any chronic pain condition; if found, even in sub-clinical severity the nonspecific effects of BF may be mobilized and directed towards improvement in pain and mood while psychotherapy remains the cornerstone of therapy.

AUTONOMIC NERVOUS SYSTEM DISORDERS

Syncope, near syncope, and dizziness are symptomatic of many primary and secondary autonomic disorders. Neurocardiogenic syncope is associated with hypotension and bradycardia; dysautonomia is characterized by progressive and gradual loss of consciousness, which commonly occurs during walking or standing. The rate and magnitude of fall in BP varies among autonomic disorders, but the disorders share the common feature of postural hypotension. Diagnosis is made by tilt table testing, and treatment usually combines pharmacotherapy and behavioral therapy.[69,70] Psychiatric disorders are common in patients with autonomic disorders. Anxiety, mood, substance abuse, and somatoform disorders are common, and evidence supports a common pathway mediated by serotonin. In the case of depression, a relationship between lower BP and depressive symptoms has been proposed.[71]

A case series of 10 patients who were tilt positive and diagnosed with one of the autonomic disorders used BF as part of overall management.

Patients had headache, lightheadedness, dizziness, near syncope, or true syncope. Therapy consisted of 10 to 12 sessions of EMG, TBF, and RT. Active relaxation and EMG BF were introduced initially, followed by TBF and passive relaxation. Five of the 10 patients obtained clinically significant improvement in each of their symptoms. Six of the seven with syncope had none at post-treatment.[72] Modifications to the standard BF protocol are necessary to address the multiple responses that comprise presyncope and syncope. In the initial stage, presyncope, when heart rate and BP are elevated, passive relaxation and hand warming are recommended. Then muscle tensing is used to counter the lightheadedness that is associated with the beginning of the syncopal episode. Patients also apply either progressive or autogenic relaxation to tension-type and migraine headache respectively.[73]

Similar behavioral techniques have been applied to individuals who demonstrate orthostatic intolerance after exposure to microgravity in space. Pilots were trained with BP BF to increase BP under supine and head-up tilt conditions.[74] Autogenic therapy and BF were applied to control motion sickness in otherwise healthy and well-conditioned astronauts. The protocol comprised training multiple physiological responses simultaneously for a total of 6 hours. Transfer of the responses learned in the laboratory to a variety of stimulus conditions, such as rotary chair, flight, and shuttle missions, was accomplished.[75]

SLEEP DISORDERS

Categories of disturbed sleep relevant to this chapter include primary insomnia (one of the dysomnias) and insomnia related to chronic pain. Patients with recurrent pain report difficulties in initiating and maintaining sleep, and the results of a poor night's sleep are daytime fatigue and problems functioning. Besides disordered sleep as a consequence of pain and psych disorders, sleep deprivation, particularly resulting from continuity problems (not simply fewer total hours), increases awareness of pain and may disrupt endogenous pain inhibitory mechanisms in the brain.[76]

Sleep hygiene is always important and should be tried first. Not only are the recommendations relatively simple, but the physician encourages the patient to begin taking responsibility for healthful sleep instead of relying on prescribed medication. Review of the literature on mind-body therapies for sleep disorders supports progressive relaxation, CBT, and stimulus control but does not favor BF alone as treatment of sleep disorders in either primary insomnia or sleep disturbance in chronic pain patients. Progressive relaxation facilitated improvements in decreasing sleep onset time.[77] In contrast, the best evidence to date does not favor

BF alone for treatment of sleep disorders in either primary insomnia or poor sleep in chronic pain patients. Stimulus control therapy is based on the premise that patients have learned to associate the bed with anxiety or stress instead of with relaxation and drowsiness. Patients are encouraged to remove any stressful stimuli from the bedroom and recondition bedtime as a time for relaxation and mental quietness.[78] Morin et al concluded from a review of two meta-analyses that progressive relaxation and stimulus control were well validated and efficacious interventions. CBT was incorporated into a multifaceted program for insomnia.[79] Fifty-eight percent were at least somewhat improved and 91% reduced medication; most encouraging was the finding that improvements were stable.[80]

EPILEPSY

Since the first case study was published in the early seventies, EEG BF has been studied as an adjunct or alternative to anticonvulsant medication. EEG BF has helped individuals with epilepsy to decrease the frequency of seizures and improve performance on neuropsychological testing, as reviewed below. Currently, there are two BF paradigms that are used to provide training in epilepsy. One is based on using the slow cortical potential shifts (SCP) and the other is configured to train with sensorimotor rhythm (SMR). Positive SCPs are associated with cortical inhibition and reduction in seizure frequency, while negativity may reflect cortical hyperexcitability.[81] Twenty-five patients with focal seizures and intractable epilepsy were offered 35 sessions of SCP BF and 20 sessions of behavioral self-control training. The patients, who evidenced fewer seizures at 1-year posttreatment compared with the 3-month baseline, evidenced less negative SCPs.[82] The use of SMR as the training module in patients with epilepsy (mostly patients that had already failed anticonvulsants) was reviewed by Sterman.[83] Eighty-two percent of 174 total patients in multiple studies achieved reduction in seizure frequency and 5% remained seizure free at 1 year. Although seizure control can be enhanced with BF, patients need to be able to transfer or generalize the training in order to use the technique outside of the clinic in order to obtain a long-term benefit. Kotchoubey et al found that successful patients were younger than age 35, were motivated, had sufficient hours of training, and were not on large doses of anticonvulsant medications.[84] Eighteen of 25 patients learned to control their SCPs with 29 one-hour sessions and obtained improvement in seizure frequency. At 1 year, 6 were free of seizures.[85] The American Academy of Child and Adolescent Psychiatry states that neurofeedback for seizure disorders meets criteria for clinical guidelines, that is, practitioners should always consider feedback as a treatment option.[83] In summary, there is supporting evidence for BF in epilepsy; however, practitioners of general BF will require an understanding of neurophysiology and the neurology of epilepsy and specialized training in neurofeedback to expand their practice into this complex area.

REHABILITATION

Based on the impact of psychological factors in patients undergoing rehabilitation, the clinician should enhance patients' motivation, reinforce positive psychological and physical change, and foster adaptation to lingering disability. BF provided to patients undergoing rehabilitation emphasizes motor learning which depends on practice and feedback (information). Using an operant conditioning paradigm, patients learn to discriminate between different levels of muscle tension. With accurate and rapid information from the BF device, higher levels of activity in specific muscles can be reinforced, while relaxation of other muscles is promoted.[86] In the rehabilitation hospital, BF equipment can be transported to the patient's bedside to avoid the counterproductive effects of transporting patients to the physical therapy clinic. Several examples of the use of BF in rehabilitation are discussed here; more extensive coverage of this topic may be found elsewhere.[87-89] One-hundred patients with spinal cord injury at C 6 or higher for longer than 1 year were offered EMG BF. The goal was to increase voluntary responses from the triceps muscles. After one to four BF sessions, a significant increase in EMG activity from the triceps muscle was observed.[90]

Patients with paretic muscles can be trained to recruit motor units and to produce a stronger voluntary contraction. In this context, BF protocols are designed to complement and build on naturally occurring sensory feedback. A three-stage process of neuromuscular reeducation is suggested. In stage one, the patient learns to contract and relax muscles voluntarily. Stage two comprises joint movement and posture. The third stage focuses on generalization of learning to the complex functions which are necessary for daily living. Improvements in stage-three skills do not occur after training directed only to stage one.[41] A group of 10 patients with hand dystonia were provided with EMG BF emanating from the proximal large limb muscles that manifested maximum tension and overactivity during writing. After a minimum of four sessions, 9 of the 10 patients reported improvement in handwriting and lessening of pain.[91]

For stroke patients in the rehabilitation setting, BF can be used to enhance the effects of exercise, to strengthen weakened muscles, and to return to more normal posture and gait. A meta-analysis was performed on data from eight studies in which EMG BF was compared to physiotherapy to improve lower extremity function in post-stroke patients. The findings pointed to EMG BF as more effective than conventional physiotherapy alone for improving ankle dorsiflexion muscle strength.[92] Phantom limb pain was treated with BF 90 minutes daily for 10 days and found to reduce pain and change the cortical reorganization that had occurred as a result of the pain.[93]

In the rehabilitation setting as well as in the BF clinic, acute pain is appropriately treated with pharmacotherapy whereas chronic pain requires a combined medical, behavioral, and psychological approach. Chronic pain is partially a learned behavior; repeated episodes of pain change the neuronal arrangement in the somatosensory cortex areas and the memory areas.[93] New applications of operant conditioning and BF may be addressed to the extinction of pain memories.[94]

ATTENTION DEFICIT/HYPERACTIVITY DISORDER

Treatment of children, adolescents, and adults with attention deficit/hyperactivity disorder (ADHD) is not founded on the lower arousal principle of BF. Rather, treatment is based on individuals learning to regulate brain wave activity in a manner similar to EEG training in epilepsy. If ADHD and ADD are associated with neurologic dysfunction in cortical and prefrontal lobe areas as summarized by Monastra and colleagues then learned control of brain wave activity can translate into improved attention, better task completion, reduced impulsiveness, and less hyperactivity.[95] Amelioration of symptoms is proposed to occur after multi-session (30–40 sessions for the inattentive type and more if hyperactivity is present) BF therapy to increase beta activity (14 hertz) and to inhibit theta (4–8 hertz).[96–98] The proximate goal of therapy is to train the patient to recognize abnormal EEG frequencies and to produce less slow wave activity.[99] For example, the beta/theta ratio was used as feedback in a 6-month training paradigm; compared with controls, the experimental group reduced inattentive behaviors and improved composite IQ scores. Therapists always remained in the room with the patients, providing additional encouragement and helping the children stay on task.[100]

EEG BF training has traditionally been used in therapists' offices and clinics. However, the large number of sessions required to learn the skill suggests that the school setting might be a practical alternative. Small numbers of students could be provided with daily EEG training sessions as part of the school day.[101] Monastra and colleagues offered 100 children between 6 and 19 years old standard treatment with medication, parent counseling and school consultation or the same plus neurofeedback.[95] One-year post training, behavior scores and TOVA (test of variable attention) remained in the normal range for the BF kids when they discontinued medication but not the non BF group. Four sessions of heart rate variability feedback were offered to children with ADHD. A significant correlation was found between heart rate variability and symptoms of ADHD, suggesting that this may be another viable feedback modality that can be effective with fewer sessions than neurofeedback. Scores on the Connors Inventory decreased after training.[102] A preliminary pilot study of 30 sessions of EEG feedback in children in a partial hospitalization program, also used the Teachers Connors Inventory as an indicator of improvement. Although scores on the hyperactivity and ADHD subscales improved after training in comparison to the control group, no significant correlations between measured brain waves and improvements were found.[103]

Home EEG equipment may be available in the future, so the required daily training sessions can be provided at home under the guidance of motivated, trained parents. Much like the limited therapist protocols for the lower arousal applications of BF, motivation and the ability to understand and follow instructions become critical factors influencing success.[104] The use of BF in ADHD remains controversial; stimulant medication is the gold standard and studies, though numerous and positive are often flawed.[105] Therefore, the consideration of BF for children and adolescents with symptoms of attention deficit with or without hyperactivity should include an accurate diagnosis, standard assessment tools such as the Connors Inventory and a well-constructed treatment plan matched to each person's ability and disability. The general BF provider will need training in the specialized equipment necessary to monitor and display the brain wave signal and a solid understanding of the characteristics of the disorder and an aptitude and desire to work with young children and adolescents.

CONCLUSION

There is strong scientific evidence for the efficacy of BF as treatment for several neurologic disorders, particularly tension-type and migraine headache. The effects of BF may be specific, nonspecific, or both. Nonspecific positive effects are mediated by gaining confidence, improving concentration, and developing more effective coping strategies. The primary effects of BF, in which control of individual physiological processes such as brain waves or muscle tension is learned, may also be specific. BF actively involves the patient in the therapeutic process; therapy is a partnership between provider and patient. Immediacy and accuracy of the BF information are critical, but the relationship between the practitioner and the patient remains important in all but a few of the treatment protocols. Patients with stress-related disorders have acquired maladaptive response patterns that have led to dysfunctional coping and oversensitivity to stress. Even neutral stimuli are perceived as threats so that, over time, risk for somatic manifestations of psychological conflict increases dramatically. Patients who react maladaptively clearly need new skills, but skills may not be enough. The assessment of a chronic pain patient must comprise psychological and emotional aspects in addition to physical aspects. The ability to self-regulate entails more than simply learning a technique. Self-regulation requires a conceptual shift towards the realization that control of physiological and psychological responses is possible. As the patient learns to self-regulate, sensory information is processed differently. For example, pain is interpreted as a message from the body, not as an inevitable prelude to an incapacitating migraine. The reply to the message involves skills only in part, but cognitive adjustments and positive psychological responses are also necessary. Although the practitioner begins with a framework and a standard treatment package in mind, the therapy should be flexible enough to be modified for individual patients. The challenges of future research are to expand the applications of BF, to develop an understanding of mechanisms, and to differentiate the subtypes of patients and disorders that are most appropriate for BF therapy.

REFERENCES

1. Schwartz NS, Schwartz MS. Definitions of biofeedback and applied psychophysiology. In: Schwartz MS, Andrasik F, eds. *Biofeedback: A Practitioner's Guide*. 3rd ed. New York, NY: Guilford Press; 2003:128–158.
2. Gilbert D, Moss D. Biofeedback and biological monitoring. In: Moss D, McGrady A, Davies TC, Wickramasekera I, eds. *Handbook of Mind-Body Medicine for Primary Care*. Thousand Oaks, CA: Sage Publications; 1994:109–122.
3. Lehrer P, et al. Stress management techniques: are they all equivalent or do they have specific effects? *Biofeedback Self Regul*. 1994;19(4):353–402.
4. Bernstein DA, Carlson CRJE. Progressive relaxation: abbreviated methods. In: Lehrer P, Woolfolk P, and Sime WE, eds. *Principles and Practice of Stress Management*. 2nd ed. New York, NY: Guilford Press; 2007;57–87.
5. Norris PA, Fahrion SL. Autogenic biofeedback in psychophysiological therapy and stress management. In: Lehrer P, Woolfolk P, eds. *Principles and Practice of Stress Management*. 2nd ed. New York, NY: Guilford Press; 2007.
6. Davis M, Eshelman E, McKay M. *The Relaxation and Stress Reduction Workbook*. 5th ed. Oakland, CA: New Harbinger; 2000.
7. Blanchard EB, Nicholson NL, Radnitz CL, Steffek BD, Appelbaum KA, Dentinger MP. The Role of Home Practice in Thermal Biofeedback. *J of Consult and Clin Psychol*. 1991;59(4):507–512.

8. Feldmen JM, Eisenberg EJ, Gambini-Suàrez E. Differential effects of stress management therapies on emotional and behavioral disorders. In: Lehrer P, Woolfolk P, and Sime WE, eds. *Principles and Practice of Stress Management.* 2nd ed. New York, NY: Guilford Press; 2007.

9. Tietjen GE, Brandes JL, Digre KB, et al. High prevalence of somatic symptoms and depression in women with disabling chronic headache. *Neurol.* 2007;68:134–140.

10. Beck AT, Rush, AJ, Shaw, BF, Emery, G. *Cognitive Therapy of Depression.* New York NY: Guilford Press; 1979.

11. Sadock BJ, Sadock VA. *Kaplan & Sadock's Synopsis of Psychiatry.* 9th ed. Philadelphia, PA: Lippincott Williams & Wilkins; 2003.

12. Dijkstra A. The validity of the stages of change model in the adoption of the self management approach in chronic pain. *Clin J of Pain.* 2005;21(1):27–37.

13. Arena JG, Schwartz MS. Psychophysiological assessment and biofeedback baselines: a primer. In Schwartz MS, Andrasik F, eds. *Biofeedback: A Practitioner's Guide.* 3rd ed. New York, NY: Guilford Press; 2003:128–158.

14. McGrady A, et al. Psychophysiologic therapy for chronic headache. Primary Care Companion. *J Clin Psychiatry.* 1999;1(4):96–102.

15. Penzien DB, Holroyd KA. Psychosocial interventions in the management of recurrent headache disorders 2: description of treatment techniques. *Behav Med.* 1994;20: 64–73.

16. Rowan AB, Andrasik F. Efficacy and cost-effectiveness of minimal therapist contact treatments of chronic headaches: a review. *Behav Ther.* 1996;27:207–234.

17. Arena J, Blanchard B. Biofeedback and relaxation therapy for chronic pain disorders. In: Gatchel R, Turk D, eds. *Psychological Approaches to Pain Management: A Practitioner's Handbook.* New York, NY: Guilford Press; 1996.

18. Earles J, Folen RA, James LC. Biofeedback using telemedicine: clinical applications and case illustrations. *Behav Med.* 2001;27:77–82.

19. deCharms RC, Maeda F, Glover GH, et al. Control over brain activation and pain learned by using real-time functional MRI. *Proc of the Natl Acad of Sci.* 2005;102(51):18626–18631.

20. Penzien DB, Rains JC, Andrasik F. Behavioral management of recurrent headache: three decades of experience and empiricism. *Appl Psychophysiol and Biofeedback.* 2002; 27(2):163–182.

21. NIH Technology Assessment Panel. Integration of behavioral and relaxation approaches into the treatment of chronic pain and insomnia. *JAMA.* 1996;276(4):313–318.

22. Bogaard MC, ter Kuile MM. (1994). Treatment of recurrent tension headache: a meta analytic review. *The Clin J of Pain.* 1994;10:174–190.

23. McGrady A, Wauquier A, et al. Effect of biofeedback assisted relaxation on migraine headache and changes in cerebral blood flow velocity in the middle cerebral artery. *Headache.* 1994;34(7):424–428.

24. Compas BE, Haaga DAF, Keefe FJ, Leitenberg H, Williams DA. Sampling of empirically supported psychological treatments from health psychology: smoking, chronic pain, cancer, and bulimia nervosa. *J of Consult and Clin Psychol.* 1998;66(1):89.

25. Holroyd K, Penzien D. Pharmacological versus non-pharmacological prophylaxis of recurrent migraine headache: meta-analytic review of clinical trials. *Pain.* 1990;42: 1–13.

26. Holroyd KA, et al. Recurrent vascular headache home-based treatment versus abortive pharmacological treatment. *J Consult Clin Psychol.* 1988;56(2):223–281.

27. Holroyd KA, et al. Enhancing the effectiveness of relaxation-thermal biofeedback training with propranolol hydrochloride. *J Consult Clin Psychol.* 1995;63:327–330.

28. Vasudeva S, Claggett AL, Tietjen GE, McGrady AV. Biofeedback-assisted relaxation in migraine headache: relationship to cerebral blood flow velocity in the middle cerebral artery. *Headache.* 2003;43:245–250.
29. Cott A, Parkinson W, Fabich M, Bedard M, Marlin R. Long-term efficacy of combined relaxation: biofeedback treatments for chronic headache. *Pain.* 1992;51(1):49–56.
30. Ham LP, Packard RC. A retrospective, follow-up study of biofeedback-assisted relaxation therapy in patients with posttraumatic headache. *Biofeedback & Self Regul.* 1996;21(2):93–104.
31. Blanchard EB, Taylor AE, Dentinger MP. Preliminary results from the self-regulatory treatment of high- medication-consumption headache. *Biofeedback Self Regul.* 1992;17(3):179–202.
32. Grazzi L, Andrasik F, D'Amico D, et al. Behavioral and pharmacologic treatment of transformed migraine with analgesic overuse: outcome at 3 years. *Headache.* 2002;42:483–490.
33. Hermann C, Blanchard EB. Biofeedback in the treatment of headache and other childhood pain. *Appl Psychophysiol and Biofeedback.* 2002;27(2):143–162.
34. Holroyd KA, Drew JB. Behavioral approaches to the treatment of migraine. *Semin in Neurol.* 2006;26(2):199–207.
35. Grazzi L, Leone M, Frediani F, Bussone G. A therapeutic alternative for tension headache in children: treatment and 1-year follow-up results. *Biofeedback and Self-Regul.* 1990;15(1):1–6.
36. Allen KD, Shriver MD. Role of parent-mediated pain behavior management strategies in biofeedback treatment of childhood migraines. *Behav Ther.* 1998;29(3):447–490.
37. Bussone G, et al. Biofeedback-assisted relaxation training for young adolescents with tension-type headache: a controlled study. *Cephalalgia.* 1998;1:463–467.
38. Andrasik F, Schwartz MS. Behavioral assessment and treatment of pediatric headache. *Behav Modif.* 2006;30:93–113.
39. Trautmann E, Lackschewitz H, Kröner-Herwig B. Psychological treatment of recurrent headache in children and adolescents—a meta-analysis. *Cephalalgia.* 2006;26:1411–1426.
40. Arena J, et al. Electromyographic biofeedback training for tension headache in the elderly: a prospective study, *Biofeedback Self Regul.* 1991;16(4):379–390.
41. Middaugh SJ. On clinical efficacy: why biofeedback does and does not work. *Biofeedback Self Regul.* 1990;15(3):191–208.
42. Flor H, Fydrich T, Tutk DC. Long term efficacy of EMG biofeedback for chronic rheumatic back pain. *Pain.* 1992;49:221–230.
43. Middaugh SJ, Pawlick K. Biofeedback and behavioral treatment of persistent pain in the older adult: a review and a study. *Appl Psychophysiol and Biofeedback.* 2002;27(3):185–202.
44. Morone NE, Greco CM. Mind-body interventions for chronic pain in older adults: a structured review. *Pain Med.* 2007;8(4):359–375.
45. Middaugh S, et al. Biofeedback assisted relaxation training for the aging chronic pain patient. *Biofeedback Self Regul.* 1991;16(4):361–377.
46. Van Tulder. 2000.
47. Kelly J, Devonshire R. *Taking Charge of Fibromyalgia.* 4th ed. Minneapolis. MN: Devonshire & Kelly; 2001.
48. Goldenberg DL, Burckhardt C, Crofford L. Management of fibromyalgia syndrome. *JAMA.* 2004;292(19):2388–2395.
49. Astin JA. Mind-body therapies for the management of pain. *The Clin J of Pain.* 2004;20(1):27–31.

50. Thieme K, Gromnica-Ihle E, Flor H. Operant behavioral treatment of fibromyalgia: a controlled study. *Arthritis Rheum.* 2003;49:314–320.

51. Sherman JJ, Turk DC. Nonpharmacologic approaches to the management of myofacial temporomandibular disorders. *Curr Pain and Headache Rep.* 2001;5(5):421–431.

52. Harris RE, Clauw DJ. The use of complementary medical therapies in the management of myofascial pain disorders. *Curr Pain and Headache Rep.* 2002;6:370–374.

53. Turner JA, Mancl L, Aaron LA. Short- and long-term efficacy of brief cognitive-behavioral therapy for patients with chronic temporomandibular disorder pain: a randomized, controlled trial. *Pain.* 2006;121:181–194.

54. Crider A, Glaros AG, Gevirtz R. Efficacy of biofeedback-based treatments for temporomandibular disorders. *Appl Psychophysiol and Biofeedback.* 2005;30(4):333–345.

55. Victor L, Richeimer SM. Psychosocial therapies for neck pain. *Phys Med and Rehabil Clin of North Am.* 2003;14(3):643–657.

56. Jensen IB, Bergstrom G, Ljungquist T, Bodin L. A 3-year follow-up of a multidisciplinary rehabilitation programme for back and neck pain. *Pain.* 2005;115:273–283.

57. Oliveira A, Gevirtz R, Hubbard D. A psycho-educational video used in the emergency department provides effective treatment for whiplash injuries. *Spine.* 2006; 31(15):1652–1657.

58. Dixon KE, Keefe FJ, Scipio CD, Perri LM, Abernethy AP. Psychological interventions for arthritis pain management in adults: a meta-analysis. *Health Psychol.* 2007;26(3):241–250.

59. Futterman AD, Shapiro D. A review of biofeedback for mental disorders. *Hosp Community Psychiatry.* 1986;37(1):27–33.

60. Wenck LS, Leu PW, D'Amato RC. Evaluating the efficacy of a biofeedback intervention to reduce children's anxiety. *J Clin Psychol.* 1996;52(4):469–473.

61. Stoyva J, Thomas B. Biofeedback methods in the treatment of anxiety and stress disorders. In: Lehrer P, Woolfolk P, eds. *Principles and Practice of Stress Management.* 2nd ed. New York, NY: Guilford Press; 2007.

62. Vanathy S, Sharma PSVN, Kumar KB. The efficacy of alpha and theta neurofeedback training in treatment of generalized anxiety disorder. *Indian J Clin Psychol.* 1998; 25(2):136–143.

63. Rice KM, Blanchard EB, Purcell M. Biofeedback treatments of generalized anxiety disorder: preliminary results. *Biofeedback Self Regul.* 1993;18(2):93–105.

64. Barlow D. *Anxiety and its Disorders: The Nature and Treatment of Anxiety and Panic.* New York, NY: Guilford Press; 1988.

65. McGrady A, Bernal GAA. Relaxation based treatment of stress induced syncope. *J Behav Ther Exp Psychiatry.* 1986;17:23–27.

66. Hammond DC. Neurofeedback with anxiety and affective disorders. *Child and Adolesc Psychiatric Clin of North Am.* 2005;1:105–123.

67. Sharp TJ. The prevalence of post-traumatic stress disorder in chronic pain patients. *Curr Pain and Headache Rep.* 2004;8(2):111–115.

68. Wickramasekera I. The placebo effect and its use in biofeedback therapy. In: Moss D, McGrady A, Davies TC, Wickramasekera I, eds. *Handbook of Mind-Body Medicine for Primary Care.* Thousand Oaks, CA: Sage Publications; 2003:69–81.

69. Grubb BP, Karas A. Clinical disorders of the autonomic nervous system associated with orthostatic intolerance: an overview of classification, clinical evaluation, and management. *PACE.* 1999;22:798–810.

70. Kosinski DJ, Wolfe DA, Grubb BP. Neurocardiogenic syncope: a review of pathophysiology, diagnosis and treatment. *Cardiovasc Rev Rep.* 1993;14:22–29.

71. McGrady A, McGinnis R. Psychiatric disorders in patients with syncope. In Grubb B, Olshansky B, eds. *Syncope: Mechanisms and Management.* 2nd ed. Malden, MA: Blackwell Futura; 2005.

72. McGrady A, Bush EG, Grubb BP. Outcome of biofeedback-assisted relaxation for neu-rocardiogenic syncope and headaches: a clinical replication series. *Appl Psychophysiol Biofeedback*. 1997;22:63–72.
73. McGrady A, Kern-Buell C, Bush E, Devonshire R, Claggett AL, Grubb BP. Biofeedback-assisted relaxation therapy in neurocardiogenic syncope: a pilot study. *Appl Psychophysiol Biofeedback*. 2003;28:183–192.
74. Cowings PS, Shapiro D, Toscano WB, Stevenson J, Miller NE. Autogenic-feedback training: a potential treatment for orthostatic intolerance in aerospace crews. *The J of Clin Pharmacol*. 1994;34(6):599.
75. Toscano WB, Cowlings PS. Reducing motion sickness: a comparison of autogenic-feedback training and an alternative cognitive task. *Aviat Space Environ Med*. 1982; 53(5):449–453.
76. Smith MT, Edwards RR, McCann UD, Haythornthwaite JA. (2006) The effects of sleep deprivation on pain inhibition and spontaneous pain in women. *Sleep*. 2006;30(4): 494–505.
77. Waters WF, Hurry MJ, Binks PG, et al. (2003). Behavioral and hypnotic treatments for insomnia subtypes. *Behav Sleep Med*. 2003;1(2):81–101.
78. Chesson ALJ, Anderson WM, Littner M, et al. (1999). Practice parameters for the nonpharmacologic treatment of chronic insomnia. *Sleep*. 1999;22(8):1128–1133.
79. Morin CM, Hauri P, Espie CA, Spielman AJ, Buysse DJ, Bootzin RR. Nonpharmaco-logic treatment of chronic insomnia: an American Academy of Sleep Medicine review. *Sleep*. 1999;22(8):1134–1156.
80. Jacobs GD, Pace-Schott EF, Stickgold R, Otto MW. Cognitive behavior therapy and pharmacoltherapy for insomnia: a randomized controlled trial and direct comparison. *Arch of Intern Med*. 2004;164(17):1888–1896.
81. Kotchoubey B, et al. Negative potential shifts and the prediction of the outcome of neurofeedback therapy in epilepsy. *Clin Neurophysiol*. 1999;110(4):683–686.
82. Strehl U, Kotchoubey B. A psychophysiological treatment of epilepsy. *Appl Psychophysiol Biofeedback*. 1999;224(2):138.
83. Sterman MB, Egner T. Foundation and practice of neurofeedback for the treatment of epilepsy. *Appl Psychophysiol and Biofeedback*. 2006;31(1):21–35.
84. Kotchoubey B, et al. Self regulation of slow cortical potentials in epilepsy: a retrial with analysis of influencing factors. *Epilepsy Res*. 1996;25(3):269–276.
85. Rockstroh B, et al. Cortical self regulation in patients with epilepsies. *Epilepsy Res*. 1993;14:63–72.
86. Barton LA, Wolf SL. Is EMG feedback a successful adjunct to neuromuscular rehabilitation? *Phys Ther Pract*. 1992;2(2):41–49.
87. Sherman RJ, Arena JG. Biofeedback in the assessment and treatment of low back pain. In: Basmajian J, Nyberg R, eds. *Spinal Manipulative Therapies*. Baltimore, MD: Williams & Wilkins; 1992.
88. Krebs DE, Fagerson TL. Biofeedback in neuromuscular re-education and gait training. In: Schwartz MS, Andrasik F, eds. *Biofeedback: A Practitioner's Guide*. 3rd ed. New York, NY: Guilford Press; 2003;485–514.
89. Wolf SL, Binder-Macleod SA. Electromyographic biofeedback in the physical therapy clinic. In: Basmajian JV, ed. *Biofeedback: Principles and Practice for Clinicians*. 3rd ed. Baltimore, MD: Williams & Wilkins; 1989.
90. Brucker B, Bulaeva N. Biofeedback effect on electromyography responses in patients with spinal cord injury. *Arch of Phys Med and Rehabil*. 1996;77:133–137.
91. Deepak KK, Behari M. Specific muscle EMG biofeedback for hand dystonia. *Appl Psychophysiol and Biofeedback*. 1999;24(4):267–280.

92. Moreland JD, Thomson MA, Fuoco AR. Electromyographic biofeedback to improve lower extremity function after stroke: a meta-analysis. *Arch Phys Med Rehabil.* 1998; 79:134–140.

93. Flor H, Diers M. Limitations of pharmacotherapy: behavioral approaches to chronic pain. *Psychiatry Relat Sci.* 2006;177:415–427.

94. Moseley GL. Graded motor imagery for pathologic pain: a randomized controlled trial. *Neurol.* 2006;67:2129–2134.

95. Monastra VJ, Lynn S, Linden M, Lubar JF, Gruzelier J, LaVaque TJ. Electroencephalographic biofeedback in the treatment of attention-deficit/hyperactivity disorder. *Appl Psychophysiol and Biofeedback.* 2005;30(2):95–114.

96. Gruzelier J, Egner T. Critical validation studies of neurofeedback. *Child and Adolesc Psychiatric Clin of North Am.* 2005;14:83–104.

97. Lubar JF, et al. Evaluation of the effectiveness of EEG neurofeedback training for ADHD in a clinical setting as measured by changes in TOVA scores, behavioral ratings, and WISC-R performance. *Biofeedback Self Regul.* 1995;20(1):83–99.

98. Lubar JF. Neurofeedback for the management of attention-deficit/hyperactivity disorders. In Schwartz MS, Andrasik F, eds. *Biofeedback: A Practitioner's Guide.* 3rd ed. New York, NY: Guilford Press; 2003:128–158.

99. Butnik SM. Neurofeedback in adolescents and adults with attention deficit hyperactivity disorder. *JCLP/In Session.* 2005;61(5):621–625.

100. Linden M, Habib T, Radojevic V. A controlled study of the effects of EEG biofeedback on cognition and behavior of children with attention deficit disorder and learning disabilities. *Biofeedback Self Regul.* 1996;21(1):35–49.

101. Boyd WD, Campbell SE. EEG biofeedback in the schools: the use of EEG biofeedback to treat ADHD in a school setting, *J of Neurother.* 1998;2(4):65–71.

102. Eisenberg J, Ben-Daniel N, Mei-Tai G, Wertman E. An autonomic nervous system biofeedback modality for the treatment of attention deficit hyperactivity disorder—An open pilot study. *Psychiatry Relat Sci.* 2004;41(1):45–53.

103. McGrady A, Fine T, Donlin J, Prodente C. The effects of neurofeedback treatment on children with behavioral, attention and concentration problems. Presented at: Association for Applied Psychophysiology and Biofeedback Annual Meeting; February 2007; Monterey, CA.

104. Rossiter TR. Patient-directed neurofeedback for AD/HD: Part I. Review of methodological issues. *J Neurother.* 1998;2(4):54–63.

105. Loo SK, Barkley RA. Clinical utility of EEG in attention deficit hyperactivity disorder. *Appl Neuropsychol.* 2005;12(2):64–76.

CHAPTER 2

Hypnosis for Pain Management

Arthur Fass

Hypnosis has earned a secure place in the modern armamentarium against pain. Given its long and somewhat checkered history this may seem an unlikely development. However, in spite of a somewhat mysterious quality, and its occasional use in some decidedly unscientific quarters, the medical community has maintained a continued interest in its clinical use.

In the course of recent years, the science of hypnosis has greatly expanded. There are now abundant reports published in the medical literature describing the benefits of hypnotherapy for a variety of medical conditions. In addition, numerous controlled studies of its effects have appeared.

The technique has found important applications in the treatment of such varied disorders as migraine headaches, irritable bowel syndrome, anxiety, phobias, as an aid to smoking cessation, as well as in the relief of chronic and acute pain.

With the advent of sophisticated brain imaging techniques, such as MRI and PET scanning, it has been possible for the first time to understand some of the physiologic changes that accompany a hypnotic state.

This chapter will deal primarily with the use of hypnosis in the management of pain. The anxiety-relieving properties of hypnosis are intimately associated with its analgesic effects and will also be discussed. Whenever possible, reference will be made to prospective, controlled studies, the foundation of clinical research, in validating therapeutic applications. We will start with a look back on the fascinating history of hypnosis and its evolution as a modern therapeutic technique.

A HISTORY OF HYPNOSIS

The origins of hypnosis will always be closely linked to the colorful career of the Austrian physician Franz Anton Mesmer (1734–1815), a charismatic and controversial figure. Mesmer used trance-like states and the power of suggestion in treating patients, giving rise to the term "mesmerism." He developed a large following of devotees who often experienced improvement in their symptoms (see chapter 5).

His ideas, however, became progressively radical even as judged by eighteenth-century standards, delving into theories of animal magnetism, astrology, and the effect of planetary tides on the body's so-called gravitational forces. Ultimately, with Mesmer having engendered the enmity of the medical establishment, a commission was assembled in France by King Louis XVI to weigh the merits of his work. The assembly included such luminaries as the chemist Antoine Lavoisier and Benjamin Franklin, who was the American ambassador to France at the time. The panel was not kind to Mesmer. They essentially labeled him a fraud and concluded that any apparent benefit of his technique was the work of the "imagination."[1]

It is likely that Mesmer had discovered the potential power of mental imagery and suggestion in modifying somatic symptoms. One of his students, Dr. Charles D'Elson, commenting after the Louis XVI committee report, opined: "If Mesmer has no other secret than that he has been able to make the imagination exert an influence upon health, would he not still be a wonder doctor? If treatment by the use of the imagination is the best treatment, why do we not make use of it?"[2(p155)]

The subject was forgotten for 50 years until interest was rekindled in the 1840s when several British surgeons employed hypnotic techniques in their clinical practices. The term "hypnotism," from the Greek *hypnos* (sleep), was coined by the English surgeon James Braid, who realized that hypnosis was not a result of external forces but of the subject's ability to summon his own powers of focus and concentration.[3]

Perhaps the most influential practitioner of early hypnosis for surgical anesthesia was the Scottish surgeon James Esdaile. In an era before chemical anesthetics, Esdaile used hypnosis as the sole method of anesthesia in over 300 major operations, receiving widespread notice in Europe and the

United States. With a relatively low mortality rate, Esdaile's efforts lent an air of respectability to the practice of hypnositic anesthesia.

Chemical anesthetic agents arrived shortly afterward, quickly supplanting hypnosis for surgical anesthesia. The chemical agents were easy to use and took less time to administer.

During the late nineteenth century, France witnessed a hypnosis revival under a different guise; an interest in the field arose among students of the nascent field of psychology. The eminent neurologist Jean Martin Charcot thought that the hypnotic state was a pathological condition akin to hysteria. Sigmund Freud met with Charcot at the Hospital Salpetriere in Paris and became fascinated with hypnosis as a tool to explore the subconscious mind in the diagnosis and treatment of neuroses. Later, however, Freud abandoned the technique, diminishing its subsequent role in psychology.[3]

After Freud's defection, interest in hypnosis in the medical community waned. However, later, amidst the suffering and trauma of the world wars, the technique proved effective in the treatment of posttraumatic stress disorder and in pain relief.[3]

The practice of hypnosis finally found its way into the medical mainstream with its endorsement by the British Medical Association in 1955 and by the American and Canadian Medical Associations in 1958. Since then, interest in hypnosis has burgeoned, and the practice of hypnosis has found myriad clinical applications. Whereas the original clinical enthusiasm was based largely on anecdotal data, there has lately been a steady flow of controlled clinical trials, putting hypnosis on a more secure scientific footing.

THEORY

The precise physiologic mechanisms of hypnosis, as with many functions of the human brain, are not fully elucidated. Though superficially resembling a sleep-like state, hypnosis is characterized by waking EEG patterns.[4] Neurologic studies using EEGs in hypnotized individuals have shown a shift of brain activity to the anterior cingulate gyrus and left prefrontal cortex.[5] Hypnotic imagination of color perception will result in measurable increases in blood flow to the visual cortex.[6] Positron emission tomography (PET scanning) has revealed early activation of the anterior cingulate gyrus in hypnotic interventions with an inhibition of neural activity between the sensory cortex and limbic system.

By most accounts, hypnosis is characterized by increased mental focus and concentration, an insouciant indifference to the external environment, and heightened receptiveness to suggestion. Most individuals will describe a pleasantly altered state of consciousness (but not sleep), an air of calmness, and a general feeling of well-being while under hypnosis. When properly performed, hypnosis is almost always accompanied by reduced perception of anxiety and stress.

The facilitation of suggestibility appears to devolve from an inclination by the hypnotized subject to suspend cortical "censoring" of received information. Hypnosis has been likened to a state of "highly focused attention with a constriction in peripheral awareness."[6]

It is widely acknowledged that there is considerable variability in individual susceptibility to hypnosis (so-called hypnotizability). This variation may occur on a genetic basis. The large majority of patients can be hypnotized to some degree. Perhaps 10% cannot be hypnotized, and 10% are particularly susceptible.[7] Women are more hypnotizable than men; children are more receptive than adults.

Speigel at Stanford has developed hypnotic susceptibility scales to provide a biostatistical basis for evaluating receptivity to hypnosis without implying any underlying mechanism. This approach could in turn provide a basis for the improved application of other complementary/ alternative modalities where the mechanism of action is controversial, obscure, or remains foreign in the view of the contemporary biomedical paradigm.

There is controversy about whether a deep level of hypnosis is required for its therapeutic effects. Most recent studies suggest that this is not necessary, and a large percentage of patients will benefit from even light levels of hypnosis. A smaller percentage of patients will be able to achieve complete hypnotic anesthesia.

HOW IS HYPNOSIS DONE?

There is no uniform method of hypnotic induction. There are elements, however, that are common to most applications of clinical hypnosis.

A state of trust and confidence must exist between hypnotist and subject. The patient often requires reassurance, especially at the first session, that there will be no loss of control or inappropriate suggestions. Medical hypnosis must be distinguished from the stage variety, which many patients are most familiar with.

The hypnosis session will usually produce immediate positive results. Almost invariably the subject will report a sense of well-being and calmness, although they will often be uncertain about their depth of hypnosis. Patients will often comment on their awareness of what was going on but with a curious unconcern about their surroundings. Subsequent sessions

The hypnosis session will usually incorporate several components:

1. **Preparation.** The patient is placed in a comfortable, secure environment, usually sitting in a quiet room. Distractions and interruptions are minimized.
2. **Induction.** The patient is guided to a state of relaxation by deep breathing, progressive muscle relaxation, and the use of imagery.
3. **Deepening.** In this phase, the hypnotic state is deepened through repetition and reinforcement. Conscious thinking is minimized.
4. **Purpose.** It is in this phase that the specific goal of the hypnotherapy session will be addressed. It is here that hypnotic suggestions are utilized to modify perceptions or behavior.[8] For example, in the case of pain management, the subject may be asked to transform the perception of pain to a numbness or tingling sensation.
5. **Awakening.** In this final phase, the patient is gradually brought out of the hypnotic state. This stage affords an opportunity to repeat and reinforce therapeutic suggestions as the level of hypnosis lightens. Final suggestions are offered to bring about a feeling of relaxation combined with energy and a vitality upon awakening.

usually produce deeper levels of hypnosis as the patient is less apprehensive about the technique. Evidence of the secondary benefits of hypnosis (i.e., pain management) must await clinical follow-up.

Effective hypnotic induction is an acquired talent. Practitioners will develop a method of using words, cadences, images, and suggestions that is most suited to their individual styles. A learning curve is required to develop best technique.

A typical hypnosis session will take 30 to 60 minutes. There are no studies or guidelines about the optimal frequency of hypnosis sessions. Practitioners must adapt to the practical realities of time constraints and scheduling limitations. A weekly session at the outset may be feasible for some caregivers. Between sessions, the patient is encouraged to practice "self-hypnosis." This method, while not quite as effective as guided therapy with a skilled hypnotist, utilizes the patients own skills at achieving a hypnotic state. They are instructed to apply breathing techniques and imagery learned during regular sessions. Self-hypnosis is a useful adjunct in hypnotherapy which can be used often and when needed by the patient.

PAIN MANAGEMENT

There is a growing body of scientific evidence on the clinical usefulness of hypnosis in pain management. Hypnosis has demonstrated a remarkable versatility in treating a variety of pain syndromes. The rising interest in hypnotherapy in the alleviation of pain coincides with the medical community's and public's increasing receptiveness to alternative medical practices.

Hypnosis in General Pain Management

Montgomery and colleagues at the Mount Sinai Medical School set out to organize and tabulate the extant medical literature on the subject of hypnosis and pain management.[9] The field to that point had been in a state of disarray, with numerous anecdotal and uncontrolled reports leaving the medical community uncertain of the clinical benefits. Montgomery's group undertook a meta-analysis of 18 previously published trials including 933 patients, nearly all of whom were divided into control groups who received standard or no treatment compared to those given hypnotic interventions for the purpose of pain management. The studies included both clinical patients as well as experimental pain groups in healthy volunteers (i.e., focal pressure). The patients included those with burn injuries, cancer, headaches, coronary disease, and painful radiologic procedures. The methods and frequency of the hypnotic interventions used in the studies are not described in detail.

The results of the meta-analysis revealed a significant beneficial effect of hypnotic interventions in the treatment of pain. Subjects in both the clinical and experimental pain categories benefited from the hypnotic intervention. Hypnoanalgesic effects were more pronounced in highly hypnotizable subjects; however, mid-range patients, making up the largest group in terms of hypnotic susceptibility did obtain significant pain relief from the hypnosis intervention. This suggests that a deep level of hypnosis is not required to achieve clinical benefit. Overall, the average individual receiving hypnotherapy experienced greater analgesic response than 75% of control subjects.

The authors conclude that hypnotherapy should be considered an effective therapeutic modality either used alone or as an adjunct to other analgesic techniques including pharmacotherapy. Moreover, the technique is effective in the majority of patients and has little downside risk.

Management of Cancer Pain

Hypnosis has a potentially important role in managing pain in cancer patients.[10] In addition to its analgesic benefits, hypnosis can provide other psychotherapeutic benefits in this patient population especially anxiety reduction and an improved outlook.

An early randomized trial examined the use of hypnosis to alleviate pain associated with metastatic breast cancer.[11] Patients were divided into three groups. Two groups were designated treatment groups, each of which received regular group therapy with psychological counseling. Part of the treatment group was also given extensive instruction in self-hypnosis. The control group received standard oncologic care with no special psychological support. Follow-up was obtained at 4-month intervals for a total of 1 year. Thirty-four patients were included in the treatment sample, with 24 controls.

The treatment patients reported no increase in pain over the course of the follow-up period, compared to a significant increase in the control group. Within the two treatment groups, those receiving hypnosis in addition to psychological counseling fared best in controlling pain intensity. Changes in pain scores correlated with self-reported levels of anxiety, depression, and fatigue reinforcing the association between mood and pain perception.

A recent, randomized trial performed by Montgomery et al. at Mount Sinai School of Medicine, New York, assessed the effects of a brief hypnosis intervention to control side effects in patients scheduled for breast surgery.[12] Two hundred patients undergoing excisional breast biopsy or lumpectomy were randomized to receive either a 15-minute preoperative hypnosis session conducted by a psychologist or to a control group of nondirective empathic listening. Following this relatively simple intervention, patients were then tracked for various postoperative indicators. Patients in the hypnosis group reported benefit in a number of clinical parameters. They experienced less pain intensity, nausea, fatigue, and emotional upset than their control counterparts. The hypnosis group required less pharmacological sedation and analgesia with propofol and lidocaine respectively. Overall costs were lower for the hypnosis group. The authors conclude that hypnosis is a valuable adjunct for breast cancer surgery patients.

General Surgery

Montgomery's group also reported a meta-analysis of the use of hypnosis for general surgical patients.[8] Twenty published studies, with over 1,600 patients were included in this analysis. All studies included a hypnosis intervention group as well as a routine care or no treatment group in patients undergoing general surgical procedures. Most, but not all, studies used a randomized design. Hypnosis was typically administered in the form of a relaxing induction phase followed by suggestions aimed at modifying postoperative side effects such as pain, nausea, or distress. Most of the interventions consisted of live sessions administered by a health care professional; the remainder utilized audiotapes.

The meta-analysis revealed a broad benefit from hypnosis intervention for a number of clinical parameters.

Overall, 89% of patients in the hypnosis groups benefited in comparison to patients receiving standard care. Positive effects were observed in all categories evaluated. These included levels of anxiety and depression, pain, pain medication, physiologic indicators (i.e., blood pressure, heart rate, and catecholamine levels). Benefit was similar between live and audiotape patient groups.

The authors conclude that the data "strongly support the use of hypnosis with surgical patients."

Obstetrics

Hypnosis has been used for over a century in the management of childbirth pain. A noninvasive method to assist in childbirth pain would be of great interest to the obstetric and anesthesia communities, particularly where epidural anesthesia is impractical or contraindicated. There have been a number or reports of the effectiveness of hypnosis in obstetric analgesia.[13-15]

Cyna and colleagues undertook a meta-analysis to assess the role of hypnosis in the pain of childbirth.[16] Trials were selected in which hypnosis was compared to a nonhypnotic intervention during pregnancy and childbirth. Three randomized, controlled trials totaling 224 patients were included in the analysis.

The results of the meta-analysis revealed a significant benefit of the hypnosis intervention. Parturient women who received hypnosis rated their labor pain less severe than controls and required less pharmacologic analgesia during labor.

Martin published a randomized, controlled trial on obstetrical hypnosis in 42 teenaged patients.[17] The treatment patients received a four-session sequence of hypnotic focused relaxation and imagery. Suggestions were directed at the patients' ability to manage stress and discomfort.

The treatment patients had a significantly lower length-of-stay than controls and fewer complications, and they required less conventional anesthesia during labor and postpartum.

Dentistry

Hypnosis has been used successfully for pain management in dentistry. Ghoneim and colleagues conducted a prospective, randomized study of

60 patients scheduled for third molar extraction.[18] The intervention group received an audiotape incorporating hypnotic induction and suggestions designed to alleviate pain and enhance healing. The treatment group listened to the tape daily in the week preceding oral surgery. Patients receiving hypnotherapy reported less anxiety before their scheduled procedure. However, there was no decrease in the consumption of analgesics and the benefit of the intervention was unclear. Other groups have discerned greater benefit from hypnosis in dental surgery patients including a diminished requirement for postoperative analgesics.[19,20]

Pediatrics and Pediatric Surgery

Given the susceptibility of children to hypnotic suggestion, the technique may hold special promise in this patient population. Butler and colleagues studied the potential usefulness of hypnosis in preparing young children for voiding cystourethrography, a particularly painful and frightening urological procedure for children.[21] The procedure involves urethral catheterization and the introduction of contrast material in the bladder under fluoroscopic imaging. Forty-four children, 29 girls and 15 boys, with an average age of 7.6 years were studied. Patients randomized to the treatment group were given a 1-hour training session in self-hypnotic visual imagery by a trained therapist, and then they practiced the technique several times a day prior to the urological procedure. The control group received no special preparation.

The results demonstrated significant benefit for the intervention group. Parents in the hypnosis group reported that the procedure was less stressful and emotionally traumatic for their children. Medical staff reported easier performance of the procedure with less distress in the hypnosis group, and the procedure time was significantly shortened.

The authors conclude that pre-procedure hypnosis may be beneficial for children undergoing urologic and other invasive or anxiety-provoking medical procedures.

CHRONIC PAIN

Jensen and Patterson performed an extensive review of published studies evaluating hypnotic treatment for chronic pain.[22] Nineteen controlled trials were reviewed, all of which involved hypnosis as a treatment arm. Patients' diagnoses included migraine headache, sickle cell disease, osteoarthritis, fibromyalgia, tension headache, and other chronic painful disorders. The hypnotic interventions, which varied considerably across studies, typically consisted of 4 to 10 hypnosis treatments administered over several weeks. Subjects were often given tapes and told to practice on their own between sessions. They were then followed for up to 12 months with periodic assessments. Comparisons were made against no treatment and nonhypnotic interventions.

The hypnotic interventions were more effective, on average, than no treatment for pain control. The degree of effectiveness varied between studies. Analgesic effects were maintained for up to 12 months when long-term follow-up was available. It was not possible to conclude whether hypnosis was particularly effective for any particular patient group.

Compared to other interventions, such as medical management and physical therapy, hypnotic intervention was often found to be superior. Other treatments employing hypnosis-like suggestions such as relaxation, progressive muscle relaxation, and biofeedback tended to produce results similar to hypnosis.

Based on the findings of this review, the authors conclude that hypnotic intervention can result in substantial and sustained benefit in the management of chronic pain.

STUDY LIMITATIONS

Studies of the benefits of hypnosis in clinical practice, although collectively persuasive, have important limitations. In many cases, the hypnotic methods are inadequately described omitting an interesting and crucial aspect of the study. For example, some authors failed to describe such basic information as the number of interventions, duration, and so forth, leaving the reader to wonder about these important details. Moreover, many studies had relatively small sample sizes, diminishing their statistical power.

Meta-analyses are subject to a number of well-known limitations including variations in study size and quality. Also, there is the real possibility that studies with negative outcomes were not submitted for publication thereby slanting the overall results.

Perhaps the most serious limitation in hypnosis trials is the lack of blinding. In most clinical trials involving placebo arms both the subjects and the caregivers are unaware of the treatment given. Because of the nature of hypnosis, and the difficulty in performing sham hypnosis, blinding is not possible. This results in an unavoidable bias.

POSSIBLE ADVERSE EFFECTS

Hypnosis is generally considered an extremely safe procedure. Adverse effects usually appear as isolated case reports in the literature. Patients with underlying psychiatric disorders should be treated with caution because of the possibility of an untoward reaction to hypnotic suggestion. A mental health professional should participate in the care of these patients. No long-term harm from hypnosis has been documented.

CONCLUSIONS

We have presented some of the recent scientific data on the use of hypnosis in pain management. Incorporating hypnosis into medical practice can be rewarding for both patient and practitioner. Patients, in general, are extremely appreciative of efforts to address their emotional as well as physical needs. Hypnosis is performed at a slow pace, a welcome respite from the hectic and sometimes frenetic tempo of modern medicine. This alone affords a degree of relaxation and stress relief.

Further light can be shed on the mechanism of hypnosis with future research. The physiologic basis can continue to unfold as brain function testing and imaging become more refined.

Additional trials could help define the effects and usefulness of hypnosis for an increasing spectrum of clinical applications. Hypnotherapy may become recognized by insurance companies as a valid and potentially cost-saving intervention.

Practitioners of hypnosis have long been convinced of its power and effectiveness. With the accumulation of clinical evidence substantiating its benefits, hypnosis is now positioned to fulfill its full promise as a modern therapeutic intervention in pain management.

REFERENCES

1. Upshaw WN. Hypnosis: medicine's dirty word. *Am J Clin Hypn.* 2006;49(2):113–122.
2. Goldsmith M. *Franz Anton Mesmer: A History of Mesmerism.* Garden City, NY: Doubleday, Doran, and Company, Inc; 1934.
3. Fass AE. Hypnosis for relief of cardiac symptomatology. In: Frishman WH, Weintraub MI, Micozzi MS, eds. *Complementary and Integrative Therapies for Cardiovascular Disease.* St. Louis, MO: Elsevier Mosby. 2005: 127–134.
4. Graci G, Sexton-Radek K. Treating sleep disorders using cognitive behavior therapy and hypnosis. In: Chapman RA, ed. *Clinical Use of Hypnosis in Cognitive Behavior: A Practitioner's Casebook.* New York, NY: Springer; 2006:296–303.
5. Gosline A. Hypnosis really changes your mind. *N Sci.* 2004;9–10.
6. Spiegel D. The mind prepared: hypnosis in surgery. *J Nat Cancer Inst.* 2007;(99): 1280–1281.
7. Rogovik AL, Goldman RD. Hypnosis for treatment of pain in children. *Can Fam Physician* 2007;53(5):823–825.
8. Montgomery GH, David D, Winkel G, et al. The effectiveness of adjunctive hypnosis with surgical patients: a meta-analysis. *Anesth Analg.* 2002;94:1639–1645.

9. Montgomery GH, DuHamel KN, Redd WH. A meta-analysis of hypnotically induced analgesia: how effective is hypnosis? *Int J Clin Exp Hypn.* 2000;48(2):138–153.
10. Barber J, Gitelson J. Cancer pain: Psychological management using hypnosis. *CA Cancer J Clin.* 1980;(30):130–136.
11. Spiegel D, Bloom JR. Group therapy and hypnosis reduce metastatic breast cancer pain. *Psychosom Med.* 1983;45(4):333–339.
12. Montgomery GH, Bovberg DH, Schnur JB, et al. A randomized clinical trial of a brief hypnosis intervention to controlside effects in breast surgery patients. *J National Cancer Inst.* 2007;99(17):1304–1312.
13. Cyna AM. Hypno-analgesia for a labouring parturient with contra-indications to central neuraxial block. *Anaesth.* 2003;(58):101–102.
14. Bonica JJ. Labour pain. In: Melzack R, Wall PD, eds. *Textbook of Pain.* New York, NY: Churchill Livingstone; 1984:377–391.
15. DeLee ST, Kroger WS. Use of hypno-anaesthesia for Caeserian section and hysterectomy. *JAMA.* 1957;163:442–444.
16. Cyna AM, McAuliffe GL, Andrew MI. Hypnosis for pain relief in labour and childbirth: a systematic review. *Br J of Anesth.* 2004;93(4):505–511.
17. Martin A. Effects of hypnosis on the labor processes and birth outcomes of pregnant adolescents. *J Fam Pract.* May 2001;50.
18. Ghoneim MM, Block RI, Sarasin DS. Tape-recorded hypnosis instructions as adjuvant in the care of patients scheduled for third molar surgery. *Anesth Analg.* 2000;90:64
19. Enqvist B, Fisher K. Preoperative hypnotic techniques reduce consumption of analgesics after surgical removal of third mandibular molars: a brief communication. *Int J Clin Exp Hypn.* 1997;45:102–108.
20. Enqvist B, Von Konow L, Bystedt H. Stress reduction, preoperative hypnosis and perioperative suggestions in maxillo-facial surgery. *Stress Med.* 1995;11:229–233.
21. Butler LD, Symons BA, Henderson MA., et al. Hypnosis reduces stress and duration of an invasive medical procedure for children. *Pediatrics.* 2005;115(1):e77–e85.
22. Jensen M, Patterson D. Hypnotic treatment of chronic pain. *J Behavioral Med.* 2006;29:95–124.

CHAPTER 3

Music Therapy

Peggy Codding and Suzanne Hanser

Music doth maketh the heart to rejoice.

—The Bible

Anthropologists and ethnomusicologists document that music has been associated with the healing of the body and mind for centuries. Since the time of early nomadic civilizations, healers have incorporated music in their rituals "to solace the sick and weary, [and] to promote unspoken emotions." In some cultures, music was used in religious and healing rituals "for entreating the gods" to "exorcise malevolent . . . demon[s]" that many believed inhabited the body of any ill person.[1] Shamans used instruments, song, and dance to call up certain melodies and rhythms as healing medicine. The music corresponded to the spirits they thought were invading the bodies of the sick.

These practices were a natural healing response to a supernatural view of illness and health. Today, trained music therapists use music experiences to promote therapeutic change in a patient's symptomatology, coping skills, and quality of life. Generally, music therapists serve as members of the patient's treatment team within the hospital unit. Some music therapists work in private practice, accepting patients by physician referral. The growing body of knowledge derived from the empiric study of music and health supports the role of music therapy as a viable treatment milieu.[2-6]

Music in some form has been used for nearly two centuries in hospitals throughout the United States. After the phonograph was invented in 1877, physicians sometimes made patient-preferred music recordings available to the sick. The music provided relief from the boredom of hospital routines and distracted patients from their physical discomfort or depression.[6] More recently, therapists have used live precomposed, improvised, or recorded music in individual or group music therapy sessions to reduce heightened feelings of fear or isolation, to promote mental focus, or to distract attention away from pain. Music therapists use music to facilitate physical activity during recuperation, to cue relaxation, and to mask unpleasant hospital sounds that cause patient stress. Some music therapists have also used music to promote essential coping strategies or to facilitate communication among family members regarding illness, treatment, or prognosis.[1]

Although acousticians frequently define music as organized sound and silence in time, twentieth-century pioneers of music therapy described the experience of music as much more. These early practitioners observed many people who were "under the influence" of music and found that listeners experienced music as a source of joy, a messenger of sadness with which they could identify, or a key to release the feelings of the moment. Music therapists have long understood that music is a powerful means of communication that is more subtle, more basic, and more personal than words. Music lyrics or melodies sometimes convey the unspeakable or the intimate that is almost inexpressible. Therapists have often seen familiar music allow an individual to elicit the memory of an important life event and to recall the very feelings that were felt at that moment. Music compels human beings to act by stimulating thought or mood, or by creating a need to move that can only be filled by the tapping of a foot or a quick step across the floor. Music, although not essential to human survival, exists and flourishes in all known cultures. It is the intimate personal expression of those who play it and sometimes the spiritual salvation of those who hear it.

Music is a natural tool for complementary or integrative medicine because it is created by human beings to speak to human beings. Music draws attention to itself and is often useful for conveying ideas that are too difficult to express by speaking them aloud. Everyone can experience music in some form and participate successfully with whatever ability that is brought to the moment. People can listen passively to music while feeling calm or light, or they can use music actively to start moving. Music can be experienced alone, with someone who is well known to the patient, or in groups.

In 1950, the National Association for Music Therapy established the field as an official discipline. The American Music Therapy Association, which was formed in 1998, along with its Standards of Practice and Code of Ethics, currently oversees 73 approved academic curricula in the United States and more than 150 approved full-time clinical internships. There are approximately 6,000 professional and student music therapists who practice in schools, clinics, and community agencies; in hospitals; and privately.[7]

Music therapy is the application of specific music techniques to meet physical, social, emotional, and psychologic goals and objectives. Music therapists are qualified to practice in the United States when they have obtained a music therapy degree from an approved college, completed an approved clinical internship, and passed a National Board Certification Examination. Continuing education is required to maintain board certification. The music therapist, after consulting with health professionals on the team, determines whether group therapy, individual work, or a bedside approach is most appropriate. In general, music therapy may be less effective for persons with hearing difficulties. However, many rhythmic and musical activities can still be enjoyed and appreciated by people with the most severe hearing loss. Because music is universal in its appeal, music therapy offers a potential methodology for individuals regardless of their functional abilities.

Music therapists assess each client's needs, establish goals and objectives consistent with the treatment team, and design strategies that incorporate nonverbal, creative ways to reach specified psychotherapeutic aims.[8] They may use any genre of music along with improvisation, singing, moving or dancing to music, playing instruments, composing music, talking about and analyzing music, learning music, or listening to music. Therapists use familiar, patient-preferred music as a nonthreatening means of establishing a clinical relationship with a new, anxious patient or as a stimulus to motivate the repetitive movement often essential to physical rehabilitation.[3] Music can encourage patients who are confused as a result of brain trauma to focus their attention on something compelling and meaningful. The music therapist might also help patients with terminal illnesses to compose lyrics and music that express their feelings. Writing the piece structures emotional release and contributes to coping; sharing the music and lyrics with family helps to communicate love and loss.

MUSIC AND THE BRAIN

For much more than a century there has been a growing literature on music and the brain. Many observations have arisen from studying patients who had suffered a change in their musical abilities after cerebral damage from stroke. Such behavioral and cognitive alterations have been termed *amusias*. These acquired impairments include diverse performance deficits, such as in singing or instrumental skills; perceptual impairments, such as in pitch and rhythm discrimination, ability to read music, and recognition of melodies; and lost talent for composing music. Perhaps the best summary of such studies is in Critchley and Henson's[9] volume titled *Music and the Brain: Studies in the Neurology of Music.*

Many earlier brain-behavior studies supported a model of a select neural substrate for musical perception and processing residing primarily in the right cerebral hemisphere. For example, Milner[10] reported impairments in discrimination of timbre, duration, and tonal patterns following right temporal lobectomy in patients with intractable epilepsy. Others have reported impaired discrimination of melodies and pitch after right hemisphere damage.[11,12] In addition, case studies of musicians with acquired aphasias after left hemisphere damage from stroke have revealed that they may continue to perceive and evaluate critically, compose, and even read music although they are no longer able to comprehend and read language in comparable fashion.[13,14] Such observations have led to an intriguing but simplistic model of cerebral dominance, specifying that language and associated verbal processes are mediated through the left cerebral hemisphere. The model says that nonverbal musical processes are mediated through right hemisphere structures, particularly the temporal lobe where primary auditory cortex and auditory association cortices are localized. This verbal/nonverbal hemispheric dichotomy, as Zatorre,[15] and Hachinski and Hachinski[16] observed, is simply not supported by available data. This evidence suggests instead that complex and diverse interactions occur between the two cerebral hemispheres during musical behaviors and experiences.

The earlier right hemisphere model of music was important for providing an initial neural linkage between music and emotion because this hemisphere has also been shown to play important roles in emotional perception and processing.[17–19] The medium of music may influence emotions in both direct and indirect ways, through overlapping or interactive neural activation and through powerful nonverbal symbolism that bypasses the pathways of language and verbal cognition. Studies in cognitive neuroscience have shown that a much broader array of neural structures participate in music behaviors and experiences than was previously thought. The most important of these structures include the frontal lobe, limbic system, and imagery-related cortical regions of the temporal, parietal, and occipital lobes.[15,20–24] These studies have been carried out in normal healthy volunteers who undergo functional brain scanning (Positron Emission Tomography, or PET) while undertaking music-related tasks. It is important to note that there is now scientific data supporting music stimulation effects in the frontal lobe and limbic system, which are key structures for emotional activation and experience of a diverse nature.[25,26] This provides a potential mechanism for musical influences on the regulation of emotions and on the autonomic centers that mediate respiration, heart rate, and so forth. Hence, there is a potential pathway for therapeutic change.

Thaut[27] has suggested that music may induce therapeutic change through its activation of affective systems. A structured approach to these systems and associated behaviors, such as through a music therapy program, may allow individuals with diverse neurologic conditions to experience, identify, express, and modulate emotions and physiologic responses in ways that are quite different from verbally mediated, insight-oriented, cognitive therapies. Moreover, music may provide a unique, complementary mode of stimulating emotions, emotional processing, and therapeutic emotional change.

MUSIC THERAPY IN MEDICAL SETTINGS

Research in music therapy as applied to medical settings has been reviewed by Standley.[2] Her recent meta-analysis suggests the following generalizations about the response to music in medical treatment:

- Based on a relatively small number of studies, women's response to music is somewhat greater than men's response.
- Children and adolescents are marginally more responsive to music than are adults. However, infants respond less to music than either of the other age groups, perhaps as a result of their having less experience with music.
- Live music performed by a music therapist results in a much greater effect on physical and psychologic states than does recorded music. However, patient-preferred music results in the greatest positive medical effect.
- Music has a greater effect when pain is present than when pain is not present; however, the positive effects of music seem to decrease as pain increases.
- The physiologic and psychologic effects of music vary according to the specific dependent measures used.
- "Greatest effects were reported for grasp strength in stroke patients, perceived effectiveness of music, EMG, self-report of pain, relaxation, and anxiety reduction. Least effects were measured by days of hospitalization, peripheral finger temperature, ease of childbirth, time of recovery from anesthesia, formula intake of neonates and neonate apnea."[2]

- "The least conservative measure of music's effect is patient self-report while systematic behavioral observation and physiological measures result in basically equivalent, conservative effect sizes. The most frequently utilized dependent variable is a physiological measure."[2]

Although a systematic review of the literature reveals somewhat inconsistent results, music therapy is generally indicated for individuals who experience pain and anxiety during the course of illness.[28]

MUSIC THERAPY TECHNIQUES FOR PAIN AND NEUROLOGIC ILLNESS

In 1994, a team of investigators at Hershey Medical Center in Pennsylvania undertook an initial research project on music therapy and brain injury that was funded through the then Office of Alternative Medicine of the National Institutes of Health.[29] It had three aims:

1. Establish a scientific framework for investigating a music therapy intervention for psychologic impairments after brain injury;
2. Examine the effects of a specific improvisational music therapy program on empiric measures of self-perception, empathy, emotional processing, and social interaction; and
3. Identify areas for future scientific study.

A stratified randomization procedure was used to assign adults with brain injuries to experimental and control groups. The 30 subjects were in the chronic phase of recovering from either traumatic brain injury (TBI) or stroke. No further medical therapies were available to address the residual social and emotional impairments that kept participants from returning to occupational activities. All subjects underwent preintervention neuropsychologic testing, with the experimental group receiving a 10-week therapy intervention and the control group meeting in similar fashion for casual support group sessions. The music therapy program was structured to address residual psychosocial impairments. Both groups were retested when the 10-week period ended. Results indicated that positive changes in emotional empathy, depression, and social behavior occurred in the music therapy group, particularly as noted by family members. Cognitive measures, as expected, did not change. The social support group also showed some positive changes in emotional empathy and a measure of daily competency, but no change was shown in depression. The findings suggested that positive changes in emotional processing, social behavior, and mood can be achieved through music therapy. Some of these effects could be achieved with socialization activities alone. However, the progress made by music therapy participants and the reports made by family members showed more evidence in social and emotional domains. Results suggested then that it may be beneficial to combine music therapy with other modes of intervention such as social support groups, preoccupational training, and even individual psychotherapy to maximize social and emotional adjustment. In the years since this study, research and clinical practice in music therapy in neuro-rehabilitation settings has expanded in scope to include a more comprehensive understanding of applications for TBI and/or stroke, physical injury in general, and individuals in low awareness states.

With patients who have neurologic illness, the research literature supports several music therapy strategies:

- Facilitating physical rehabilitation and communication;
- Coping with pain by using music as a focus of attention and distraction;
- Relieving anxiety and depression through music-facilitated stress management and coping techniques; and
- Improving orientation for people with dementia using structured, success-oriented musical experiences.

Facilitating Physical Rehabilitation and Communication

As human knowledge about the relationship of brain function and psychophysiologic activity increases, so does the understanding of music perception and active response. Music therapists have used this developing knowledge to determine effective strategies for using music in the rehabilitation of persons with neurologic dysfunction attributed to traumatic brain or spinal cord injury.[30–33] In this setting, music applications are coordinated with other therapies to assist patients in reaching the sensory-motor, cognitive, communication, social, and emotional goals of rehabilitation.

Research in music therapy is active in the area of TBI. Two reviews of literature in music therapy and neurological rehabilitation are notable in recent years. A review of American and British journals by Paul and Ramsey examined music applications in music and physical therapy in the modalities of neurology, orthopedics, rehabilitation and pediatrics. Results suggest that the pairing of music and physical therapies can improve participation in therapy, ease discomfort and improve cognition, communication, balance, range of motion, strength and balance.[34]

Gilbertson published the most comprehensive review of literature describing music therapy techniques for TBI populations and age groups using the Music Therapy World Journal Index. The review included experimental studies of therapeutic applications of music to TBI from 12 music therapy journals and 20 databases worldwide. Studies were analyzed for type of study, music application/techniques, population characteristics, and age. Each was also categorized according to music use, that is, whether the focus of music was improvisation or music was precomposed and used in some other way. All studies were analyzed for gender, trauma, primary diagnosis, clinical symptoms, timescale, assessment, concurrent therapies, musical biography, and specific results. Individual studies are described in the review.

Clinical music techniques identified in the review across studies were defined as auditive music therapy, auditory stimulation, improvisation, composition, instructional song, instrumental playing, melodic intonation therapy, intonation exercises, music reception, rhythmic auditory stimulation, singing instruction, song creation, song listening, song text writing, song reminiscing, song story, traditional oriental music therapy, and vocalization exercises. Critical themes in the literature were that the key and role of the music therapist in the weeks following head injury was clinical assessment. Primary responses of head injured clients to stimuli were minimal and described as a lack of interaction to the environment, and an absence of vocalization and movement.[35]

During music therapy sessions, the music therapist would often begin by responding through musical improvisation to any sounds or movements made by the client. The therapist would then build upon these early developmental steps as they occurred through continued improvisation, music listening, vocalization, and reality orientation. Later, experiences such as lyric substitution in songwriting would be used for emotional expression to introduce clients to their feelings, then clients to each other as a means of encouraging a return to social life. Results of the 2005 review suggest the following core aspects of music in therapy with clients having experienced TBI:

- Music therapy provides a unique nonverbal assessment strategy in initial phases of rehabilitation following TBI.
- Music, in a therapeutic setting, is an integrative medium that provides a logical context for initial attempts towards orientation and cognition following trauma.
- People who have experienced TBI have used music therapy to redevelop some aspects of the personal identity.
- Music therapy may offer a relevant and appropriate therapeutic resource in the future for family members of people with TBI.[35]

Music strategies have also had many positive effects when applied to the broader range of patients served in physical rehabilitation. A review of the experimental research available in English regarding music applications in rehabilitation generated 120 studies between 1950 and 1993.[3] According to this review, the settings in which music therapy has been implemented most frequently are general hospitals with rehabilitation units, state hospitals and schools, special education classes within public schools, and comprehensive rehabilitation centers or nursing/retirement centers. In these settings, music therapy has been implemented primarily for patients with cerebral palsy, developmental disabilities, orthopedic impairments, paralysis, and poliomyelitis. Other studies describe the effects of music in acute or chronic neurologic rehabilitation.[3] Purdie reviewed music uses in neuro-rehabilitation in music therapy literature between 1981 and 1996 and observed applications of music in Parkinson's disease, stroke, TBI, Huntington's chorea, multiple sclerosis, brain disorders, coma, and spinal cord injury. Positive clinical outcomes were reported for self esteem, fine and gross motor recovery, social interaction, and motivation.[36]

Patients in rehabilitation commonly present a myriad of physical disorders. Brain injury may be considered a factor in the patient's disorder or it may not. Music therapy in the rehabilitation of individuals with brain injury involves substantial research in music in the restorative development of muscle control and movement. The neurologic music therapy model (NMT) was developed at the Center for Biomedical Research in Music at Colorado State University in Fort Collins. The model emphasizes sensorimotor training using music in a medical model to promote physical rehabilitation in two ways: "movement *to* music" and "movement *through* music." Rhythm or beat is used to organize movement in "movement to music" training.[37] For example, rhythmic auditory stimulation may be used to improve the uneven gait of the individual with TBI. Patterned sensory enhancement, which incorporates additional elements of music such as harmony, melody, and dynamic variations in addition to rhythm, may also be used to cue temporal or spatial change in support of the activities of daily.[38] "Movement through music" experiences for physical rehabilitation involve therapeutic instrumental music playing in which the playing of instruments provides the structure for therapeutic exercise and endurance.[39]

Music therapy interventions in physical rehabilitation are most often used for two purposes: to distract the patient's attention away from the pain and to decrease the monotony of repetitive movements associated with rehabilitation while sustaining the patient's interest in the specific activities and their repetition. Music motivates. Common uses of music therapy in rehabilitation include the following:

- Promoting neuromuscular coordination;
- Structuring movement or muscle stimulation, such as in stretching, exercise, vestibular stimulation, and proprioceptive responses to stimulation;

- Enhancing muscular and motor control, for example, with tremors;
- Reestablishing neuromotor patterns to include basic motor skills or movement in rhythm;
- Structuring muscular relaxation, including tension release of rigid or spastic muscles;
- Improving joint mobility and agility, and preventing stiffness;
- Improving muscle and joint strength;
- Improving respiratory capacity and rate;
- Improving balance and posture;
- Increasing range of motion and the extension and flexion of limbs;
- Enhancing muscle tone and counteracting atrophy; and
- Improving muscular endurance and reaction time.[3]

Core aspects of music in therapy with clients having experienced traumatic brain injury and in need of physical rehabilitation include:

- Music therapy can lead to an increase in the level of involvement in therapy and rehabilitation in general.
- By focusing on social and psychological areas, music therapy enhances rehabilitation success and, in turn, provides a balance to therapies focused on physical function.
- Music therapy can lead to an increase in independence in activities of daily life.
- Music therapy has been used in therapy to influence gait positively, particularly with patients presenting a static level of disability.
- Music therapy is appropriate for patients of many ages and has been applied with patients between 3 and 84 years of age.[35]

Music has been described as a sensory medium capable of arousing the nervous system and cueing altered states of awareness in human beings.[40] A patient's state of awareness at any moment is influenced by the focus of his or her attention. The individual's focus is altered by the characteristics of the presented stimulus as perceived, and finally he or she reacts to the sensory information.[35] When the most desirable sensory stimuli available to a patient at a particular moment is patient-preferred music, and when that music is presented at an amplitude that is pleasing to the ear, the music serves as a catalyst to do the following:

- Alter the patient's emotions by calling upon previous associations with the particular piece;

- Channel the patient's cognitive focus away from hospital sounds and physical preoccupation and toward more pleasing and normalizing music stimuli; and
- Either command an immediate physical response to the music, with little to no preparatory thought, or facilitate more purposeful movement over extended periods of time.[3,28,47]

Music therapy is an effective treatment modality for some individuals in low awareness states whose receptive and expressive communication skills are severely compromised.[41] Those in a minimally conscious state or vegetative state may be aware of a range of emotions but unable to respond or do so in a severely limited way. Music therapists consider that the fundamentals of communication are also those of music.[41,42] Patients in low awareness states may respond to music for four reasons. They respond to vocal dynamics, pitch, articulation, melodic contour, phrasing, and timing regardless of stage of life or level of awareness because these are the powerful elements of both music and communication. Music motivates regardless of culture; it begins to do so at birth and continues to stimulate and arouse until the end of life. Music can communicate and stimulate feeling without relying on language. Finally, music assists with neurological development and neuroplasticity as it supports the connections to be made between unhealthy and healthy tissue in individuals with brain damage.[41]

The overall goal of music therapy with minimally conscious patients is to demonstrate that the client can respond differently and purposefully to contrasting stimuli. Additional goals are:

1. To assess behavioral responses to (motivating) musical stimuli;
2. To provide a forum to reinforce yes/no;
3. To assess whether movement is purposeful;
4. To provide a framework for developing voice; and
5. To assist relatives having difficulty interacting due to communication impairment.[43]

Core aspects of music in therapy with clients having experienced traumatic brain injury who may be minimally responsive include:

- Music therapy offers musical dialogue-based interaction for patients emerging from coma or who are initially diagnosed as minimally responsive.
- Music therapy provides a unique therapeutic possibility for patients with severe TBI (Glasgow Coma Score 3–8).[35]

Music motivates by arousing the human will to act. Human will is a key factor in physical rehabilitation and a possible predictor of patient success. It serves as the primary catalyst for actions that bring about desired physical change and psychologic health. Music has the power to focus attention, and to elicit, drive, and regulate movement.[43] Music therapists use music in rehabilitation to cue physical response, structure response completion, or reinforce occurrences of a particular nonmusic behavior.[44-47]

Music used as therapy can be directed toward the specific goals of physical rehabilitation. Preferred music accompanied by a verbal suggestion of progressive relaxation might be used to calm an anxious or distracted patient. Alternatively, music might be prescribed for the chronically fatigued or unresponsive patient to direct mental focus, motivate action, and structure repetitions of physical exercise. For example, as described earlier in the neurologic music therapy model, when carefully selected rhythms are used to accompany gait irregularities in stroke patients, the structure provided by the repeated rhythm enables the patient to anticipate and thereby to prepare for movement structured in time, much like in dancing. In other words, rhythms at movement-appropriate tempi are introduced to a patient to stimulate movement response or to reinforce patient gait. When movement begins, the repeated rhythm or beat helps structure repeated movements so the movements become synchronous with the rhythmic sound.[48] Although music therapists use the process of successive approximations to bring this about, the structure of the music, especially the beat and anticipation of the next beat, often forces physical precision in musical time for at least the duration of the musical stimulus, or physical *entrainment* with the aural stimulus. Gait-appropriate rhythms can be embedded in patient-preferred live or recorded music and then played at a tempo that forces increasing precision in locomotor movement. This can result in more fluid and efficient movement. Rhythmic auditory stimulation a music entrainment technique used to facilitate movement by providing an auditory structure to force precision, has been used to improve gait velocity, cadence, stride length, and symmetry in patients suffering TBI.[48] After repeated use and patient improvement, the music structure is withdrawn from walking activities using fading techniques. The patient has then relearned the essential skill of walking as well as possible.[3,41,48]

Patient-preferred music is also used in physical rehabilitation to sustain physical posture. In this case, preferred-music listening is contingent upon the patient's initiation and maintenance of a desired posture, such as holding the head up. For example, when the patient's head falls, the music stops; when the head position is returned voluntarily to the designated posture, the music begins again and continues to play until the head again drops.[49]

Music therapy interventions can be applied to the neuro-rehabilitation patients presenting with TBI and speech dysfunction.[50-54] Subjects in the modicum of studies available are primarily diagnosed with aphasia. The identified music intervention is predominantly Melodic Intonation Therapy.[55-58] The literature regarding music and TBI primarily describes use of music in speech and language rehabilitation, the models of interventions used, and music-based clinical assessment of TBI.[30,55-58]

Melodic Intonation Therapy (MIT) is a primary strategy used by physicians, speech therapists, and music therapists for speech and language rehabilitation. MIT is a structured music/language model which combines basic language with music forms to facilitate cooperation between left and right brain hemispheres in the processing and expression of speech through sung syllables. Primarily successful with people having expressive aphasia, MIT involves the embedding of short functional words or phrases into brief melodies with special attention to rhythm. Intoned syllables, then words, and finally phrases are used to gradually reintroduce simple speech, inflection, and rhythm to aphasic patients. As the patient experiences success in using expressive language by "singing" or intoning functional words and phrases, the music element is faded and speech often improves. MIT techniques can generate improvement in speech rate, clarity, vocabulary, and inflection.[52,53]

The theory behind MIT is that speech functions that have been impaired by damage to one hemisphere of the brain might be relearned by other cells, possibly in the other hemisphere. If this is the case, return of speech capability might be a matter of retraining brain cells. Some patients maintain musical capacity, especially singing abilities, following TBI.[59-62] Techniques of MIT are used to retrain speech through simplified singing experiences in which singing is the obvious link to eventual speech.

One study of MIT in neuro-rehabilitation involved eight patients presenting a variety of speech disorders resulting from left-hemisphere lesion. Three experiments were completed. During Experiment 1, patients recalled new words from lists and notes of familiar material such as proverbs or prayers. Recall of familiar chanted prayers and proverbs was better than the recall of word lists. In Experiment 2, patients with aphasia repeated, then recalled, the lyrics from new songs and did not reproduce more words when singing than when speaking. During Experiment 3 an auditory model was provided while the patient learned new songs. When asked to recall the words, patients were able to recall more words and exhibited greater recall when singing the words than when speaking them. Choral singing of the words was more effective than choral speaking.[63]

A second study describes the use of MIT with aphasic patients. In a single case study, MIT was used with a male singer with severe Broca's aphasia. Thirty new phrases were presented in one of three experimental conditions: unrehearsed, rehearsed with repetition, or rehearsed with verbal production with melody (MIT). Results after 5 weeks of intense therapy demonstrated superior vocal production of MIT phrases during therapy, a benefit for all rehearsal conditions and longer term phrase production for the MIT condition after 5 weeks. MIT seemed to contribute to improved speech praxis and promoted separate storage and/or access to phrase information.[64] Core aspects of music therapy with clients experiencing TBI and in need of speech rehabilitation are:

- Music therapy offers a strategy to positively influence mood state often affected by TBI.
- In therapy, music provides an adequate field of interaction for emotional expression, communication of feelings, and validation of emotionality.
- Music therapy leads to improvements in vocal ability, and some aspects of speech ability including voice control, intonation, rate of speech, and verbal intelligibility.
- Music therapy provides a strategy to enhance memory of events and information during phases of posttraumatic amnesia and neuropsychological disorder.[35]

Coping With Pain

According to the gate-control theory of pain, a competing stimulus might be able to direct a person's concentration away from pain. Listening to music or, better yet, engaging in focused musical activity guides the attention to a positive stimulus. In this way, music is effective in distracting from pain. Pain mechanisms may be considered psychologic events that translate incoming pain signals in the spinal and thalamic areas of the brain.[65] Music and other stimuli that change the sensation, affect, and motivation associated with pain are capable of diffracting the perception of pain.[66] Music also alters pain perception by changing the mood, diverting attention, focusing on taking control of pain, and using relaxation skills.[67] Therefore, cognitive and behavioral strategies that condition a relaxation response to music have been successful.[68,69]

Music techniques have had many positive effects when applied to the pain and anxiety associated with a neurologic illness. A meta-analysis of music therapy research through 1996 included 92 empiric studies. In these studies, patients who had been diagnosed with a variety of illnesses or who experienced pain were exposed to music or music techniques.[70] These data yield effect sizes of 1.72 for headache patients, 1.26 for chronic pain patients, and 1.17 for physical rehabilitation patients. The effectiveness of music in diminishing pain decreases with the intensity of pain. More recent reviews of the effects of music on pain and stress reduction also support the overall efficacy of music strategies.[71-73]

Controlled experimentation with hospitalized patients reveals many successful applications of music listening strategies, but there are some mixed results. In general, music listening alone is effective in reducing pain and anxiety even when little emphasis is placed on the choice of music for a particular individual. Listening to recorded music has been shown to reduce pain during such diverse medical procedures as laceration repair,[74] abdominal surgery,[75] inguinal hernia repair,[76] hysterectomy,[77] orthopedic surgery,[78] and coronary artery bypass graft.[79] Considerable empiric evidence exists to support the use of music therapy in managing pain and symptoms of cancer and in palliative care.[80,81] Other applications of music and music therapy are indicated for such varied conditions as chronic pain of rheumatoid and osteoarthritis,[82,83] debridement procedures,[84] and anxiety of patients in a rehabilitation unit.[85] Research on music listening for other painful procedures, like chest-tube removal, lumbar microdiscectomy, procedural pain, and renal lithotripsy has failed to demonstrate significant effects.[86-89] However, these studies were not performed by music therapists and did not attend to patient preference, conditioning of a positive and relaxing response to the music, and other significant details in a therapeutic music process.

Certain music therapy procedures designed to reduce pain have been particularly effective. Vibroacoustic therapy has been applied successfully in a large number of studies[90] as have other interventions by music therapists involving live music[91] and individualized approaches.[92,93]

Music therapy protocols for pain are diverse and incorporate techniques ranging from passive listening to active music making. Selected music therapy techniques include the following:

- *Movement to music.* Exercising muscles affected by pain while listening to music often creates a positive mood, distracts from physical discomfort, and structures exercise so that patients report a quick and pleasant passage of time. Performing physical therapy regimens while listening to preferred music or playing simple percussion instruments focuses attention on a stimulus that evokes pleasure and relaxation.
- *Breathing to music.* Pairing deep, relaxed breathing with rhythmic music provides cues for a regular breathing tempo. This, in turn, encourages the patient to maintain even respiration, which facilitates a relaxed body.

- *Imagery to music.* Guided imagery involves preparing patients by having them relax to programmatic music, close their eyes, and visualize various scenes and images. The music might take individuals to places where they would like to go, or it might conjure a familiar, soothing environment like home.
- *Listening to music.* Much of the research by professionals who are not music therapists involves having patients listen to music that is either self-selected or chosen by the researcher. Listening alone has been shown to be effective in reducing pain. Listening to music is a natural leisure activity used by people to enhance their daily lives. When a hospitalized patient listens to preferred music, its familiarity often results in feelings of comfort and normalcy. When possible, music therapy procedures include listening to music and inducing relaxation training procedures before the onset of pain.
- *Improvising to music.* To break the cycle of recurring pain, music therapists use a projective technique of expressing feelings by playing music. Some patients find it cathartic to express themselves in this way. The complex process of creating and performing music may mediate pain perception and can be used with children as well as adults. Playing instruments that do not require previous training, such as drums, xylophones, hand chimes, rain sticks, and other percussion, may result in instant success. Keyboards and other instruments that require more dexterity provide a rich source of creativity for those who are capable of producing an aesthetically pleasing sound. As the attention is focused on multiple areas, pain perception fades.
- *Composing songs.* Writing about the experience of coping with pain is similar to communicating the feelings surrounding the experience of pain. Music therapists facilitate the process of songwriting or musical composition by probing for content and structuring the melodic, harmonic, and rhythmic aspects of the music.
- *Vibroacoustic therapy.* This technique involves providing the patient with low frequency vibrations along with music, via speakers embedded in a chair or bed. For stimulation, loud music with a strong beat is administered; for relaxation, soft music with a slower tempo and less pronounced rhythm is indicated. Currently, compact discs with pulsed sinusoidal tones provide the physical stimulus. The treatment plan, duration and choice of music are based on the desired outcomes of the session and the individual needs of the patient.

Relieving Anxiety and Depression

Having a neurologic illness may mean living with pain, worry, and uncomfortable treatment, and the prospect of living with a severe or chronic condition. The following techniques may help to relieve anxiety and depression:

- *Taking control of feelings.* When patients find a piece of music that moves them deeply, relaxes them completely, or distracts them actively, they see how they can control their feelings quickly and relatively easily. Attending concerts, enrolling in a choir or community ensemble, or learning to play a musical instrument redirects attention to interests and skills.
- *Increasing pleasant events and mood.* Engaging in pleasant music-related activities has been shown to reduce depression when it is applied with other behavior therapy techniques.[94]
- *Focusing on abilities, talents, and strengths.* Retraining musical competencies or introducing new ones offers the patient with a degenerative condition the opportunity to witness growth and potential in contrast to the loss of abilities. Engaging in any form of preferred music activity in which the patient can demonstrate competence and mastery is indicated.[95]

Improving Orientation and Success

Loss of cognitive function occurs in age-related memory loss as well as in more devastating progressive illnesses such as Alzheimer's disease and Parkinson's disease. Music therapy is often considered the treatment of choice for cognitively impaired older adults who respond to music but little else. Many individuals who are in advanced stages of dementia participate actively in music therapy using preserved skills such as singing familiar songs, performing well-known compositions, and providing rhythmic accompaniment to pieces of music. This ability to retain music competencies has been documented in several studies.[96–99]

Music therapy is used widely in long-term care settings with great success. There is a growing body of evidence supporting the efficacy of music therapy. Brotons and colleagues[100] reviewed 69 studies published between 1987 and 1997. A meta-analysis of this research[101] reveals an effect size of 0.79, thereby demonstrating a significant effect of music therapy on a variety of symptoms. Music therapy has been used to improve socialization,[102] cognition,[103] and quality of life,[104] and to manage disruptive and inappropriate behaviors such as agitation,[105–110] physical aggression,[111] wandering,[112,113] and sleeplessness.[114] It has been applied at all levels of care, from community senior centers to assisted and long-term care facilities. Techniques are diverse and depend on a comprehensive assessment of functional needs, musical abilities, and interests in music. The following are ways that music therapy is used both in groups and individually:

- *Music therapy in groups.*[115] When applied in groups, structured musical experiences offer a way for people with dementia to experience success and to orient to reality. Group participants may master and demonstrate musical skills such as singing, playing instruments, improvising, creating new songs or compositions, moving or dancing to music, and accompanying a song. Through this process, they are able to experience a sense of competence, which they may not feel in other areas of their lives. Music therapists create failure-free environments by demanding only what each participant is capable of performing. This may be accomplished by asking specific individuals to provide a steady beat on percussion instruments, to sing along, to solo, or to create new rhythms or simple patterns (ostinati) on tuned instruments. The success of a musical creation that can be recorded and played back for the group may lead to group cohesiveness, positive affect, and self-esteem while focusing attention on positive, creative actions.
- *Individual behavior management strategies.* Music is effective in decreasing agitation[87] when its use is contingent upon appropriate behavior, when it is used as a comforting stimulus, or when it is used to attract attention. Music therapists may sing or play music for an individual to maintain a calm mood while the individual is engaged in activities of daily living. They may also redirect the attention of an agitated person who is in the throes of a catastrophic reaction by clapping and singing, thereby engaging the individual in a constructive and acceptable activity.[116,117]

CASE STUDIES

CASE ONE

Mary B. is a 59-year-old woman diagnosed with fibromyalgia. She has impaired mobility and experiences difficulty in performing many daily living skills, including dressing herself. She is extremely fragile and presents a rigid posture and gait, creating the appearance that she can hardly move. The severe, chronic pain throughout her body has contributed to her diagnosis of major depressive disorder. Her symptoms include hopelessness, insomnia, and dysphoria. Diabetes and allergies prevent her from taking medications for her condition.

Mary has little motivation to attend classes or support groups at the hospital, but she enjoys listening to music at home and reports this activity as her only consolation. Her physician referred Mary to music therapy when he learned that music calmed her enough to lull her to sleep at night. The music therapy assessment revealed that Mary had enjoyed piano lessons and had played frequently for friends until hand pain had incapacitated her. The music therapist taught Mary relaxation techniques that were cued by her favorite music. She resumed piano lessons on an electronic keyboard that enabled her to play with minimal pressure on the keys. Mary also began exercising to music in the morning and practicing deep muscle relaxation accompanied by a different kind of music at night.

Six months later, Mary still suffers from fibromyalgia, but she deals with her pain using music to relax her muscles and control her movements. She is motivated to dress and move more freely now that she attends weekly matinees and concerts. Other patients like Mary are also using music as therapy to facilitate their living with pain and neurologic illness. Many of these patients experience relief from various symptoms and are able to comply more easily with treatments that are paired with musical.

CASE TWO

Ann C. is a 44-year-old woman who was admitted for evaluation after falling backwards from a 20-foot ledge in the mountains and landing on her back. The patient exhibited difficulty breathing and heart irregularities at the scene of the accident. Further diagnosis indicated a collapsed left lung, premature ventricular contractions, and rapid changes in blood pressure. Computerized tomography (CT) scan of the spine showed significant anterior column damage to thoracic vertebrae T7, T8, T9, T11, and T12 with compression. Also presented were a 3 to 4 mm retropulsion of the inferior portion of T7 at the spinal canal, and a 2 to 3 mm retropulsion of T9. A small linear fracture was observed at T1. Magnetic Imaging Resonance (MRI) scan of the thoracic spine indicated some compromise in the motion of her fractures, but no cord compression or gross intrinsic cord edema or hemorrhage. Ann reported that she had no feeling in her chest or in the area of her back surrounding the point of contact. Fractures were evident in posterior ribs 5, 6, and 7. There was no evidence of deep vein thrombosis of the lateral lower extremities. Hematoma was present in the right shoulder, and use of both arms was limited. There were contusions on the back of the skull and probable coronary contusions but no evidence of internal hemorrhage.

Following examination in the emergency room, the patient was transferred by air to a multi-trauma hospital where she was reexamined and admitted to the critical care unit for a period of one week. Once stabilized, Ann was fitted for a Thoraco Lumbar Sacral Orthotic (TLSO) brace, admitted to a multi-trauma unit for an additional week, and finally released to a rehabilitation hospital for an additional 8 days of physical rehabilitation. Inpatient treatment occurred in three distinct phases:

Phase I: Critical care
Phase II: Multi-trauma
Phase III: Physical rehabilitation

Music therapies, physical therapies, and occupational therapies were incorporated into the treatment protocol. Sessions with a neuro-psychologist were designed to support the development and use of the patient's coping skills.

Phase I: The patient was heavily medicated and disoriented for the first week following injury. Ann was unaware of the day, time, or place, and unresponsive when verbally prompted with questions or with commands to act. Staff reported one incidence of a panic attack in which Ann quickly attempted to remove medical apparatus from her body.

Phase II: When the patient's cognitive disorientation decreased and vital signs were stable, she was admitted to the multi-trauma unit of the hospital. Treatment objectives changed during this phase from stabilization to improvement of cognitive focus, increased physical exercise (first in bed) as a means of reducing muscle atrophy, and increased use of the upper body and limbs. Treatment objectives also included relearning daily living skills such as dressing; putting on her TLSO brace while lying down; eating using arms and hands; and moving, standing, and walking in her brace. Adaptive devices and strategies for accomplishing these skills were addressed in each therapy session. In all activities, purposeful and efficient use of movement and increased physical endurance were emphasized.

Pain management strategies first used by the patient during Phase II were intravenous administration of a combination of drug therapies followed by patient use of a morphine pump. However, allergy to selected drugs and their replacements resulted in severe and unrelenting nausea, vomiting, dehydration, and physical weakness shortly after introduction. The patient refused medication for pain management early in Phase II of treatment. She indicated that she would rather experience pain alone than pain with accompanying nausea. Ann was moved to a private room at this time to minimize environmental stressors resulting from the treatment activities and responses of patients in the same room.

Music therapy was used by Ann through all phases of hospitalization. Initially, she listened to music that was identified as preferred by a family member. Music listening was introduced during critical care as a means of assessing cognitive function and to cue any kind of response to stimuli. Familiar music was then used to stimulate long term memory and, thus, improve cognitive function. During Phase I, the patient, who is a musician herself, responded increasingly to music listening experiences and to topic-related questions with brief, but topic-specific verbalizations.

During Phase II, active music listening was used as a pain management strategy to focus attention away from pain and nausea for brief periods of time, and as a means of normalizing the hospital environment by masking stress-generating hospital sounds. Music used as a distractor from pain was an essential alternative to medication because it was implemented in the absence of medication for pain. Music listening was also used to calm the patient, reducing the possibility of an anxiety attack while intubated. No further anxiety attacks were observed. Additionally, music listening was employed to cue relaxation prior to sleep and whenever new IV lines were introduced, which occurred frequently.

As Phase II progressed, the strategies previously mentioned were continued. However, additional music applications were also implemented. Music was used to focus Ann's attention on herself and her use of coping skills. This was important during the intensive daily 4-hour physical and occupational therapy sessions. Music was used prior to respiratory therapy to relax her for machine-accompanied deep breathing activities. Tempo-appropriate music was also used intermittently during respiratory therapy to structure continued deep breathing and stamina during the procedure and to minimize anxiety. These activities were designed to improve respiratory capacity that had been reduced as a result of the lung collapse and from being bedridden. Successful respiratory therapy was essential to this phase of treatment so that the patient could be removed from oxygen and become mobile.

Phase III: During physical rehabilitation, music was added to the treatment protocol to motivate gross, fine motor and locomotor movement, and to promote Ann's use of her upper body, especially her arms. Occupational therapists used tempo-appropriate music as a rhythmic structure for upper body movements during in-bed exercises. This music was also used to lengthen the time spent exercising and the fluidity of movement in space. Improvised piano music played by the music therapist was used to structure pacing in walking activities and to increase the amount of time spent walking.

An important use of music during physical rehabilitation was aiding psychological counseling. The neuropsychologist used music lyrics and recorded music to introduce topics for discussion that were designed to promote Ann's acceptance of her injury and its implications for the future. Additionally, the trained music therapist introduced songwriting to encourage active verbal and musical expression of emotion about the accident during recovery. Through music experiences and counseling, Ann was encouraged to integrate the accident into her life experience and to make decisions aimed at improving her quality of life. For example, Ann reported that she felt emotionally "numbed" by the experience. With Ann's help, meaningful, client-preferred music was selected that would cue or "trigger" feelings allowing her to release and express emotion when and where she felt safe to do so. The neuropsychologist and music therapist were able to work together to promote Ann's psychological well-being as her physical health stabilized.

Near the end of her hospitalization, Ann was introduced to group music therapy to promote social interaction following the isolation of some therapy and prior to her release. Music therapy sessions were designed to expose Ann to appropriate peer role models who were further along in the process of rehabilitation. After 3 weeks of hospitalization and rehabilitation, Ann was released to continue her recuperation as an outpatient. She remained in her TLSO brace for several months and continued physical therapy under the care of her neurologist. One year later, Ann was walking, actively engaged in physical therapy, and involved in a pain management program. She had returned to work full time in her continuing career as a music therapist.

In this case study, music therapy was used as a treatment alternative to do the following:

1. Assess cognitive function;
2. Reduce patient stress;
3. Distract attention from physical pain;
4. Mask undesirable hospital sounds;
5. Relax the patient prior to stressful procedures;
6. Provide intermittent rhythmic structure for exhalation during respiratory therapy;
7. Structure gross motor movement in marked time by forcing movement to (eventual) precision and prolonging time spent in repetitive exercise;

8. Facilitate patient self-disclosure, initiate the grieving process, and/or provide an avenue for creative self-expression when used as a cue in psychotherapy; and

9. Provide a transitional structure for patient reintroduction into a social group; peer support through modeling and interaction.

This final step is one of the many small steps that physically injured persons must first choose to take, and then take, in the slow and arduous journey to improved health after trauma.

CONCLUSION

This chapter has reviewed the literature on music therapy and provided an overview of evidence-based techniques in neurologic disorders and pain management. The authors recommend that music therapy be included in treatment plans as part of a comprehensive approach to meeting patient needs for pain management.

REFERENCES

1. Davis WB, Gfeller KE, Thaut MH. *An Introduction to Music Therapy.* 2nd ed. Boston, MA: McGraw-Hill; 1999.
2. Standley JM. Music research in medical/dental treatment: an update of a prior meta-analysis. In: Furman CE, ed. *Effectiveness of Music Therapy Procedures: Documentation of Research and Clinical Practice.* Silver Spring, MD: National Association for Music Therapy; 2000.
3. Staum MJ. Music for physical rehabilitation: an analysis of the literature from 1950–1993. In: Furman CE, ed. *Effectiveness of Music Therapy Procedures: Documentation of Research and Clinical Practice.* Silver Spring, MD: National Association for Music Therapy; 1996.
4. Standley JM, Prickett CA, eds. *Research in music therapy: a tradition of excellence: outstanding reprints from the Journal of Music Therapy 1964–1993.* Silver Spring, MD: National Association for Music Therapy; 1994.
5. Radocy RE, Boyle JD. *Psychological foundations of musical behavior.* Springfield, IL: Charles C Thomas; 1997.
6. Taylor DB: Music in general hospital treatment from 1900 to 1950. *J Music Ther.* 1981;(18):62–73.
7. American Music Therapy Association (AMTA). *AMTA Member Sourcebook.* Silver Spring, MD: American Music Therapy Association; 1998.
8. Hanser SB. *The Music Therapist's Handbook.* Boston, MA: Berklee Press; 1999.
9. Critchley M, Henson RA, eds. *Music and the Brain: Studies of the Neurology of Music.* London, England: Heinemann; 1977.
10. Milner B. Laterality effects in audition. In: Mountcastle VB, ed. *Interhemispheric Relations and Cerebral Dominance.* Baltimore, MD: Johns Hopkins University Press; 1962.

11. Samson S, Zatorre RJ. Melodic and harmonic discrimination following unilateral cerebral excision. *Brain Cogn.* 1988;7:348–360.

12. Peretz M. Processing of local and global musical information by unilaterally brain damaged patients, *Brain.* 1990;(113):1185–1205.

13. Luria AR, Tsvetkova LS, Futer DS. Aphasia in a composer. *J Neurol Sci.* 1965;2:288–292.

14. Gardner H. *Art, Mind and Brain: A Cognitive Approach to Creativity.* New York, NY: Basic Books; 1982.

15. Zatorre RJ. Functional specialization of human auditory cortex for musical processing. *Brain.* 1998;(121):1817–1818.

16. Hachinski KV, Hachinski V. Music and the brain. *CMAJ.* 1994;(151):293–296.

17. Blonder LS, Bowers D, Heilman KM. The role of the right hemisphere in emotional communication. *Brain.* 1991;(114):1115–1127.

18. Borod JC. Interhemispheric and intrahemispheric control of emotion: a focus on unilateral brain damage. *J Consult Clin Psychol.* 1992;60:339–348.

19. Adolphs R, et al. Cortical systems for the recognition of emotion in facial expressions. *J Neurosci.* 1996;(16):7678–7687.

20. Sergent J, et al. Distributed neural network underlying musical sight-reading and keyboard performance. *Science.* 1992;(257):106–109.

21. Tramo MJ. Music of the hemispheres. *Science.* 2002;291:54–56.

22. Zatorre RJ, Evans AC, Meyer E. Neural mechanisms underlying melodic perception and memory for pitch. *J Neurosci.* 1994;(14):1908–1919.

23. Platel H, et al. The structural components of music perception: a functional anatomical study. *Brain.* 1997;(120):229–243.

24. Levitin DJ. *This is Your Brain on Music: The Science of a Human Obsession.* New York, NY: Dutton; 2006.

25. Blood AJ, et al. Emotional responses to pleasant and unpleasant music correlate with activity in paralimbic brain areas. *Nat Neurosci.* 1999;2:382–387.

26. Eslinger PJ, Leder L. Behavior and emotional changes after focal frontal lobe damage. In: Bogorisslavsky J and Cummings JL, eds. *Behavior and Mood Disorders in Focal Brain Lesions.* Cambridge: Cambridge University Press; 2000.

27. Thaut MH, et al. The connection between rhythmicity and brain function. Institute of Electrical and Electronic Engineering. *Eng Med Biol.* 1999;18:101–108.

28. Evans D. The effectiveness of music as an intervention for hospital patients: A systematic review. *J Adv Nurs.* 2002;(37):8–18.

29. Eslinger P, Stouffer J, Rohrbacher M, Grattan L. *Music Therapy and Psychosocial Adjustment to Brain Injury: Report to the National Institutes of Health, Office of Alternative Medicine.* Grant Number 1-R21RR009415-01. Hershey, PA: Pennsylvania State University, Hershey Medical Center; 1993.

30. Adamek MS, Shiraishi IM. Music therapy with traumatic brain-injured patients: speech rehabilitation, intervention models, and assessment procedures (1970–1995). In: Furman CE, ed. *Effectiveness of Music Therapy Procedures: Documentation of Research and Clinical Practice.* Silver Spring, MD: National Association for Music Therapy; 1996.

31. Gilbertson S. Music therapy in neurosurgical rehabilitation. In: Wigram T, Backer JD, eds. *Clinical Applications of Music Therapy in Developmental Disability, Paediatrics and Neurology.* London, England: Jessica Kingsley; 1999.

32. Staum MJ. Music for physical rehabilitation: an analysis of the literature from 1950–1993. In: Furman CE, ed. *Effectiveness of Music Therapy Procedures: Documentation of Research and Clinical Practice.* Silver Spring, MD: National Association for Music Therapy; 1996.

33. Tomaino CM. Music and memory. In: Tomaino CM, ed. *Clinical Applications of Music in Neurologic Rehabilitation.* St Louis, MO: MMB Music; 1998.
34. Paul S, Ramsey D. Music therapy in physical medicine and rehabilitation. *Australian Occup Ther J.* 2000;(47):111–118.
35. Gilbertson SK. Music therapy in neurorehabilitation after traumatic brain injury: A literature review, In: Aldridge, D, ed. *Music therapy and neurological rehabilitation,* St. Louis, 2005, Jessica Kingsley Publishers.
36. Purdie H. Music therapy with adults who have traumatic brain injury and stroke, *British J of Music Ther.* 1997;11(2):45–50.
37. Thaut MH, Schleiffers S, Davis W. Analysis of EMG activity in biceps and triceps muscle in an upper extremity gross motor task under the influence of auditory rhythm. *J of Music Ther.* 1991;28(2):64–88.
38. Hurt CP, Rice RR, McIntosh GC, Thaut MH. Rhythmic auditory stimulation in gait training for patients with traumatic brain injury. *J of Mus Ther.* 1998;25(4):228–241.
39. Magee W, Wheeler B. Music therapy for patients with traumatic brain injury. In: Murrey GJ, ed. *Alternate Therapies in the Treatment of Brain Injury and Neurobehavioral disorders: A Practical Guide.* New York, NY: Hawthorne Press; 2006.
40. Sacks O. Music and the brain. In: Tomaino CM, ed. *Clinical Applications of Music in Neurologic Rehabilitation.* St Louis, MO: MMB Music; 1998.
41. Magee W. Music therapy with patients in low awareness states: Approaches to assessment and treatment in multidisciplinary care. *Neuropsychol Rehab.* 2005;15(3–4): 522–536.
42. Aldridge D. Music, communication and medicine [discussion paper]. *J of the Royal Society of Med.* 1989;(82):743–746.
43. Magee W. Clinical music therapy in neurological setting. Paper presented at the Berklee College of Music; Feb. 1–5, 2007; Boston, MA.
44. Madsen CK. Focus of attention and aesthetic response. *J Res Music Educ.* 1997;45(1): 80–89.
45. Hurt CP. Rhythmic auditory stimulation in gait training for patients with traumatic brain injury. *J Music Ther.* 1998;35(4):228–241.
46. Madsen CK. *Teaching Discipline: A Positive Approach for Educational Development.* Raleigh, NC: Contemporary Publishing Company of Raleigh; 1998.
47. Madsen CK. *Music Therapy: A Behavioral Guide for the Mentally Retarded.* Lawrence, KS: National Association for Music Therapy; 1981.
48. Staum MJ. Music and rhythmic stimuli in the rehabilitation of gait disorders. *J Music Ther.* 1983;22(2):69–87.
49. Wolfe DE. The effect of automated interrupted music on head posturing of cerebral palsied individuals. *J Music Ther.* 1980;17(4):184–206.
50. Thaut MH. Music therapy in neurological rehabilitation. In: Davis WB, Gfeller KE, Thaut MH, eds. *An Introduction to Music Therapy Theory and Practice.* Boston, MA: McGraw-Hill; 1999.
51. Barker VL, Brunk B. The role of creative arts group in the treatment of clients with traumatic brain injury. *Music Ther Perspect.* 1991;9:26–31.
52. Cohen NS. The effect of singing instruction on the speech production of neurologically impaired persons. *J Music Ther.* 1992;24(2):87–102.
53. Cohen NS. The use of superimposed rhythm to decrease the rate of speech in a brain-damaged adolescent. *J Music Ther.* 1988;25(2):85–93.
54. Cohen NS. The application of singing and rhythmic instruction as a therapeutic intervention for persons with neurogenic communication disorders. *J of Mus Ther.* 1993; 30(2):81–99.
55. Schaefer S, Murrey MA, Magee W, Wheeler B. Melodic intonation therapy with brain-injured patients (pp. 75–87). In: Murrey GJ, editor. *Alternate Therapies in the*

Treatment of Brain Injury and Neurobehavioral Disorders: A Practical Guide. New York, NY: Hawthorne Press; 2006.

56. Magee W, Brumfitt S, Freeman J, Davidson J. The role of music therapy in an interdisciplinary approach to address functional communication in complex neuro-communication disorders: a case report. *Disability and Rehab.* 2006;28(19):1221–1229.

57. Goldfarb R, Bader E. Espousing melodic intonation therapy in aphasia rehabilitation: a case study. *International J of Rehab Res.* 1979;2(3):333–342.

58. Belin P, Van Eeckhout P, Zilbovicius M, Remy P, Francois C, Guillaume S. Recovery from nonfluent aphasia after melodic intonation therapy: a PET study. *Neurology.* 1996;47(6):1504–1511.

59. Galloway H. A comprehensive bibliography of musical studies referential to communication development, processing disorders and remediation. *J Music Ther.* 1975;12:164–197.

60. Kinsella G, Prior MR, Murray G. Singing ability after right and left sided brain damage: a research note. *Cortex.* 1988;24(1):165–169.

61. Jacome DE. Aphasia with elation, hypermusia, musicophilia and compulsive whistling. *J Neurol Neurosurg.* 1984;47(3):308–310.

62. Brust JC. Music and language: musical alexia and agraphia. *Brain.* 1980;103(2):367–392.

63. Racette A, Bard C, Peretz I. Making non-fluent aphasics speak: sing along! *Brain: A J of Neur.* 2006;129(Pt 10):2571–2584.

64. Wilson S, Parsons K, Reutens D. Preserved Singing in aphasia: a case study of the efficiency of melodic intonation therapy, *Music Percep.* 2006;24(1):23–35.

65. Filippini JF. Some useful basics of functional anatomy for a better understanding of the pain phenomenon. *Rev Laryngol Otol Rhinol.* 1996;117:75–78.

66. Wall PD. On the relation of injury to pain: the John J. Bonica lecture. *Pain.* 1979;6:253–264.

67. Magill-Levreault L. Music therapy in pain and symptom management. *J Palliat Care.* 1993;9:42–48.

68. Wolfe DE. The effect of automated interrupted music on head posturing of cerebral palsied individuals, *J Music Ther.* 1978;15:162–178.

69. Brown CJ, Chen ACN, Dworkin SF. Music in the control of pain, *Music Ther.* 1989;8:47–60.

70. Standley JM. Music research in medical/dental treatment: an update of a prior meta-analysis. In: Furman CE, editor. *Effectiveness of music therapy procedures: documentation of research and clinical practice,* Silver Spring, MD: National Association for Music Therapy; 1996.

71. Maslar P. The effect of music on the reduction of pain: a review of the literature. *Art Psychother.* 1986;13:215–219.

72. Hanser SB. Music therapy and stress reduction research, *J Music Ther.* 1985;22:193–206.

73. Dileo C, Bradt J. *Medical Music Therapy: A Meta-Analysis and Agenda for Future Research.* Cherry Hill NJ: Jeffrey Books; 2005.

74. Menegazzi JJ, et al. A randomized, controlled trial of the use of music during laceration repair. *Ann Emerg Med.* 1991;20(4):348–350.

75. Good M et al. Relaxation and music to reduce postsurgical pain. *J Adv Nurs.* 2001;33(2):208–215.

76. Nilsson U, Rawal N, Unosson M. A comparison of intra-operative or post-operative exposure to music—a controlled trial of the effects on postoperative pain. *Anaesth.* 2003;58(7):699–703.

77. Eisenman A, Cohen B. Music therapy for patients undergoing regional anesthesia. *AORN J.* 1995;62:947–950.

78. Lukas LK. Orthopedic outpatients perception of perioperative music listening as therapy. *J Theory Construct & Testing*. 2004;8(1):7–12.
79. Zimmerman L, Nieveen J, Bernason S, Schmaderer M. The effects of music interventions on postoperative pain and sleep in coronary artery bypass graft (CABG) patients. *Scholarly Inquiry for Nurs Prac*. 1996;10(2):153–170.
80. Hanser S. Music therapy in adult oncology: research issues. *J Soc Integrative Onc*. 2006;4(2):62–66.
81. Hilliard RE. Music therapy in hospice and palliative care: a review of the empirical data. *Evidence Based Compl Altern Med*. 2005;2:173–178.
82. Schorr JA. Music and pattern change in chronic pain. *Adv Nurs Sci*. 1993;15:27–36.
83. Zelazny CM. Therapeutic instrumental music playing in hand rehabilitation for older adults with osteoarthritis: four case studies. *J Music Ther*. 2001;38(2):97–113.
84. Daveson BA. A model of response: coping mechanisms and music therapy techniques during debridement. *Music Ther Perspect*. 1999;17:92–98.
85. Mandel SE. Music for wellness: music therapy for stress management in a rehabilitation program, *Music Ther Perspect*. 1996;14:38–43.
86. Brocious SK. Music: An intervention for pain during chest tube removal after open-heart surgery. *Am J Crit Care*. 1999;8(6):410–415.
87. Heiser RM, Chiles K, Fudge M, Gray SE. The use of music during the immediate postoperative recovery period. *AORN J*. 1997;65(4):777–778, 781–795.
88. Kwekkeboom, KL. Music versus distraction for procedural pain and anxiety in patients with cancer. *Onc Nurs Forum*. 2003;30(3):433–440.
89. Cepeda MS, Diaz JE, Hernandez W, Daza E, Carr DB. Music does not reduce alfentanil requirement during patient-controlled analgesia (PCA) use in extracorporeal shock wave lithotripsy for renal stones. *J Pain Symptom Manage*. 1998;16:382–387.
90. Skille O, Wigram T. The effects of music, vocalization, and vibration on brain and muscle tissue: studies in vibroacoustic therapy. In: Wigram T, Superstar B, West R, eds. *The Art and Science of Music Therapy: A Handbook*. Chur, Switzerland: Harwood Academic; 1995.
91. Malone AB. The effects of live music on pediatric patients receiving intravenous starts, venipunctures, injections, and heel sticks. *J Music Ther*. 1996;33:19–33.
92. Standley JM, Hanser SB. Music therapy research and applications in pediatric oncology treatment. *J Pediatr Oncol Nurs*. 1995;12:3–8.
93. Michel DE, Chesky KS. A survey of music therapists using music for pain relief. *Art Psychother*. 1995;22:49–51.
94. Hanser SB, Thompson LW. Effects of a music therapy strategy on depressed older adults. *J Gerontol*. 1994;49:265–269.
95. Hanser SB. Music therapy with depressed older adults. *J Int Assoc Music Handicap*. 1989;4:16–27.
96. Crystal HA, Grober E, Masur D. Preservation of musical memory in Alzheimer's disease. *J Neurol Neurosurg*. 1989;52:1415–1416.
97. Beatty W, Zavadil K, Bailly R, et al. Preserved musical skill in a severely demented patient. *Int J Clin Neuropsychol*. 1988;10:158–164.
98. Swartz KP, Hartz EC, Crummer LC, Walton JP, Frisina RD. Does the melody linger on? music cognition in Alzheimer's disease. *Seminar on Neurology*. 1989;9:152–158.
99. Swartz KP, Walton J, Crummer, Hartz E, Frisina R. P3 event-related potentials and performance of healthy older adults and AD subjects for music perception tasks. *Psychomusicol*. 1992;11:96–118.
100. Brotons M, Koger SM, Pickett-Cooper P. Music and the dementias: a review of literature. *J Music Ther*. 1997;34:204–245.

101. Koger SM, Chapin K, Brotons M. Is music therapy an effective intervention for dementia?: a meta-analytic review of literature. *J Music Ther.* 1999;36:2–15.

102. Pollack NJ, Namazi KH. The effect of music participation on the social behavior of Alzheimer's disease patients. *J Music Ther.* 1992;29:54–67.

103. Smith G. A comparison of the effects of three treatment interventions on cognitive functioning of Alzheimer patients. *Music Ther.*1986;6A:41–56.

104. Lipe A. Using music therapy to enhance the quality of life in a client with Alzheimer's dementia: a case study *Music Ther Perspect.* 1991;9:102–105.

105. Brotons M, Pickett-Cooper P. The effects of music therapy intervention on agitation behaviors of Alzheimer's disease patients. *J Music Ther.* 1996;33:2–18.

106. Clair AA, Bernstein B. The effect of no music, stimulative background music and sedative background music on agitation behaviors in persons with severe dementia. *Activities Adaptation Aging.* 1994;19:61–70.

107. Gerdner LA, Swanson EA. Effects of individualized music on confused and agitated elderly patients. *Arch Psychiatr Nurs.* 1993;7:284–291.

108. Goddaer J, Abraham I. Effects of relaxing music on agitation during meals among nursing home residents with severe cognitive impairments. *Arch Psychiatr Nurs.* 1994;8:150–158.

109. Tabloski P, McKinnon-Howe L, Remington R. Effects of calming music on the level of agitation in cognitively impaired nursing home residents. Am J Alzheimer Care Relat Disord Res. 1995;10:10–15.

110. Ward CR, Los Kamp L, Newman S. The effects of participation in an intergenerational program on the behavior of residents with dementia. Activities Adaptation Aging. 1996;20:61–76.

111. Thomas DW, Heitman RJ, Alexander T. The effects of music on bathing cooperation for residents with dementia. *J Music Ther.* 1997;34:246–259.

112. Fitzgerald-Cloutier ML. The use of music therapy to decrease wandering: an alternative to restraints. *Music Ther Perspect.* 1992;11:32–36.

113. Groene RW II. Effectiveness of music therapy: 1:1 interventions with individuals having senile dementia of the Alzheimer's type. *J Music Ther.* 1993;30:138–157.

114. Lindenmuth GF, Patel M, Chang PK. Effects of music on sleep in healthy elderly and subjects with senile dementia of the Alzheimer's type. *Am J Alzheimer Dis Relat Disord Res.* 1992;2:13–20.

115. Hanser SB, Clair AA. Retrieving the losses of Alzheimer's disease for patients and caregivers with the aid of music. In: Wigram T, Saperston B, West R, eds. *The Art and Science of Music Therapy: A Handbook.* Chur, Switzerland: Harwood Academic; 1995.

116. Hanser SB. Music therapy with individuals with advanced dementia. In: Volicer L, Bloom-Charette L, eds. *Enhancing the Quality of Life in Advanced Dementia.* Philadelphia, PA: Brunner/Mazel; 1999.

117. Hanser SB. Music therapy to reduce anxiety, agitation, and depression. *Nurs Home Med.* 1996;10:286–291.

CHAPTER 4

Laser Biostimulation (Phototherapy)

Michael I. Weintraub

The creation of a thousand forests is in one acorn.

—*Ralph Waldo Emerson*

Knowledge, once gained, casts a faint light beyond its own immediate boundaries. There is no discovery so limited as not to illuminate something beyond itself.

—*John Tyndall*

As the circle of light increases, so does the circumference of darkness around it.

—*Albert Einstein*

The application of light for medicinal purposes (healing) has been used for thousands of years. The ancient Greeks believed that sunlight exposure induced strength and health. During the middle ages, the disinfectant properties of sunlight were used to combat plague and other illnesses, and in the nineteenth century, cutaneous tuberculosis (scrofula) was treated with ultraviolet light exposure. Currently light therapy is used to treat psoriasis, hyperbilirubinemia, and seasonal affective disorder (SAD).

Light has one identity as electromagnetic waves consisting of photonic energy bundles that are divisible into wave lengths. Visible light, called the visual spectrum, is 400 to 700 nanometers (nm) appreciated by the human eye. The human eye is sensitive to approximately 90% of the spectrum of electromagnetic radiation that propagates through the atmosphere and reaches the earth's surface. As a sensory organ, the eye evolved to detect that portion of the spectrum that is there to be seen in the terrestrial environment.

One nanometer (nm) equals one billionth of a meter. The smaller the wave length, the higher the energy (from Planck's Law, the energy level is the inverse of the wavelength multiplied by Planck's Constant), and the greater its ability to penetrate tissues. For example, a blue-violet light is a shorter wave length while a red light has a longer wave length. Infrared is even longer (lower energy) and ultraviolet is even shorter (higher energy) than the visible spectrum. Dermatologists are therefore concerned that the DNA-causing damage of ultraviolet light with a shorter wavelength and higher, "ionizing" energy is dangerous. The fact that infrared light has a longer wavelength and lower energy state has also been used as an argument for using infrared light as a safer form of tanning.

X-rays, gamma rays, ultraviolet rays, cosmic rays, and others all fall below visible light on the electromagnetic spectrum. Longer wave lengths such as infrared rays, microwaves, television transmissions, and FM/AM radio waves have different characteristics.

HISTORY

The atomic models that lead to the discovery of lasers were theorized and established in 1917 by Albert Einstein. His discovery became known as LASER for Light Amplification by Stimulated Emission of Radiation. When an atom is in an excited state and then an incoming light particle reaches it, it may eject an additional photon instead of being absorbed. This theory was a revolutionary concept that proved to be true, and Einstein received the Nobel Prize for describing the photoelectric effect. By 1960, the first practical ruby red laser was developed by T. H. Maiman[1] who used crystals and mirrors to produce a monochromatic, nondivergent light beam in which all waves were parallel and in phase. These characteristics were subsequently referred to as monochromaticity, collimation, and coherence, respectively. The original ruby red beam was a visible red light with a wave length of 694 nm. Since then, various crystals and gases have been used to expand the electromagnetic spectrum into the infrared and visible light lasers.

DEFINITIONS

LASER (Light Amplification by Stimulated Emission of Radiation). When light is directed onto an object, one of the following occurs:

1. The light is reflected.
2. The light is transmitted.
3. The light is scattered.
4. The light is absorbed.

Every object has optic properties that determine the effectiveness of light and the reaction of light with that object. For example, mid-infrared and far-infrared lasers, such as carbon dioxide (CO_2) and holmium, or yttrium-aluminum garnet (YAG), are primarily absorbed by water in the tissues. This absorption of the infrared light energy converts to heat, which leads to local vaporization that does not spread. Near infrared and visible-light lasers such as neodymium, YAG, and argon are poorly absorbed by water but are rapidly absorbed by pigment such as hemoglobin and melanin. This optic property makes these lasers effective in the destruction of tissues that are rich in pigment such as retina, gastric mucosa, and pigmented cutaneous lesions. It is easy to see how these so-called high-powered surgical lasers, using heat and energy, lead to specific tissue changes. During the past 30 years, numerous animal and laboratory experiments were carried out using these high-energy lasers. These experiments produced results that have ultimately led to human testing and approval by the Food and Drug Administration (FDA) of the use of lasers on humans.

Despite more than 30 years of similar experiments using weak or low-level, nonthermal lasers, that is, low level laser therapy (LLLT), there is still controversy concerning its effectiveness as a treatment modality due to lack of randomized, double-blind, placebo-controlled trials and peer-reviewed publications. Various articles exist that make claims yet many have flawed methodology, various time and dosage schedules, and absence of strict placebo design. Despite all these shortcomings, several studies were brought to the attention of the FDA and in 2002 they approved an application for laser light for pain relief as a therapeutic device.

THEORY

Cold laser, or LLLT, is based on the idea that monochromatic light energy, which is wave length–dependent for its penetration, can alter cellular functions. Because the original European studies on wound healing in animals was positive, it was described as a biostimulation. Mester and colleagues[2] and Lyons[3] found that light could be stimulatory at low powers and could elicit an opposite inhibitory effect at higher powers. In addition, the cumulative dosages of the radiation could sometimes be inhibitory. Today there are a variety of lasers, but the two most popular are helium-neon (He-Ne) and gallium aluminum arsenide (GaAlAs [830 nm]). In practice, these visible and infrared lasers have powers of 30 to 90 mW and deliver from 1 to 9 J/cm^2 (Joules/Square centimeters) to treatment sites. To date, they have been shown to be safe within this spectrum but they have also been used at higher dosages.

MECHANISMS OF ACTION

Musculoskeletal tissues appear to have optic properties that respond to light between 500 and 1,000 nm. The sufficient specific laser dosage and the number of treatments needed are still the subject of controversy. It is hypothesized that light-sensitive organelles, or chromatophores,[4] absorb light and that ultimately the energy produces a biologic reaction. It has been suggested that chromatophores exist on the myelin sheath and mitochondria, and that it is the monochromatic wave length properties, rather than coherency and collimation, that induce biologic changes. It is presumed that the collimation and coherency lead to rapid degradation by scatter. Others have theorized that primary photoreceptors represent flavins and porphyrins and that the therapeutic benefit of pain reduction by a combination of red and near infrared light is due to combination of increased beta endorphins, blocking depolarization of C-fiber afferents, reduced bradykinin levels, and ionic channel stabilization.

TISSUE PENETRATION

Tissue penetration is a reflection of the wavelength. The shorter He-Ne laser beam (632 nm) penetrates several millimeters into tissue whereas the GaAlAs 830 nm/30 mW allows photons to penetrate more than an inch (3 cm). Several authors have stated that an infrared laser beam travels about 2 mm into tissue and that this represents one penetration depth with loss of 1/e (37%) of its intensity.[5] However, the shorter, visible, He-Ne red beam is attenuated the same amount in 0.5 to 1 mm.[6-8] How does one measure the decay in the amount of energy with distance? At the surface of the skin, the laser delivers from 1 to 9 J/cm^2. Karu[9] has demonstrated that 0.01 J/cm^2 can alter cellular processes. As a result, approximately six penetration depths (3 to 6 mm for He-Ne red light and about 24 mm for GaAlAs IR) are possible before the strength of the beam stream drops from 9 J/cm^2 to 0.01 J/cm^2. Thus, the threshold and specific therapeutic amount needed to stimulate the superficial nerve and tissues differs from the deeper structures. There is also a scattering of energy that influences nonneural adjacent tissues (i.e., flexor tendons in forearm/wrist with stimulation at level of carpal tunnel).

It has been stated that tissue penetration and saturation with pulsed frequency settings of 1–100 Hz influenced pain and neuralgia whereas 1,000 Hz influenced edema and swelling and that 5,000 Hz influenced inflammation. Superpulsed laser with gallium arsenide (GaAs) infrared diode provides the deepest penetration in body tissues. It operates at a wavelength of 904 nm. Superpulsing is defined as a mechanism whereby there are continuous bursts of very high power pulses of light energy (10–100 Watts) that are of extremely short duration (100–200 nanosec/ Hz). This allows GaAs penetration to tissue depths of 3–5 cm and deeper. Some versions of GaAs therapeutic lasers actually penetrate to tissue depths of 10–14 cm.[10]

LASER RESEARCH

There have been many claims and studies regarding LLLT, but the varied quality of trials has led to controversy. Basford,[5,8,11] a major critic of the deficiencies of many studies, describes that LLLT research has developed along the following three separate lines:

1. Cellular function
2. Animal studies
3. Human trials

Perhaps the strongest and most well-established research has been on changes in cellular functions.

There is a strong body of direct evidence indicating that LLLT can significantly alter cellular processes (Table 4.1). Following are specific areas of treatment that have been cited:

- Stimulation of collagen formation leading to stronger scars[12]; increased recruitment of fibroblasts and formation of granulation tissue[13]; increased neovascularization[14]; and faster wound healing[3,15,16]
- Pain relief analgesia and reduced firing frequency of nociceptors[17]

- Enhanced remodeling and repair of bone[4,16]
- Stimulation of endorphin release[18]
- Modulation of the immune system via prostaglandin synthesis[2,19]

ANIMAL AND LABORATORY STUDIES

Basic animal and cellular research with red-beam, low-level laser has produced both positive and negative results. Passarella[20] believes that the optic properties of mitochondria are influenced by He-Ne laser irradiation, producing new mitochondrial conformations that ultimately lead to increased oxygen consumption. Walker[21] has suggested that He-Ne laser affects serotonin metabolism, and Yu[22] has demonstrated an increased phosphate potential and energy charge with light exposure. Further research continues at the cellular level. Fibroblast, lymphocyte, monocyte, and macrophage cells have been studied, and bacterial cell lines of E. coli have served as models of investigation.[23] The most popular laser in such cellular research has been the He-Ne laser with a wave length of 632.8 nm. However, some major discrepancies among the existing literature lie in the wide variation of laser parameters employed, particularly dose and treatment time. Because imprecise dosimetry has clouded the issues, the optimal dose for achieving a biologic benefit has yet to be determined.

Despite the problems posed by a lack of standardization, lack of controls, and imprecise dose and treatment schedules for in vivo experimental work, results from cellular research were extrapolated into

TABLE 4.1 Cellular Effects Altered by Low-Energy Irradiation

Phenomenon	Effect	
Collagen and protein Synthesis	↑↑	↓↓
Cell Proliferation and Differentiation	↑↑	↓↓
Cell Motility	↑↑	
Membrane potential and binding Affinities	↑↑	
Neurotransmitter Release	↑↑	
Prostaglandin Synthesis	↑↑	
ATP Synthesis	↑↑	
Phagocytosis	↑↑	
Oxyhemoglobin Dissociation	↑↑	

research on animals. Subsequently, a wide variety of animal models were employed to assess the putative biostimulatory effects of laser irradiation on wound healing. Small, loose-skinned rodents, such as mice, rats, or guinea pigs have been used most often, but models using pigs have led to different results. It has been argued that pigskin represents a more suitable model for extrapolation to humans because it is similar in character to human skin, thus leading to its use in human skin grafts, for example.[11,24]

Baxter[25] provides an excellent review of the animal models used in the wound-healing literature. The details of experimental and irradiation procedures are so numerous and variable, however, that reproducibility and intertrial comparisons are usually not practical. Research groups reported either an acceleration in healing or no effect on the healing process. Two frequent criteria for assessing wound healing were collagen content and tensile strength. Rochkind[26] conducted one of the largest series of controlled animal trials on crushed sciatic nerves versus normal nerves in rats. Constant low-intensity laser irradiation (7.6 to 10 J/cm^2 daily for up to 20 days) with recording of compound action potentials demonstrated highly beneficial effects. Wound-healing rates in both irradiated and nonirradiated wounds were accelerated, but the amplitude of action potentials in crushed sciatic nerves were raised substantially only in the irradiated groups. The laser treatment also greatly reduced the degeneration of motor neurons and suggested that these results might be extrapolated for application in human research trials.

The information gained from in vivo animal trials exposed to laser photo biostimulation indicated that in certain animal models, wound healing could be achieved. The reader is cautioned to remain both critical and skeptical because variations exist as to methodology, techniques, dosimetry, exposure time, and frequency of treatments.

HUMAN CLINICAL TRIALS

Despite the above controversy and limitations, many clinicians were persuaded by the cellular and animal data to attempt human trials. A number of disorders, including neurologic, rheumatologic, and musculoskeletal conditions, have been treated with LLLT with various claims. The FDA has previously been a major obstacle due to the absence of randomized, placebo-controlled trials with varied methodology; varied dosages and techniques, and the absence of objective parameters. However, in February 2002 it approved the aforementioned application for pain relief.

CARPAL TUNNEL SYNDROME

Carpal Tunnel Syndrome is a common clinical disorder seen in 5%–10% of the population with compression of the median nerve at the wrist. Acroparesthesia in the first three fingers (numbness, tingling and burning) often arises and may interfere with sleep. When resistant to conservative treatment, the disorder often progresses with weakness and atrophy. There are nine flexor tendons adjacent to the median nerve and they often intersect the nerve fascicles in the carpal tunnel. Thus, nerve compression or tendonitis may serve as a cause as well as narrow the canal diameters.

Basford,[27] utilizing only 1 J of energy, found that he could statistically influence both sensory and motor distal latencies in normal volunteers. Basford's study was a double-blind controlled study using a GaAlAs percutaneous laser. Weintraub[28] used a similar laser, but at higher energy levels of 9 J, and Compound Motor Action Potential/Sensory Nerve Action Potential (CMAP/SNAP) electrophysiologic parameters to achieve a nearly 80% success rate in resolving the symptoms of carpal tunnel syndrome. There were no controls in the study, but almost 1,000 sensory and motor latencies of nerves were studied before and after each treatment. Particularly interesting was the fact that the distal latency was prolonged in 40% of subjects, yet they remained asymptomatic. This prolonged latency suggests that nonneural tissues were stimulated and could be responsible for symptoms of tendonitis. With this dosage, a significant number of individuals had immediate slowed prolongation of distal latency (nerve conduction). However, they remained asymptomatic and by the next visit, the distal latency was back to baseline or improved. This observation has also been noted by others.[29] For example, Padua[30] has validated Weintraub's study, and currently three placebo-controlled studies are being performed with preliminary results of 70% success (personal communication, 1999). Additionally, there are two reports using higher doses of 10–12 J of IR diode (40 to 50 mW) revealing alterations of both the median and superficial radial nerve.[31-33]

Naeser[34] and Branco[35] used a combination of two noninvasive, painless treatment modalities, namely, red-beam laser and microamps transcutaneous electrical nerve stimulation (TENS), to stimulate acupuncture points on the affected hand. Sham controls were used. A significant reduction in median nerve sensory latencies in the treated hand and a 92% reduction in pain were observed. Postoperative failures also improved with this protocol. Weintraub (personal observation) utilized his original protocol (9 J/cm^2) plus stimulation of various acupressure points as per Naeser[34] and Branco[35] as well as the flexor tendons in the upper wrist, achieved up to 85% improvement.

NEURALGIAS

Other superficial nerves also respond to laser biostimulation. Disorders such as meralgia paresthetica, cubital tunnel syndrome, tarsal tunnel syndrome, radial nerve palsy, and traumatic digital neuralgias have responded to this treatment.[36] Due to the small number of individuals treated, these observations are to be considered anecdotal. However, Weintraub believes that his observations of nonneural structures playing an important yet unappreciated role in symptomatic carpal tunnel syndrome, and probably other nerve entrapments, is indeed important. For example, the distal latency of the median nerve could be greater than 5 ms in patients who have become asymptomatic with laser treatment. Either a threshold exists for the median nerve, or the tendons and blood vessels surrounding the median nerve exert some influence. Franzblau and Werner[37] raised similar issues in a provocative editorial titled, "What is carpal tunnel syndrome?"

NEUROGENIC PAIN

The efficacy of laser therapy in various pain syndromes has been investigated by several groups. Preliminary double-blind studies by Walker[21] demonstrated improvement in seven out of nine patients with trigeminal neuralgia. Two out of five patients improved with postherpetic neuralgia and five out of six patients improved with radiculopathy. Baxter[38] also believed that laser was effective for postherpetic neuralgia. Moore[39] investigated the efficacy of using GaAlAs laser in the treatment of postherpetic neuralgia in a double-blind, crossover trial on 20 patients. The result was an apparently significant reduction in pain. Hong[40] validated this study with 60% of the patients feeling improvement within 10 minutes. Friedman[41] used an intraoral He-Ne laser directed at a specific maxillary alveolar tender point to significantly abort atypical facial pain.

Trigeminal neuralgia was successfully treated with He-Ne laser by Walker.[42] In the 35 patients studied in this double-blind, placebo-controlled trial, he found a significant difference in visual analog scale (VAS) ratings between active and placebo-treated patients.

Using an intraoral He-Ne laser directed at the specific maxillary alveolar tender point (Figure 4.1), Weintraub was able to abort acute migraine headaches in 85% of cases with sham controls. These findings support the trigeminovascular theory of migraine with a maxillary (V2) provocative site.[43] These results rival pharmacotherapeutical results. Interestingly, Friedman[44] used the same maxillary alveolar tenderness (MAT) point (Figure 4.1) to treat atypical facial pain and migraine headache cryotherapy (cold water). The treatment achieved a striking reduction in discomfort.

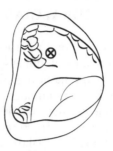

FIGURE 4.1   Laser site for migraine headache.

RADICULITIS

Several groups have investigated the efficacy of laser therapy in the treatment of radicular and pseudoradicular pain syndromes. Bieglio[45] and Mizokami[46] reported positive effects. Low-power laser has also been used successfully to induce preoperative anesthesia in both veterinary practice and dental surgery.[47] In contrast to the numerous clinical human studies of laser-mediated analgesia, there have been relatively few laboratory studies. Most of the experiments have been completed in China using a variety of animals including rats, goats, rabbits, sheep, and horses. There are no English abstracts or translations of most of these works. Other studies published in English have reported variable findings using the tail-flick methodology in animals.

Laser acupuncture using an He-Ne diode was reported to be successful in the treatment of experimental arthritis in rats. Vocalization and limb withdrawal were the parameters used in response to noxious stimulation.[48] Although it is clear that problems exist in extrapolating the findings of laboratory work to humans, Naeser[34] and Branco[35] were successful with this procedure in carpal tunnel syndrome (CTS). Similarly, Weintraub[28] saw additional improvement when he incorporated Naeser's acupressure points (Figure 4.2) with his protocol (Figure 4.3).

SOFT TISSUE HEALING

One of the major economic burdens in the United States has been caused by the high incidence of soft tissue injuries and low back pain and subsequent work disability l. Numerous studies using He-Ne and infra-red (IR) laser diodes (830 nm range) have reported varying results,[8,11,49,50] but randomized controlled and blinded studies have been difficult to carry out.

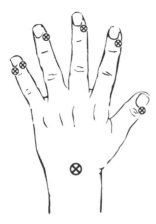

FIGURE 4.2   Dorsal hand.

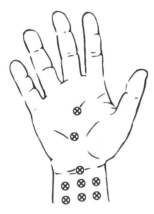

FIGURE 4.3   Volar wrist, palm.

Rheumatologists in the United States have identified encouraging results in rheumatoid arthritis,[51] with similar results being reported in the Soviet Union/Russia, Eastern Europe, and Japan. Walker reported success after a 10-week course of treatment with He-Ne units. Using a GaAlAs 830 nm, Asada[52] found 90% improvement in an uncontrolled trial on 170 patients. Despite these generally positive results, Bliddal[53] did not see any significant change in symptoms of morning stiffness or joint function; however, there was slight improvement in pain scales. Similar positive results have been reported for osteoarthritis and other pseudoarthritic conditions. Critics have argued, however, that because rheumatoid arthritis is a disease of exacerbation and remission, it is difficult to assess efficacy.

A number of reports document the apparent efficacy of laser therapy in reducing pain associated with sports injuries. These reports initially came from Russia and Eastern Europe and were subsequently confirmed by Morselli[54] and Emmanoulidis.[55] It is notable that in the latter study improvement was accompanied by a decrease in thermographic readings.

Tendinopathies, especially lateral humeral epicondylitis (tennis elbow), have been studied by numerous groups as well as the author. There has usually been a relatively rapid response to therapy; however, Haker[56] failed to show any effect with laser acupuncture treatment for tennis elbow.

CHRONIC NECK PAIN

This problem is common and is often associated specifically with a herniated disk, degenerative disk disease, degenerative spine disease, spinal stenosis, or facet joint dysfunction. The small C-nociceptive afferents and the larger myelinated A-delta fibers usually innervate these areas. Local chemical dysfunction with release of Substance P, phospholipase A, cytokines, nitric oxide, and so forth are probably also involved. It is theorized that direct photoreceptors of photons by cytochromes produce elevated ATP production and changes in the cell membrane permeability. Antiedema affects and anti-inflammatory responses have been alleged to occur by reduced bradykinin levels and increased beta endorphins. The depth of the penetration as well as the total dosage influences the success of the treatment at the target tissue level. Thus, combinations of high output (CW) gallium aluminum arsenide (GaAlAs) and gallium arsenide (GaAs) (superpulsing) can achieve penetration of 3–5 cm and even deeper (10–14 cm). Additionally acupressure point stimulation (2–4 J of energy) to the ear, hand, or body should also be utilized.

LOW BACK PAIN

This chronic pain syndrome is the most common cause of disability in the United States affecting 75%–85% of Americans at some point in their lifetimes. Common causes include herniated disks, spinal stenosis, spondylosis, facet joint dysfunction, as well as failed back syndrome secondary to surgery. Similarly, the small C-nociceptive afferents and A-delta fibers are involved with localized chemical dysfunction producing altered signal transduction. A combination of high-output gallium aluminum arsenide infrared lasers with 9 J/cm and/or gallium arsenide superpulsed infrared laser may be effective in treating the deeper tissues. Usually the nerve irritation occurs deep around 60 mm secondary to herniated disk. Acupressure point stimulation should also be utilized.

CEREBRAL PALSY IN BABIES AND CHILDREN

Asagai[57] performed LLLT on acupressure points in 1,000 babies and children with cerebral palsy. The LLLT effectively suppressed tonic muscle spasms.

STROKE

Naeser[58] improved blood flow in stroke patients using laser acupuncture treatment and noted improvement in symptomatology.

VERTIGO

Weintraub has achieved benefit by stimulating Naguien acupressure points with an 830-nm laser (see Figure 4.4). Naeser[59] in a review of the highlights of the Second Congress, World Association for Laser Therapy, reported that Wilden treated inner ear disorders, including vertigo, tinnitus, and hearing loss, with a combination of 630 to 700 nm and 830 nm laser.

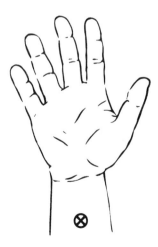

FIGURE 4.4   Naguien.

The total dosage was at least 4000 J. Daily 1-hour laser treatments to both ears were performed for at least 3 weeks. The lasers were applied to the auditory canal and the mastoid and petrosal bone. Wilden said that he used this approach for more than 9 years with 800 patients and, except in very severe cases, most patients reported improvement in hearing.

ACUTE MIGRAINE HEADACHE

Laser applied to the Hegu point (see Figure 4.5) on the contralateral side may be effective for treating migraine headaches. Intraoral He-Ne along the zone of maxillary alveolar tenderness (see Figure 4.1) also achieves success in the range of 78%. Stimulation is repeated three times at 1 to 1 1/2-minute intervals.

MERALGIA PARESTHETICA

Meralgia paresthetica is an often-disabling symptom that is due to compression of the lateral anterior femoral cutaneous nerve at the level of the inguinal ligament. The author has treated 10 patients with this condition by stimulating from the level of the inguinal ligament to the level of the knee anterolaterally (see Figure 4.6). Significant pain reduction has been noted in 8 of the 10 patients by the fourth treatment, but there have been recurrences.

CUBITAL TUNNEL SYNDROME

Compression of the ulnar nerve in the cubital tunnel may be associated with an epicondylitis. Anecdotal experience by the author has produced benefit in six patients.

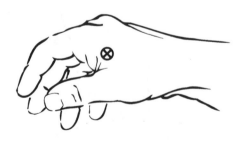

FIGURE 4.5   Hegu.

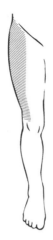

FIGURE 4.6   Laser site for Meralgia paresthetica.

FACIAL PALSY

Idiopathic Bell's palsy or facial palsy secondary to Lyme disease has been treated anecdotally with an 830-nm laser by the author. It is unclear whether this treatment has accelerated healing since there is a high incidence of spontaneous resolution.

TARSAL TUNNEL SYNDROME

Compression of the medial and lateral plantar nerves at the level of the ankle has been attempted in two cases using 830 nm laser. There were no significant results.

PERIPHERAL NEUROPATHY AND NEURITIS

The soles of the feet and various acupressure points were stimulated without relief in 10 cases of nondiabetic peripheral neuropathy; however, Anodyne utilizing monochromatic infra-red and visible light phototherapy in diabetic peripheral neuropathy has been reported as successful inducing temporary or permanent relief from pain and inflammation.[60]

TRAUMATIC NEURITIS

Traumatic neuritis secondary to dog bites in the limbs has been found to be sensitive to laser therapy in two cases by the author.

SAFETY

No detrimental effects are produced by low-output, nonthermal lasers, although it is obvious that direct retinal exposure is to be avoided. Pregnancy does not appear to be a contraindication with LLLT, but investigators have been advised to avoid treating pregnant women and individuals with local tumors in the area of treatment. Individuals taking photosensitizing drugs such as tetracycline, or having photosensitive skin, should probably avoid this treatment. It has also been suggested that phototherapy applications following steroid injections are contraindicated since anti-inflammatory medicine is well documented to reduce the effectiveness of photobiostimulation.[61]

CONCLUSIONS

The neurologic community is faced with many conditions that respond poorly or marginally to pharmacologic therapy. Thus, the appeal of non-invasive therapeutic laser and other phototherapy devices that are both effective and safe is evident, and they are a most welcome to the physician's armamentarium. Therapeutic laser treatment has been used successfully in a number of fields and is a popular modality worldwide. Critical analysis of the literature indicates that the majority of the studies suffer from methodological flaws such as absence of controls, variable duration and intensity of laser treatment, and poor quality. Consequently, the majority of observations are to be considered anecdotal in nature until appropriate randomized control trials have been undertaken. In the interim, laser therapy appears to be safe and worthy of further investigation for the management of pain.

REFERENCES

1. Maiman TH. Stimulated optical radiation in ruby [letter]. *Nature.* 1960;187:493–494.
2. Mester E, Toth N, Mester A. The biostimulative effect of laser beam. *Laser Basic Biomed Res.* 1982;22:4–7.
3. Lyons RF et al. Biostimulation of wound healing in vivo by a helium-neon laser. *Ann Plast Surg.* 1987;18:47–50.
4. Walsh J. The current status of low level laser therapy in dentistry: part I—soft tissue applications. *Aust Dent J.* 1997;42:247–254.
5. Basford J. Laser therapy. Paper presented at: 50th Annual Meeting of the American Academy of Neurology; April 27, 1998; Minneapolis, MN.
6. Anderson RR, Parrish JA. The optics of human skin. *J Invest Dermatol.* 1981;77:13–19.

7. Kolari PJ. Penetration of unfocused laser light into the skin. *Arch Dermatol Res.* 1985;277:342–344.

8. Basford JR. Low intensity laser therapy: still not an established tool. *Lasers Surg Med.* 1995;16:331–342.

9. Karu TI. Photobiological fundamentals of low power laser therapy. *IEEE J Quantum Electron.* 1987;QE-23:1703–1717.

10. Kneebone WJ. Treatment of chronic neck pain utilizing low-level laser therapy. *Practical Pain Management.* 2007;64–66.

11. Basford J. Low-energy laser treatment of pain and wounds: hype, hokum? *Mayo Clin Proc.* 1986;61:671–675.

12. Mester E, Mester AF, Mester A. The biomedical effects of laser applications. *Lasers Surg Med.* 1985;5:31–39.

13. Mester E, Jaszsagi-Nagy E. The effect of laser radiation on wound healing and collagen synthesis. *Stud Biophys.* 1973;35:227–230.

14. Mester E, Toth N, Mester A. The biostimulative effect of laser beam. *Laser Basic Biomed Res.* 1982;22:4–7.

15. Lam TS et al. Laser stimulation of collagen synthesis in human skin fibroblast cultures. *Lasers Life Sci.* 1986;1:61–77.

16. Rochkind S et al. Stimulating effect of HeNe low dose laser on injured sciatic nerves of rats. *Neurosurgery.* 1987;20:843.

17. Mezawa S et al. The possible analgesic effect of soft-laser irradiation on heat nociceptors in the cat tongue. *Arch Oral Biol.* 1988;33:693–694.

18. Yamada K. Biological effects of low-power laser irradiation on clonal osteoblastic cells (MC3T-E1). *Nippon Siekeigeka Gakkai Zasshi.* 1991;65:787–799.

19. Kubasova T, Kovacs L, Somosy Z. Biological effect of He-Ne laser investigations on functional and micromorphological alterations of cell membranes, in vitro. *Lasers Surg Med.* 1984;4:381–388.

20. Passarella S. HeNe laser irradiation of isolated mitochondria. *J Photochem Photobiol.* 1989;31:642–643.

21. Walker JB. Relief from chronic pain by low-power laser irradiation. *Neurosci Lett.* 1983;43:339–344.

22. Yu W et al. Photomodulation of oxidative metabolism and electron chain enzymes in rat liver mitochondria. *Photochem Photobiol.* 1997;66:866–871.

23. Karu TI. Molecular mechanisms of the therapeutic effect of low intensity laser irradiation. *Lasers Life Sci.* 1988;2:53–74.

24. Hunter J, Leonard L, Wilson R, et al. Effects of low energy laser on wound healing in a porcine model. *Lasers Surg Med.* 1984;3:285–290.

25. Baxter GD. *Therapeutic Lasers: Theory and Practice.* New York, NY: Churchill Livingstone; 1997.

26. Rochkind S et al. Systemic effects of low-power laser irradiation on the peripheral and central nervous system, cutaneous wounds and burns. *Lasers Surg Med.* 1989;9:174–182.

27. Basford J et al. Effects of 830 nm continuous wave laser diode irradiation on median nerve function in normal subjects. *Lasers Surg Med.* 1993;13:597–604.

28. Weintraub MI. Non-invasive laser neurolysis in carpal tunnel syndrome. *Muscle Nerve.* 1997;20:1029–1031.

29. Snyder-Mackler L, Bork CE. Effect of helium-neon laser irradiation on peripheral sensory nerve latency. *Phys Ther.* 1988;68:223–225.

30. Padua L et al. Laser bio-stimulation: a reply. *Muscle Nerve.* 1998;21:1232–1233.

31. Walsh DM, Baxter GK, Allen JM. The effect of 820 nm laser upon nerve conduction in the superficial radial nerve. Abstract presented at: Fifth International Biotherapy Laser Association Meeting; 1991; London, England.

32. Baxter GD et al. Effects of low intensity infrared laser irradiation upon conduction in the human median nerve in vivo. *Exp Physiol.* 1994;79:227–234.

33. Bork CE, Snyder-Mackler L. Effect of helium-neon laser irradiation on peripheral sensory nerve latency. *J Am Phys Ther Assoc.* 1988.68:223.

34. Naeser MA, Hahn KK, Lieberman B. Real vs. sham laser acupuncture and microamps TENS to treat carpal tunnel syndrome and worksite wrist pain: pilot study. *Lasers Surg Med Suppl.* 1996;8:7.

35. Branco K, Naeser MA. Carpal tunnel syndrome: clinical outcome after low-level laser acupuncture, microamps transcutaneous electrical nerve stimulation and other alternative therapies: an open protocol study. *J Alt Comp Med.* 1999;5:5–26.

36. Weintraub MI. Reply to Padua et al. *Muscle Nerve.* 1998;21:1233.

37. Franzblau A, Werner RA. What is carpal tunnel syndrome? *JAMA.* 1999;282:186–187.

38. Baxter GD et al. Low level laser therapy: current clinical practice in northern Ireland. *Physiotherapy.* 1991;77:171–178.

39. Moore KC et al. A double-blind crossover trial of low level laser therapy in the treatment of post-herpetic neuralgia. *Lasers Med Sci.* 1988;301.

40. Hong JN, Kim TH, Lim SD. Clinical trial of low reactive level laser therapy in 20 patients with post-herpetic neuralgia. *Laser Ther.* 1990;2:167–170.

41. Friedman MH, Weintraub MI, Forman S. Atypical facial pain: a localized maxillary nerve disorder? *Am J Pain Manage.* 1994;4:149–152.

42. Walker JB, Akhanjee LK, Cooney MM. Laser therapy for pain of rheumatoid arthritis, *Lasers Surg Med.* 1986;6:171.

43. Weintraub MI. Migraine: a maxillary nerve disorder? A novel therapy: preliminary results. *Am J Pain Manage.* 1996;6:77–82.

44. Friedman MH. Intra-oral maxillary chilling: a non-invasive treatment in acute migraine and tension-type headache treatment. *Headache Q Curr Treat Res.* 1998;9:274.

45. Bieglio C, Bisschop C. Physical treatment for radicular pain with low-power laser stimulation. *Lasers in Surg Med.* 1986;6:173.

46. Mizokami et al. Effect of diode laser for pain: a clinical study on different pain types. *Laser Ther.* 1990;2:171–174.

47. Christensen P. Clinical laser treatment of odontological conditions. In: Kert J, Rose L, eds. *Clinical Laser Therapy: Low Level Laser Therapy.* Copenhagen, Denmark: Scandinavian Medical Laser Technology; 1989.

48. Zhu L et al. The effect of laser irradiation on arthritis in rats. *Pain.* 1990;5 (suppl): 385.

49. Klein RG, Eek BC. Low-energy laser treatment and exercise for chronic low back pain: double-blind control trial. *Arch Phys Med Rehabil.* 1990;71:34–37.

50. Gam AN, Thorsen H, Lonnberg F. The effect of low-level laser therapy on musculoskeletal pain: a meta-analysis. *Pain.* 1993;52:63–66.

51. Goldman JA, et al. Laser therapy of rheumatoid arthritis. *Lasers Surg Med.* 1980;1:93–101.

52. Asada K, Yutani Y, Shimazu A. Diode laser therapy for rheumatoid arthritis: a clinical evaluation of 102 joints treated with low reactive laser therapy (LLLT). *Laser Ther.* 1989;1:147–151.

53. Bliddal H, et al. Soft laser therapy of rheumatoid arthritis. *Scand J Rheumatol.* 1987; 16:225–228.

54. Morselli, et al. Very low energy-density treatment by CO_2 laser in sports medicine. *Lasers Surg Med.* 1985;5:150.

55. Emmanoulidis O, Diamantopoulos C. CW IR Low-power laser applications significantly accelerates chronic pain relief rehabilitation of professional athletes: a double-blind study. *Lasers Surg Med.* 1986;6:173.

56. Haker E, Lundberg T. Laser treatment applied to acupuncture point in lateral humeral epicondylalgia: a double-blind study. *Pain.* 1990;43:243–248.
57. Asagai Y et al. Application of low reactive-level laser therapy (LLLT) in the functional training of cerebral palsy patients. *Laser Ther.* 1994;6:195–202.
58. Naeser MA et al. Laser acupuncture in the treatment of paralysis in stroke patients: a CT scan lesion site study. *Am J Acupuncture.* 1995;23:13–28.
59. Naeser MA. Review of second congress: World Association for Laser Therapy (WALT) meeting. *J Alt Comp Ed.* 1999;5:177–180.
60. Leonard DR, Farooqi MH, Myers S. Restoration of sensation, reduced pain and improved balance in subjects with diabetic peripheral neuropathy: a double-blind, randomized, placebo-controlled study with monochromatic near-infra-red treatment. *Diabetes Care.* 2004;27:168–172.
61. Lopes-Martins RA, Albertini R, Lopes-Martins PS, et al. Steroid receptor antagonist M. Fepristone inhibits the anti-inflammatory effect of photoradiation. *PhotoMed Laser Surg.* 2006;24:197–201.

CHAPTER 5

Magnetic Field Biostimulation Therapy

Michael I. Weintraub

It is better to understand a little than to misunderstand a lot.

—Anatole France

Human fascination with magnetism transcends time with extravagant claims of magnetic healing traced back more than 4,000 years. Attempts to explain this invisible force's efficacy by utilizing unique and unfounded scientific principles and claims as well as the commercial efforts to sell these products has produced an interesting history of pseudoscience, quackery, sensationalism, and controversy. Despite the fact that permanent magnets and electromagnetic therapies are currently riding the crest of public enthusiasm as an alternative and complementary medical treatment, it is not surprising that the scientific community in the twenty-first century remains somewhat skeptical of the current widespread claims. A major obstacle has been an inability to determine mechanism of action. Additionally, fundamental questions regarding efficacy can only be determined by rigorous, randomized, double-blind, placebo-controlled trials, which have only recently come into vogue in the scientific community. Therefore, the goal of this chapter is to give the reader a brief historical perspective as well as provide a critical assessment of the literature. The scientific community should look at this subject objectively and perhaps reverse the entrenched skepticism.

HISTORICAL PERSPECTIVE

There are several excellent reviews of this rich history. Claims of magnetic healing can be traced back more than 4,000 years.[1-8] According to the *Yellow Emperor's Canon of Internal Medicine* (or the *Yellow Emperor's Inner Classic*), magnetic stones (lodestones) were applied to acupressure points as a means of pain reduction. Similarly, the ancient Hindu Vedas ascribed therapeutic powers of Ashmana and Siktavati (instruments of stone). In fact, the term "magnet" was probably derived from Magnes, a shepherd who, according to legend, was walking on Mt. Ida when the metallic tacks in his sandals were drawn to specific rocks. These rocks were mineral lodestones that contained magnetite, a magnetic oxide of iron (Fe_3O_4). These natural magnetic stones were noted to influence other similar adjacent stones that were brought into close proximity, producing movement, Thus, the ancients called them "live stones" or "Herculean stones" as they were meant to lead the way. Various powers were attributed to these stones as noted in the writings and artifacts of the ancient Greek and Roman civilizations. For example, Plato, Euripides, and others indicated that these "invisible powers of movements" could be put to practical use such as building boats with iron nails and destroying opposition boats by bringing them close to magnetic mountains or magnetic rock. Medicinal and healing properties were also attributed to these lodestones and in fact, various magnetic rings and necklaces were sold in the marketplace in Samothrace around 200 A.D. to treat arthritis and pain. Similarly, lodestones were ground up to make powders and salves to treat various conditions. Numerous claims and anecdotal stories persisted leading to the public embrace of these "so-called magical devices." In 1289, the first major treatise on magnetism was written by Peter Peregrinus. He ascribed lodestone curative properties for gout, baldness, and arthritis and spoke about strong aphrodisiac powers. He also described drawing poison from wounds with close application. His work contains the first drawing and description of a compass in the Western world.

The Middle Ages witnessed a dark period for science and the emergence of numerous myths that persist in certain segments of society. For example, it was believed that magnets could extract gold from wells and that application or ingestion of garlic could neutralize magnetic properties. The idea that magnets could be used therapeutically began in the early sixteenth century when Paracelsus, considered to be one of the most influential physicians and alchemists of his time, used lodestones (magnets) to treat conditions such as epilepsy, diarrhea, and hemorrhage. He believed that every person is a magnet, that they could attract good and evil and that magnets are an important elixir of life.

Scientific enlightenment in the sixteenth century firmly began with work of Dr. William Gilbert, physician to Queen Elizabeth I of England. He wrote his classic text *DeMagnete* in 1600 describing hundreds of detailed experiments concerning electricity and also terrestrial magnetism. He debunked many quack medicinal applications and was responsible for laying the groundwork for future research and study. Despite the fact that Galvani and Volta made significant contributions for the next 100 years there were no major advancements in the study of magnetism.

In the early eighteenth century, there was significant interest in both magnetism and electricity. Francis Hauksbee, in 1705, invented an electrostatic engine that by rotating and spinning an attached globe, could transfer an electronic charge to various metallic objects brought close, that is, chain, wire, metal. This procedure induced electrical shocks. Refinements in this machine led to more general usage, and in 1743, traveling circuses throughout Europe and the American colonies provided individuals with shocks for a small fee. Legend suggests that Benjamin Franklin witnessed an "electrified boy exhibition" and became interested in both electricity and magnetic phenomena. Franklin is famed for his experiments on electricity using lightning by attaching a key to an airborne kite in a thunderstorm (as depicted in the heroic portrait by Benjamin West. See Figure 5.1). In fact, it was actually Franklin's young son who was sent out into the lightening storm with the kite, risking the exhibition of Franklin's own version of the electrified boy.

Much of the current magnetic terminology regarding electricity (e.g., charge, discharge, condenser, electric shock, electrician, positive, negative, plus and minus, etc.) originated with Franklin. Franklin distinguished himself in studies primarily of electric fluid and charges and concluded that all matter contained magnetic fields that are uniformly distributed throughout the body. He believed that when an object is magnetized, the fluid condenses in one of its extremities. That extremity becomes positively magnetized whereas the donor region of the object becomes negatively magnetized. He felt that the degree to which an object can be magnetized depends on the force necessary to start the fluid moving within it.

The scientific revolution came to Europe with the development of carbon-steel magnets (1743–1751). Father Maximilian Hell and later his student, Anton Mesmer, applied these magnetic devices to patients, many of whom were experiencing hysterical or psychosomatic symptomatology. Specifically in his major treatise "On the Medicinal Uses of the Magnet," Mesmer described how he fed a patient iron filings and then applied specially designed magnets over the vital organs to generally stop uncontrolled seizures. His cures were not only astounding, but also good theater since they were performed in front of large groups (see Figure 5.2).

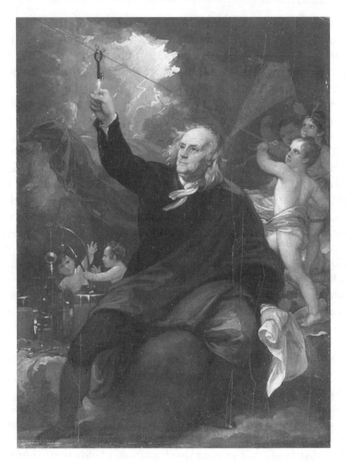

FIGURE 5.1   Portrait of Benjamin Franklin.

The power of suggestion was clearly being displayed and ultimately transferred to nonferric objects such as paper, wood, silk and stone. Mesmer reasoned that he was not dealing with ordinary mineral magnetism but rather with a special "animal magnetism." The term "mesmerization" is often attributed to his displays of people overcoming illness and disease by "mesmerizing" their bodies' innate magnetic poles to induce a crisis, often in the form of convulsions. After this crisis, health would be restored. He hailed this as a specific natural force of healing. His exaggerated claims of success infuriated his conservative colleagues and forced the French Academy of Science under King Louis VI to convene a special study in 1784. The panel for this study included Anton Lavoisier, J. R. Guillotin, and Benjamin Franklin. In a controlled set of

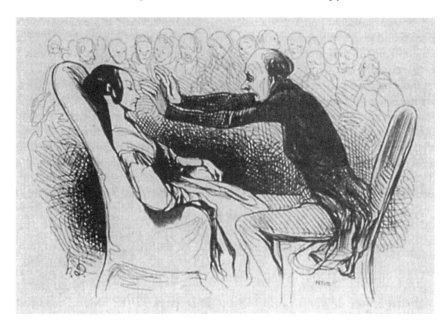

FIGURE 5.2   Mesmerism and hypnotism were the object of criticism during the nineteenth century.

experiments, blindfolded patients were exposed to a series of magnets or sham-magnetic objects and were asked to describe the induced sensation. The committee concluded that the efficacy of the magnetic healing resided entirely within the mind of the individual and that any healing was due to suggestion. Based on these conclusions, the medical establishment declared Mesmer's theories fraudulent and that mesmerism was equated with medical quackery. Mesmer left France in disgrace. Others from the panel who remained in France lost their heads. However, in the United States, magnetic therapy flourished with significant sales of magnets, magnetic salves, and liniments by traveling magnetic healers. Later in the nineteenth century David Daniel Palmer, the founder of chiropractic and self-described "magnetic healer," stated that putting down his hands for physical manipulation of the patient obtained better results than the "laying on of hands."

Hans Christian Oersted (1777–1851), a physicist, continued his studies and noted that a compass needle was deflected when a current flowed through a nearby wire. He also discovered that not only did a current-carrying wire coil exert a force on a magnet, but a magnet exerted a force on the coil of wire inducing an electrical current. The coil behaved like a magnet, as if it possessed magnetic north and south poles. Magnetism and electricity were somehow connected. Oersted was instrumental in creating a proper scientific environment that led to further study with Ampere deducing the quantitative relationship between a magnetic force and electric current. In the 1820s, Michael Faraday and Joseph Henry (later founding Secretary of the Smithsonian Institution in the 1850s) demonstrated more connections between magnetism and electricity demonstrating that a changing magnetic field could induce an electric field perpendicularly.

In 1886, the Sears catalog advertised numerous magnetic products such as magnetic rings, belts, caps, soles for boots, girdles, etc. In the 1920s, Thacher created a mail-order catalog advertising over 700 specific magnetic garments and devices and products that he described as a "plain road to health without the use of medicine and was dependent on the magnetic energy of the sun." He believed that the iron content of the blood made it the primary magnetic conductor of the body and thus the most efficient way to "recharge" the body's magnetic field was by wearing his magnetic garments. The complete set was said to "furnish full and complete protection of all the vital organs of the body." *Collier's Magazine* dubbed Thacher the "king of the magnetic quacks." There was no governmental regulation of these devices or claims and thus these types of promotion fueled skepticism. The FDA did not exist at that time, and there were no good scientific trials yet the unsubstantiated claims led to the passage of the Pure Food and Drug Act of 1906 and the subsequent formation of the FDA.

In 1896, D'Arsonval reported to the Société de Biologie in Paris that when a subject's head was placed in a strong time-varying magnetic field, phosphenes (retinal stimulation) were perceived. Some 15 years later, Sylvanus P. Thompson (1910) confirmed not only could phosphenes be induced, but that exposure to a strong alternating magnetic field also produced taste sensation. Various coils were constructed by Dunlap and later Magnusson and Stevens. They noted that magnetophosphenes were brightest at a low frequency of about 25 Hz and became fainter at higher frequencies.

After World War II, there was heightened interest and research in magnetotherapy in Japan and the former Soviet Union. Specifically in Japan, magnetotherapeutic devices were accepted under the Drug Regulation Act of 1961 and by 1976, various devices were commonly and commercially employed to treat various illnesses and promote health. Similar interests from Bulgaria, Romania, and Russia led to various therapeutic approaches so that the physician had available the use of magnetic fields to assist in treating disease. Today, Germany, Japan, Russia, Israel, and at least 45 other countries consider magnetic therapy to be an official medical procedure for the treatment of various neurological and inflammatory conditions.[9] By contrast, magnetotherapy had limited acceptance in Western medicine. Unwarranted claims as well as charlatans only further led to public and scientific skepticism.

The modern era of magnetic stimulation began with the work of R. G. Bickford (1965) who considered the possibility of stimulation of the nervous system (frog nerve and human peripheral nerves). He also discussed the generation of eddy currents in the brain that could reach a certain magnitude to stimulate cortical structures through an intact cranium.[10] Barker and colleagues at the University of Sheffield developed the first commercial cranial magnetic stimulator in 1985.[11,12] They gave a practical demonstration at Queen's Square by stimulating Dr. Merton's brain which caused muscle twitches. As might be expected, the physiological and clinical possibilities became obvious.[13] While there were technical challenges, they were met with the development of devices capable of stimulating brain focally at frequencies of up to 100 Hz with specific coil configurations (i.e., circular and figure 8). Adaptations for focal therapy were created. Thus, a new discipline developed using high and low repetitive stimulation frequencies directed to previously inaccessible areas of the brain and body.[14–16] As of July 1998, over 6,000 publications exist that deal with basic neurophysiology, clinical syndromes and therapeutic implications. While most of the initial papers were the results of open-label (non-placebo) observations, many current publications represent rigorous, randomized, double-blind, placebo-controlled trials. Thus, pooling all of this information, both experimental and clinical, strongly suggests that the application of exogenous magnetic fields at low levels does indeed induce a biological effect on a variety of systems, especially pain reduction and the musculoskeletal system.

TERMINOLOGY AND MAGNETIC PRINCIPLES

In order to understand the role of magnetism, essential terms must be defined. "Biomagnetics" refers to the field of science dealing with the application of magnetic fields to living organisms. Basic research on cells in culture as well as clinical trials have provided a better understanding of mechanisms of action.[17–25] Human tissues are dielectric and conductive and therefore can respond to electric and magnetic fields that are oscillating or static. Cell membranes consist of paramagnetic and diamagnetic lipoprotein materials that respond to magnetic fields and serve as signaling (transduction) pathways by which external stimuli are sent and conveyed to the cell interior. Calcium ions are very important in transduction coupling at the cell membrane level. Electromagnetic fields can also alter the configuration of atoms and molecules in dielectric and para/diamagnetic substances. Thus atoms in these substances polarize, to some degree, when placed in an electromagnetic field and act as a dipole and align accordingly.[26-33] Adey feels that free radicals are important for signal transduction. Chemical bonds are essentially electromagnetic bonds formed between adjacent atoms. The breaking of the chemical bonds of a singlet pair allows electrons to influence adjacent electrons with similar or opposite spins thereby becoming triplet pairs, etc. Thus, by imposing magnetic fields in this medium, one may influence the rate and amount of communication between cells. At the cell membrane level, free radicals of nitric oxide (NO) may play an essential role in this regulation of receptors specifically.[17,23,29] It is known that free radicals are involved in the normal regulatory mechanisms in many tissues and that certain disorders are associated with disordered free radical regulation producing oxidative stress. These include Alzheimer's, Parkinson's disease, cancer, coronary artery disease, etc. This entire area is still incompletely understood yet under intense research scrutiny.

UNITS OF MEASURE

The magnetic field strength is indicated by magnetic flux density, which is the number of field lines (flux) that cross a unit of surface area. It is usually described as Gauss (G) or Tesla (T). There are 10,000 G in each Tesla. Because there is an exponential decay of field strength with distance from a magnetic source, the objective is to apply a static magnetic device as close to the skin as possible and to assure that a magnet of sufficient size and surface field is utilized when the target is in deep tissue areas, such as lumbar back.

PROFESSIONAL AND SCIENTIFIC ORGANIZATIONS

There are at least five major professional and scientific societies[25] involved in the study of the biological and clinical effects of EMF:

1. Bioelectromagnetic Society (BEMS).
2. European Bioelectric Association (EBEA).
3. Bioelectrochemical Society (BES).
4. Society for Physical Regulation in Biology and Medicine (SPRBM).
5. Engineering in Medicine and Biology (IEEE).

TERMINOLOGY

Magnetotherapy

Magnetotherapy is defined as the use of time-varying magnetic fields of low-frequency values (3 Hz–3 KHz) to induce a sufficiently strong current to stimulate living tissue.

Faraday's Law (1831)

Faraday's Law provides the fundamental relationship between a changing magnetic field and a conductor (any medium that carries electrically charged particles). Using a wire as an example of a conductor, Faraday's Law basically states that any change in the magnetic environment of the coil of wire with time will cause a voltage to be induced in the wire. No matter how the change is produced, a voltage will be generated. Thus, magnetic field amplitude may be varied by powering the electromagnet with sinusoidal or pulsing current or by moving a permanent magnet or away from the wire, moving the wire toward or away from the magnetic field, rotating the wire relative to the magnet, etc.[33–37]

Lenz's Law

Lenz's Law states that the polarity of the voltage induced according to Faraday's Law is such that it produces a current whose magnetic field opposes the applied magnetic field (back emf). Therefore, if a current is passed through a coil which creates an expanding magnetic field around the coil, the induced voltage and associated current flow produce a magnetic field in opposition to the directly induced magnetic field.

Eddy Current

Eddy currents are currents induced by the voltage generated according to Faraday's Law in any conducting medium. When the conducting medium does not contain defined current pathways, there is no induced current, only induced voltage. There is movement in a spiral, swirling fashion and this in turn potentially penetrates the membranes of the neurons. If the induced current is of sufficient amplitude, an action potential or an excitatory or inhibitory postsynaptic potential may be produced.

Lorentz Force and Hall Effect

The Hall Effect and the Lorentz Force are related to the same physical phenomenon of electromagnetism. In the Hall Effect, when charged particles in a conductor move along a path that is transverse to a magnetic field, the particles experience a force that pushes them towards the outer walls of the conductor. The positively charged particles move to one side and the negatively charged particles move to the other side. This produces a voltage across the conductor known as the Hall Voltage. Because the human body is replete with charged ions, the Hall Effect would certainly take place to varying degrees when a magnetic field is passed through the body. The strength of the Hall Voltage produced depends on three factors: (a) the strength of the magnetic field, (b) the number of charged particles moving transverse to the magnetic field, and (c) the velocity of movement of the charged particles (ions). The pulsing and static magnetic fields in current therapeutic applications are much too weak and the endogenous currents much too small for the Hall Effect to be of any significance in magnetic field bioeffects.[38,39] However, this is somewhat controversial and not universally accepted. Clearly, cellular and neural components in the body provide conductive pathways for ions, so it is reasonable to assume that these components would be prime objects of attention to observe the Hall Effect. It is presumed that this voltage might add to the nerve's resting potential of −70 mV and make it harder to depolarize. Once the resting potential rises from its normal undisturbed voltage of about −70 mV to a voltage of approximately −55 mV (threshold potential), an action-potential spike is initiated. When ions move under the influence of a voltage, they become an electric current in which magnitude is determined by Ohm's Law, which states that electric current equals voltage divided by resistance.

Larmour Precession (lpm)

This phenomenon predicts the effects of ions exposed to a combination of exogenous AC/DC magnetic fields at approximately 0.1 G and the dynamics of ions in a binding site. A bound ion in a static magnetic field will precess at the Larmour frequency and will accelerate faster to preferred orientations in the binding site with increased magnetic field strength. Thus, an increased binding rate can occur with a resultant acceleration in the downstream biochemical cascade.[40]

TYPES OF MAGNETIC FIELDS

Magnetic fields can penetrate all tissues including epidermis, dermis, subcutaneous tissue as well as tendons, muscles and even bone. The specific amount of magnetic energy and its effect at the target organ depends on the size, strength, and duration of contact of the device.

Magnetic fields fall into two broad categories: static (DC) and time-varying (AC).

The strength of static magnetic devices varies from 1–4,000 G. Static fields have zero frequency because the polarity and field strength does not change with time but rather remains constant. Permanent magnets only produce static fields unless they are rotated or otherwise moved causing the magnetic field amplitude to change with time at the tissue target. Static magnetic fields that are either permanent or electromagnetic are in the range of 1–4,000 G and have been reported to have significant biological effects.[22,24,25,41,42] The most common static magnets sold to the public are known as refrigerator or flat-button magnets. They are made of various materials and also have different designs. Configuration can be unidirectional where only one magnetic pole is represented on one side of the surface (while the opposite pole is on the opposite side away from the applied surface) or the surface can have a bipolar north/south design that appears repetitively as concentric ring, multi-triangular, and quadripolar configurations.

Geometric Patterns

Bipolar magnets refer to a repetitive north/south polarity created on the same side of a ceramic or plastic alloy or neodymium material, whereas the term "unipolar" refers to only one magnetic pole at a given surface, that is, north or south. Multipolar alterations of north and south have also been employed. Each specific manufacturer makes claims as to the superiority of their product; however, the most important characteristic of the magnetic field is the field strength at the target site and also the duration of exposure leading to biological effect. It is believed that tissue, cells, etc., have a so-called biological window that can interact with these invisible fields. Static magnetic fields of 5–20 G have been felt to be pertinent. Thus, the Gauss rating and field strength at the surface are irrelevant in predicting biological response. Bipolar magnets, using a small arc, are capable of inducing biologically significant fields at a relatively short distance from the surface (1–1.5 cm) whereas the unipolar magnet penetration is much deeper (4–8 cm).[8]

Review of the literature reveals that static magnetic fields in the 1–4,000 G range have been reported to have significant biological effect. Basic science has demonstrated that static magnetic fields ranging from 23–3,000 G can alter the electrical properties of solutions. Additionally, weak static magnetic fields can modulate myosin phosphorylation at the molecular level in a cell-free preparation enzyme assay mixture.[43] At a cellular level, exposure to 300 G doubled alkaline phosphatase activity in osteoblast-like cells.[44] Neurite outgrowth from embryonic chick ganglia was significantly increased using 225–900 G exposure.[45,46] In several experiments using unidirectional and multipolar magnets, McLean and colleagues demonstrated a blockade of sensory nociceptive neuron action potentials by exposure to a static magnetic field in the 10 mT range. A minimum magnetic field gradient of 15 G/mm was required to cause approximately 80% action potential blockade in isolated nerve preparations.[47] This blockade reversed when the magnetic exposure was removed. Protection against kainic acid-induced neuronal swelling was also demonstrated with magnetic exposure.[48] Others have demonstrated a biphasic response of the acute microcirculation in rabbits by exposure to static magnetic fields (10 G).[49,50] Despite all this provocative and promising data in both in vitro and in vivo studies, skepticism prevails due to design flaws.[51,52] Specifically, the lack of a rigorous, randomized, double-blind, placebo-controlled trials design, lack of basic mechanisms of action, lack of optimum target dosage and optimum polarity are yet to be defined. Additionally, the absence of nonmagnetic placebos as controls has also been described as a problem. Over the past 3 years, there have been attempts to properly address these criticisms with randomized placebo-control trials.

Clinical Applications

Colbert has reviewed 22 therapeutic trials published in the American literature from 1982 to 2002.[42] Clinical improvement in subjects who wore permanent magnets on various parts of their bodies was demonstrated in 15 studies whereas 7 reported limited or no benefit. Magnetic field strength varied from 68–2,000 G with variable time exposure varying from 45 minutes to constant wearing over 4 months. Thus the optimum treatment duration has yet to be established as well as the optimal polarity (unidirectional, multipolar, etc.). Complicating the issue even further is the observations by Blechman and colleagues[53] that a significant number of the static magnets sold to the public had lower field flux density measurements compared to the manufacturers' claims. It is known that a large amount of cancellation occurs in multipolar arrays. Similarly, Eccles[54] did a critical review of the randomized controlled trials utilizing static magnets for pain relief. He found a 73% statistical reduction in pain. He also commented on the difficulty performing double-blind studies using static magnets because of the obvious interaction with metallic objects.

Specific clinical trials utilizing double-blind, placebo design include Vallbona and colleagues,[55] who applied 300–500 G concentric circle bipolar magnets over pain pressure joints in post-polio patients for 45 minutes and reduced pain by 76%. Carter and colleagues[56] applied unipolar

1000 G static magnets and placebos over carpal tunnel for 45 minutes and both groups had significant pain reduction. This was felt to represent placebo effect. Unidirectional magnetic pads (150–400 G) ceramic magnets were placed over liposuction sites immediately postoperatively and kept in place for 14 days producing 40%–70% reduction of pain, edema, and discoloration.[57] Brown and colleagues in 1999 demonstrated statistical reduction of pelvic pain.[58] Patients with fibromyalgia slept on a unidirectional mattress pad (800 G ceramics magnets) for a four-month period with a 40% improvement.[59] Weintraub noted 90% reduction of neuropathic pain with DPN occurring with constant wearing of multipolar 475 G insole devices. There was also a 30% reduction of neuropathic pain in the nondiabetic peripheral neuropathy.[57,60] A nationwide study also confirmed the above in 275 cases with placebo controls (2003).[61]

Hinman and colleagues found a 30% response to magnetic application of unipolar static magnets positioned over painful knees with short-term application.[62] Greater movement was also noted. Holcomb using a quadripolar array of static magnets with alternating polarity demonstrated analgesic benefit in patients with low back pain and knee pain.[51]

Saygili and colleagues[63] failed to detect changes in capillary blood flow after continuous exposure to a magnetic field for 45 days. Hong and colleagues[64] used magnetic necklaces and placebos in 101 patients with chronic neck and shoulder pain for three consecutive weeks following baseline electrodiagnostic studies with no significant improvement. Martel and colleagues[65] could not identify any change in forearm blood flow with randomized placebo cross-over design with 30 minutes of magnetic exposure (bipolar). Other negative randomized, placebo-controlled, clinical trials should also be mentioned, including Collacott's study of bipolar devices in chronic low back pain[66] and Winemiller's study of plantar fasciitis.[67] Weintraub and colleagues commented on design flaws in both of these studies.[68,69] Simultaneous application of static magnets to the back and feet in failed back syndrome was also ineffective.[70] Pilla[53] independently assessed the strength of the magnetic devices and found them to be less than the manufacturer claims thereby confirming Bleckman's observations.

It is assumed that the biological benefits from static magnetic fields are similar to pulsed electromagnetic fields but the link has been imperfect. The specific mechanism of biological benefit remains to be determined. At present, the most generally accepted theory is that static magnetic fields on the order of 1–10 G could affect ion-ligand binding producing modulation.[19,22,41] There may also be physical realignment and translational movement of diamagnetically anisotropic molecules. Despite these theoretical and scientific rationales for benefit, criticism and skepticism prevail. Critics allege that it is all placebo, yet a more enlightened and open-minded appraisal would accept the positive in vitro and in vivo observations. Ramey,[52] a veterinarian, has been a noted critic of static magnets yet these devices are used extensively in veterinary medicine (i.e., magnetic blankets for race horses, etc.).

The World Health Organization has stated that there are no adverse effects on human health from exposure to static magnetic fields, even up to 2 T which equals 20,000 G.[71] Similarly, the United States FDA in 2003 extended nonsignificant risk status for MRI up to 8 T.[72]

Pulsed Electromagnetic Fields

Pulsed electromagnetic fields (PEMF) require an electric current to produce its pulsating (time-varying) magnetic field. This is because the coil that produces the magnetic field is stationary. Regardless of how the waveforms are transmitted through the coil, the ensuing magnetic flux lines appear in space in exactly the same manner as the flux lines appear from a permanent magnet. The magnetic field penetrates biological tissues without modification and the induced electric fields are produced at right angles to the flux lines. The ensuing current flow is determined by the tissue's electrical properties (impedance) and will determine the final spatial dosimetry. Peak magnetic fields from PEMF devices are typically 5–30 G at the target tissue with varying specific shapes and amplitudes of fields.

Basic Science

Cellular studies (in vitro, in vivo) have been most provocative. Markov, in a review article,[24,25] has summarized various cellular and structural changes to this PEMF exposure. Specifically, fibrinogen, fibroblasts, leukocytes, platelets, fibrin, cytokines, collagen, elastin, keratinocytes, osteoblasts, free radical changes are noted. Additionally, magnetic fields also influence vasoconstriction, vasodilatation, phagocytosis, cell proliferation, epithelialization, and scar formation.

Similarly, in a review article, Pilla has summarized the effects of these weak PEMF on both signal transduction and growth factor synthesis as it relates to fractures.[22,38,39,41] He noted that there is up regulation of growth factor production, calcium ion transport, cell proliferation, IGF-II release, and IGF-II receptor expression in osteoblasts as a mechanism for bone repair. He also cited an increase in both TGF-$b1$ mRNA and protein in osteoblast cultures producing an effect on a calcium/calmodulin-dependent pathway. Other studies with chondrocytes confirm similar increases in TGF-$b1$ mRNA and protein synthesis from PEMF suggesting a therapeutic application to joint repair.[73,74] PEMF has also been successfully applied to stimulate nerve regeneration. Neurite outgrowth has been demonstrated in cell cultures exposed to EMF. Eddy currents are generated that can depolarize, hyperpolarize, and repolarize nerve cells suggesting a potential neuromodulation can arise.

Clinical Applications

In 1979, the FDA approved the use of PEMF as a means of stimulating and recruiting osteoblast cells at a fracture site. By applying coils around the cast, it would induce current flows through the fracture site producing 80% success. It became apparent after early testing that intermittent exposure as compared to continuous exposure was the optimal technique. Currently, there are four FDA-approved devices for treatment of nonunion fractures and each has specific signal parameters, treatment time, etc. It is not yet clear how long PEMF exposure must last in order to trigger a bioelectric effect. Wave forms tend to be asymmetric, biphasic and quasi-rectangular, or quasi-triangular in shape. This indicates that tissues have various windows of vulnerability and susceptibility to PEMF. Based on the high success of PEMF, it is currently considered part of the standard armamentarium of orthopedic spine surgeons and is recommended as an adjunct to standard fracture management. Additionally, the results are equivalent to surgical repair with minimal risk and are more cost effective.

PEMF has also been directed to other orthopedic conditions as well as painful musculoskeletal disorders. These include aseptic necrosis of hips, osteoporosis, osteoarthritis, osteogenesis imperfecta, rotator cuff dysfunction, low back pain, and so forth.[75–84] Markov, in his reviews,[8,24,25] stated that with the exception of periarthritis, which reported no difference between treatment and control groups, reduced pain scores were noted in carpal tunnel pain (93%),[85] rotator cuff (83%),[81] and 70% of MS patients had reduced spasticity.[86] Pilla reports double-blind studies claiming benefit for chronic wound repair,[85,87–89] acute ankle sprain[73,74] and acute whiplash injuries.[90,91]

Pujol and colleagues[75] targeted musculoskeletal pain using magnetic coils with benefit compared to placebo controls. Weintraub used nine consecutive 1-hour treatments directed to patients with peripheral neuropathy inducing greater than 50% reduction of neuropathic pain. This was an open-label, non-placebo trial.[92]

Pickering[93] demonstrated that gentamicin effect against staph epidermidis could be augmented by exposure to PEMF. Pulsed high frequency (27 MHz) electromagnetic therapy in a double-blind, placebo-controlled study, directed for persistent neck pain produced significant improvement by the second week of therapy.[90,91]

Raji and Boden in 1983 applied a 27 MHz signal to a transected common peroneal nerve of a rat and with daily 15 minutes of treatment produced accelerated healing with reduced scar tissue, increased blood vessels, and maturation of myelin.[76] Despite all the convincing data, the use of PEMF does not enjoy universal acceptance. Additionally, the large number of different commercially available PEMF devices that generate different shaped and amplitude low-frequency fields presents a major variable in attempting to understand and analyze the putative biological clinical effects. It has been speculated that the target area receives 5–30 G and each tissue has its own biophysical window and specific encoding susceptibility.[41]

Despite all this provocative data, there is considerable uncertainty about the specific mechanisms involved as well as the optimal approach of frequency, amplitude, and duration of exposure. Of course, this issue may be moot based on available data since several different devices generate different frequencies, amplitudes, and duration and have been successful in similar nonunion fracture healing. Additionally, there is an abundance of experimental and clinical data that have demonstrated that ELF and static magnetic fields can have a profound effect on a large variety of biological systems, organisms, and tissues as well as cellular and subcellular structures. It is assumed that the target is the cell membrane with ion/ligand binding and that even small changes in transmembrane voltage could induce a significant modulation of cellular function. In a recent review, Pilla has attempted to provide a unifying approach for static and pulsating magnetic fields, as well as weak ultrasound which also induces electric fields comparable to PEMF.[22] Pilla also utilized radiofrequency 27.12 Hz when pulsed (nonthermal) and has achieved soft tissue healing, reduction of edema and postoperative pain relief. This has recently been approved by the FDA.[89]

A novel device has now been developed with time-varying, biaxial rotation which generates simultaneous static (DC) and oscillating fields (AC). They are constantly changing and thus produce variable exposure to tissues and amplitudes at the target tissue. Weintraub and colleagues have recently found this to be effective in reducing neuropathic pain from diabetic peripheral neuropathy and carpal tunnel syndrome.[94,95]

Transcranial Magnetic Stimulation (TMS) is a specific adaptation of PEMF which creates a time-varying magnetic field over the surface of the head and depolarizes underlying superficial neurons that induce electrical currents in the brain. Hi-intensity current is rapidly turned on and off in the electromagnetic coil through the discharge of capacitors. Thus, brief (micro seconds) and powerful magnetic fields are produced which in turn induce current in the brain. Two magnetic stimuli delivered in close sequence to the same cortical region through a single stimulating coil are utilized. The first stimulation is a conditioning submotor subthreshold intensity that influences the intracortical neurons and exerts a significant modulating effect on the amplitude of the motor evoked potential (MEP) evoked by the second, supramotor threshold stimulus. This modulating effect depends on the interval between the stimuli. Cortical inhibition consistently occurs at intervals between 1 and 5 msec and facilitation at intervals between 10 and 20 msec. This is simple to perform, inexpensive, generally safe, and it provides useful measures of neuronal excitability. It has also been used along the neuraxis and continues to provide important insights into basic neurological functions, neurophysiology, and neurobiology. While usually used as a research tool, it has been proposed that TMS should be considered therapeutically. The abnormalities that are revealed by TMS are not disease specific and need clinical correlation. Initially, stimulation directed to the primary motor cortex in a number of movement disorders helped appreciate the role of the basal ganglia. Specific TMS studies included Parkinson's disease, dystonia, Huntington's chorea, essential tremor, Tourette's syndrome, myoclonus, restless legs, progressive supranuclear palsy, Wilson's disease, stiff-person syndrome, Rett's syndrome, and so forth. The results were promising suggesting that future large multicenter trials are warranted.

TMS has also proved useful in investigating the mechanisms of epilepsy, and repetitive TMS may prove to have a therapeutic role in the future.[96]

TMS also is used in preoperative assessment of specific brain areas so as to optimize the surgical procedure. Both inhibitory and facilatory interactions in the cortex can be studied by combining a subthreshold conditioning stimulus with a suprathreshold test stimulus at different short (1–20 msec) intervals through the same coil. Additionally, this paired-pulsed TMS approach is used to investigate potential CNS activating drugs, various neurological and psychological diseases, and so forth. Left and right hemispheres often react differently.[97] The clinical utility of this aspect has not yet been demonstrated. If TMS pulses are delivered repetitively and rhythmically, the process is called repetitive TMS (rTMS) and can be modified further to induce excitatory or inhibitory effects. Rarely seizures may be provoked in epileptics as well as normal volunteers.[14,98–109]

Repetitive TMS leads to modulation of cortical excitability. For example, high frequency repetitive TMS (rTMS) of the dominant hemisphere, but not the nondominant hemisphere, can induce speech arrest.[110] It also correlates with the Wada test. The higher the stimulation frequency the greater the disruption of cortical function. Lower frequencies of rTMS in a 1 Hz range can suppress excitability of the motor cortex while 20 Hz stimulation trains lead to temporarily increased cortical excitability.

Pascual-Leone et al have been studying these effects in neurological disorders such as Parkinson's disease, dystonia, epilepsy, stroke. Osenbach[96] provides a comprehensive review of motor cortex stimulation for intractable pain concluding that MCS (Magnetic Cortical Stimulation) provides relief in carefully selected patients with a variety of neuropathic pain but leaves many unanswered questions. Tinnitus has been recalcitrant to many therapies but there has been increasing utilization of magnetic and electrical stimulation of the auditory cortex with benefit.[9,111] Other psychiatric conditions including anxiety, mania, depression, and schizophrenia are also being treated with TMS.[15,99,112] Nonetheless, these early observations and data suggest a rich potential therapeutic utility heretofore not known. The underlying neurobiology is still a work in progress in various neuropsychiatric syndromes. Sham TMS is difficult and there is some evidence to suggest that there is some biological effect on the brain with tilting of the coils.[112]

Safety

A controversial and legitimate concern relates to the possible role of malignancy and birth defects by exposure to EMF on living tissue. Specifically, this concern has been raised due to the foci of childhood leukemia cases reported adjacent to high power lines. During a 5-year period (1991–1996), Congress appropriated $60 million for dedicated research to look for a causal association. The result was no significant risk from power line frequencies has been able to be confirmed or justified. *No funding* was made available to explore and expand the beneficial effects of magnetics and EMF fields! The facts are there is now a 30-year experience and history of approved use of PEMF for recalcitrant fracture repair with not one adverse effect reported. Similarly, static magnetic fields have been employed for therapeutic uses for centuries, and there have also been no adverse effects reported.

The FDA has received a number of reports and complaints through its Medical Device Reporting System (MDR) concerning EMF interference with a variety of medical devices, such as pacemakers and defibrillators. Additionally advances in MR technology, using ultra-high MF systems >3 T, while safe, led to a reassessment of biomedical implant devices that were previously considered safe at 1.5 T. The technology demonstrated of the 109 implants/devices, 4% were considered to have a MF interaction at 3 T and were potentially unsafe.[113] Because of potential concerns regarding radio frequency induced MF with thermal effects at the cellular and molecular levels, the FDA has limited switching rates necessary to generate these gradient fields to a factor of 3 below the mean threshold of peripheral nerve stimulation.[113] Recently, Weintraub and colleagues[40] looked at the role of biologic effects of 3 T MRIs and found that there was 14% of subjects experiencing sensory symptoms (new or altered) with both 3 T or 1.5 T.

CONCLUSION

The study of magnetic fields (static, pulsed) has evolved from a medical curiosity into significant and specific medical applications. That PEMF and TMS can influence biological functions and serve as a therapeutic intervention is not in dispute; however, judging the efficacy of static magnets for various clinical conditions remains challenging, particularly since the important dosimetry component has not been documented. The ultimate question is what will it take to convince the scientific community of the merits of static magnetotherapy? While the debate continues, more attention must be focused on creating strong randomized, placebo-controlled designs and on looking for biological markers. This step should help reduce the skepticism of the medical community. A major obstacle for future progress has been the lack of research funding, especially NIH funding. When Senator Arlen Specter (R-Pennsylvania), a senior member of the Senate Appropriations Subcommittee on Health and Education, which makes the NIH budget, asked the leadership of NIH about funding research on bioenergy he was told that NIH "does not believe in bioenergy." Perhaps the U.S. Department of Energy should sponsor research in this field. They can not respond that they don't believe in energy. Industry, that is, device makers, have been willing to support many innovative studies but if major advancement in knowledge is to occur regarding magnetotherapy, recent history shows that it must be with a combination of support by government and industry.

ACKNOWLEDGMENTS

I wish to thank Begell House, Inc., for permission to update my prior article on Magnetotherapy[7] that appeared in *Critical Reviews in Physical and Rehabilitation Medicine 2004*. I also wish to thank A. A. Pilla, PhD, Paul Rosch, MD, Marko Marcov, MD, PhD, and Vincent Ardizzone, EE, for their prior assistance and enhancing my understanding of the topic.

REFERENCES

1. Mourino MR. From Thales to Lauterbur, or from the lodestone to MR imaging: magnetism and medicine. *Radiol.* 1991;180:593–612.

2. Geddes L. History of magnetic stimulation of the nervous system. *J Clin Neurophysiol.* 1991;8:3–9.

3. Macklis RM. Magnetic healing, quackery and the debate about the health effects of electromagnetic fields. *An Intern Med.* 1993;118:376–383.

4. Armstrong D, Armstrong EM. *The Great American Medicine Show.* New York, NY: Prentiss Hall; 1991.

5. Weintraub, MI. Magnetic biostimulation in neurologic illness. In Weintraub MI, Micozzi, MS, eds. *Alternative and Complementary Treatment in Neurologic Illness.* New York: Churchill Livingstone; 2001;278–286.

6. Rosch P. Preface: a brief historical perspective. In: Rosch PJ, ed. *Bioelectromagnetic Medicine.* New York: Marcel Dekker, Inc; 2004;III–VII.

7. Weintraub MI. Magnetotherapy: historical background with a stimulating future. *Crit Rev in Phys and Rehab Med.* 2004;16:95–108.

8. Markov MS. Magnetic field therapy: a review. *Electromagnetic Biol and Med.* 2007; 26:1–23.

9. Whitaker J, Adderly B. *The Pain Relief Breakthrough.* Little Brown & Co. 1998; 24–38.

10. Bickford RG, Fremming BD. Neuronal stimulation by pulsed magnetic fields in animals and man. In: *Digest of Sixth International Conference on Medical Electronics and Biological Engineering.* 1965;112.

11. Barker AT, et al. Magnetic stimulation of the human brain and peripheral nervous system: an introduction and the results of an initial clinical evaluation. *Neurosurgery.* 1987;20:100–109.

12. Barker AT. Introduction to the basic principles of magnetic nerve stimulation. *J Clin Neurophysiol.* 19918:26–37.

13. Merton PA, Morton, MA. Stimulation of the cerebral cortex in the intact human subject. *Nature.* 1980;285:227.

14. Kobayashi M, Pascual-Leone A. Transcranial magnetic stimulation in neurology. *Lancet Neurol.* 2003;2:145–156.

15. George MS, Nahas Z, Kozel FA, et al. Mechanisms and the current state of transcranial magnetic stimulation. *CNS Spectr.* 2003;8:496–502, 511–514.

16. Pascual-Leone A, Valls-Sole J, Wasserman EM, Hallett M. Responses to rapid-rate transcranial magnetic stimulation of the human motor cortex. *Brain.* 1994; 117:847–858.

17. Adey WR. Ramel C, Norden B, eds. *Resonance and Other Interactions of Electromagnetic Fields With Living Organisms.* Oxford, UK: Oxford University Press; 1992.

18. Lednev LL. Possible mechanism of weak magnetic fields on biological systems. *Bioelectromagnetics.* 1991;12:71–75.

19. Pilla AA, Muchsam DJ, Markov MS. A dynamical systems/larmor precession model for weak magnetic field bioeffects: ion binding and orientation of bound water molecules. *Bioelectro Chemistry.* 1997;43:241–252.

20. Engstrom S, Fitzsimmons R. Five hypotheses to examine the nature of magnetic field transduction in biological systems. *Bioelectromagnetics.* 1999;20:423–430.

21. Timmel CR, Till U, Brocklehurst B, et al. Effects of Weak Magnetic Fields on Free Radical Recombination Reactions. *Molecular Physics.* 1998; 95: 71–89.

22. Pilla AA. Weak time-varying and static magnetic fields: from mechanisms to therapeutic applications. In: Stavroulakis P, ed. *Biological Effects of Electromagnetic Fields.* New York: Springer Verlag; 2003:34–75.

23. Adey WR. Potential therapeutic applications of non-thermal electromagnetic fields: ensemble organization of cells in tissue as a factor in biological field sensing. In: Rosch, PJ, Markov MS, eds. *Bioelectromagnetic Medicine.* New York: Marcel Dekker, Inc; 2004:1–15.

24. Markov MS. Magnetic and electromagnetic field therapy: basic principles of application for pain relief. In: Rosch, PJ, Markov MS, eds. *Bioelectromagnetic Medicine*. New York: Marcel Dekker, Inc; 2004::251–264.
25. Markov MS, Colbert AP. Magnetic and electromagnetic field therapy. *J Back Musculoskel Rehab*. 2001;15:17–29.
26. Farndale RW, Maroudas A, Marsland TP. Effects of low-amplitude pulsed magnetic fields on cellular ion transport. *Bioelectromagnetics*. 1987;8:119–134.
27. Maccabee PJ, Amassian VE, Cracco RQ, et al. Stimulation of the human nervous system using the magnetic coil. *J Clin Neurophysiol*. 1991;8:38–55.
28. Rossini PM, Barker AT, Berardelli A, et al. Non-Invasive electrical and magnetic stimulation of the brain, spinal cord and roots: basic principles and procedure for routine clinical application: report of an IFCN Committee. *Electroencephalogr Clin Neurophysiol*. 1994;91:79–92.
29. Adey WR. Physiological signaling across cell membranes and cooperative influences of extremely low frequency electromagnetic fields. In: Frohlich H, ed. *Biological Coherence and Response to External Stimuli*. New York: Springer-Verlag; 1988: 148–170.
30. Rosen AD. Magnetic field influence on acetylcholine release at the neuromuscular junction. *Am J Physiol*. 1992;262: 1418–1422.
31. Repacholi MH, Greenebaum B. Interaction of static and extremely low frequency electric and magnetic fields with living systems: health effects and research needs. *Bioelectromagnetics*. 1999;20:133–160.
32. Blumenthal NC, Ricci J, Breger L, et al. Effects of low intensity ac and/or dc electromagnetic fields on cell attachment and induction of apoptosis. *Bioelectromagnetics*. 1997;18:264–272.
33. DeLoecker W, Cheng N, Delport PH. Effects of pulsed electromagnetic fields on membrane transport. *Emerging Electromagnetic Med*. 1990;45–57.
34. Serway RA. *Principles of Physics*. 2nd ed. Philadelphia: Saunders College Publishing; 1998:636–669.
35. Smith WF. *Principles of Materials Science and Engineering*. 3rd ed. New York: McGraw-Hill; 1996:659–706.
36. Wittig JE, Engstrom S. Magnetism and magnetic materials. In: McLean MJ, Engstrom S, Holcomb RR, eds. *Magnetotherapy: Potential Therapeutic Benefits and Adverse Effects*. 2002:3–18.
37. Goodman R, Blank M. Insights into electromagnetic interaction mechanisms. *J Cell Physiology*. 2002;192:16–22.
38. Pilla AA, Nasser PR, Kaufman JJ. The sensitivity of cells and tissues to therapeutic and environmental EMF. *Bioelectrochem and Bioenergetics*. 1993;30:161–169.
39. Pilla AA, Nasser PR, Kaufman JJ. The sensitivity of cells and tissues to weak electromagnetic fields. In: Allen MJ, Cleary SF, Sowers AE, Shillady DD, eds. *Charge and Field Effects in Biosystems—3*. Boston, MA: Birkhauser; 1992:231–241.
40. Weintraub, MI, Khoury A, Cole SP. Biologic effects of 3 Tesla (T) MR imaging comparing traditional 1.5 T and 0.6 T in 1023 consecutive outpatients. *J Neuro Imaging*. 2007;17:241–245.
41. Pilla AA, Muehsam DJ. Pulsing and static magnetic field therapeutics: from mechanisms to clinical application. In: McLean MJ, Engstrom S, Holcomb RR, eds. *Magnetotherapy: Potential Therapeutic Benefits and Adverse Effects*. 2002:119–144.
42. Colbert AP: Clinical Trials Involving Static Magnetic Field Applications. In: Rosch PJ, Markov MS, eds. *Bioelectromagnetic Medicine*. New York: Marcel Dekker, Inc; 2004:781–796.
43. Markov MS, Pilla AA. Weak static magnetic field modulation of myosin phosphorylation in a cell-free preparation: calcium dependence. *Bioelectrochem and Bioenergetics*. 1997;43:233–238.

44. McDonald F. Effect of static magnetic fields on osteoblasts and fibroblasts in vitro. *Bioelectromagnetics*. 1993;14:187–196.
45. Sisken BF, Walker J, Orgel M. Prospects on clinical applications of electrical stimulation for nerve regeneration. *J Cellular Biochem*. 1993;52:404–409.
46. Macias MY, Buttocletti JH, Sutton CH, et al. Directed and enhanced neurite growth with pulsed magnetic field stimulation. *Bioelectromagnetics*. 2000;21:272–286.
47. McLean MJ, Holcomb RR, Wamil AW, et al. Blockade of sensory neuron action potentials by a static magnetic field in the mT range. *Bioelectromagnetics*. 1995;16:20–32.
48. McLean M, Holcomb RR, Engstrom S, et al. A static magnetic field blocks action potential firing and kainic acid-induced neuronal injury in vitro. In: McLean MJ, Engstrom S, Holcomb RR, eds. *Magnetotherapy: Potential Therapeutic Benefits and Adverse Effects*. 2002:29–40.
49. Ohkubo C, Xu S, Acute effects of static magnetic fields on cutaneous microcirculation in rabbits. *In Vivo*. 1997;11:221–226.
50. Okano H, Gmitrov J, Ohkubo C. Biphasic effects of static magnetic fields on cutaneous microcirculation in rabbits. *Bioelectromagnetics*. 1999;20:161–171.
51. Holcomb RR, McLean MJ, Engstrom S, et al. Treatment of mechanical low back pain with static magnetic fields: result of a clinical trial and implications for study design. In: McLean MJ, Engstrom S, Holcomb RR, eds. *Magnetotherapy: Potential Therapeutic Benefits and Adverse Effects*. 2002;171–189.
52. Ramey DW. Magnetic and electromagnetic therapy. *Sci Rev Alt Med*. 1998;2:13–19.
53. Blechman AM, Oz MC, Nair V, Ting W. Discrepancy between claimed field flux density of some commercially available magnets and actual gaussmeter measurements. *Altern Ther Health Med*. 2001;7:92–95.
54. Eccles NJ. A critical review of randomized controlled trials of static magnets for pain relief. *J Altern Complimen Med*. 2005;11:495–509.
55. Vallbona C, Hazelwood CF, Jurida G. Response of pain to static magnetic fields in post-polio patients: a double-blind pilot study. *Arch Phys Med and Rehabil*. 1997;78:1200–1203.
56. Carter R, Aspy CB, Mold J. The effectiveness of magnet therapy for treatment of wrist pain attributed to carpal tunnel syndrome. *J Fam Pract*. 2002;51:38–40.
57. Man D, Man B, Plosker H. The influence of permanent magnetic field therapy on wound healing in suction lipectomy patients: a double-blind study. *Plast and Reconstr Surg*. 1999;104:2261–2296.
58. Brown CS, Ling FW, Wan JY, Pilla AA. Efficacy of static magnetic field therapy in chronic pelvic pain: a double-blind, pilot study. *Am J Obs Gyn*. 2002;187:1581–1587.
59. Colbert AP, Markov MS, Banerij M, Pilla AA. Magnetic mattress pad use in patients with fibromyalgia: a randomized, double-blind pilot study. *J Back Musculoskel Rehabil*. 1999;13:19–31.
60. Weintraub, MI. Magnetic bio-stimulation in painful diabetic peripheral neuropathy: a novel intervention. A randomized, double-blind, placebo, cross-over study. *Am J Pain Manage*. 1999;9:8–17.
61. Weintraub MI, Wolfe, GI, Barohn RA, et al. Static magnetic field therapy for symptomatic diabetic neuropathy: a randomized, double-blind, placebo-controlled trial. *Arch Phys Med Rehabil*. 2003:84:736–746.
62. Hinman MR, Ford J, Heyl H. Effects of static magnets on chronic knee pain and physical function: a double-blind study. *Altern Ther Health Med*. 2002;8:50–55.
63. Saygili G, Aydinlik E, Ercan MI, et al. Investigation of the effect of magnetic retention systems used in prostheses on buccal mucosal blood flow. *Int J Prosthodont*. 1992;5:326–332.

64. Hong CZ, Lin JC, Bender LF, et al. Magnetic necklace: its therapeutic effectiveness on neck and shoulder pain. *Arc Phys Med Rehab.* 1982;63:462–466.

65. Martel GF, Andrews SC, Roseboom CG. Comparison of static and placebo magnets on resting forearm blood flow in young, healthy men. *J Orthop Sports Phys Ther.* 2002;32:518–524.

66. Collacott EA, Zimmerman JT, White DW, Rindone JP. Bipolar permanent magnets for the treatment of low back pain: a pilot study. *JAMA.* 2000;283:1322–1325.

67. Winemiller MH, Billow RG, Laskowski ER, Harmsen WS. Effect of magnetic vs. sham-magnetic insoles on plantar heel pain: a randomized controlled trial. *JAMA.* 2003;290:1474–1478.

68. Weintraub, MI. Magnets for patients with heel pain. *JAMA.* 2004;291:43.

69. Weintraub, MI. Are magnets effective for pain control? *JAMA.* 2000;284:565.

70. Weintraub, MI, Steinberg RB, Cole SP. The role of cutaneous magnetic stimulation in failed back syndrome. *Sem in Integrative Med.* 2005;3:101–103.

71. United Nations Environment Programme MF. The International Labour Organization. World Health Organization,United Nations, Geneva. Switzerland; 1987.

72. U.S. Food and Drug Administration, Center for Devices and Radiological Health. MDR Data File. www.FDA.gov/CDRH/MDRFILE/html. Accesed April 1, 2003.

73. Ciombor D, Lester G, Aaron R, et al. Low-frequency EMF regulates chondrocyte differentiation and expression of matrix proteins. *J Orthopaedic Res.* 2002;20:40–50.

74. Pilla AA, Martin DE, Schuett, AM, et al. Effect of pulsed radiofrequency therapy on edema from grades i and ii ankle sprains: a placebo-controlled, randomized, multi-site, double-blind, clinical study. *J Athl Train.* 1996;S31:53.

75. Pujol J, Pascual-Leone A, Dolz C, et al. The effect of repetitive magnetic stimulation on localized musculoskeletal pain. *Neuro Rep.* 1998;9:1745–1748.

76. Raji ARM, Bowden REM. Effects of high pulsed power electromagnetic field on the degeneration and regeneration of the common personal nerve in rats. *J Bone Joint Surg.* 1983;65:478–492.

77. Mooney V. A Randomized, double-blind, prospective study of the efficacy of pulsed electromagnetic fields for interbody lumbar fusions. *Spine.* 1990;15:708–715.

78. Zdeblic TD. A prospective randomized study of lumbar fusion: preliminary results. *Spine.* 1993;18:983–991.

79. Linovitz RJ, Ryaby JT, Magee FP, et al. Combined magnetic fields accelerate primary spine fusion: a double-blind, randomized, placebo-controlled study. *Proc Am Acad Orthop Surg.* 2000;67:376.

80. Aaron RK, Lennox D, Bunce GE, Ebert T. The conservative treatment of osteonecrosis of the femoral head: a comparison of core decompression and pulsing electromagnetic fields. *Clin Orthopaed.* REL RES. 1989;249:209–218.

81. Binder A, Parr G, Hazelman B, Fitton-Jackson S. Pulsed electromagnetic field therapy of persistent rotator cuff tendonitis: a double-blind, controlled assessment. *Lancet.* 1984;8179:695–697.

82. Wilson DH, Jagadeesh O. The effect of pulsed electromagnetic energy on peripheral nerve regeneration. *Ann of N Y Acad of Sci.* 1974;238:575–580.

83. Jacobson JI, Gorman R, Yamanashi WS, et al. Low-amplitude, extremely low frequency magnetic fields for the treatment of osteoarthritic knees: a double-blind clinical study. *Altern Ther Health Med.* 2001;7:54–64.

84. Pipitone N, Scott DL. Magnetic pulsed treatment for knee osteoarthritis: a randomized, double-blind, placebo-controlled study. *Curr Med Res Opin.* 2001;17:190–196.

85. Battisti E, Fortunato M, Giananneshi F, Rigato M. Efficacy of the magnetotherapy in idiopathic carpal tunnel syndrome. In: Suminic D, ed. Proc IV EBEA Congress Zagreb, Yugoslavia, 1998;34–35.

86. Lappin MS, Lawrie FW, Richards TL, Kramer ED. Effects of a pulsed electromagnetic therapy on multiple sclerosis, fatigue and quality of life: a double-blind, placebo-controlled trial. *Alt Thera.* 2003;9:38–48.

87. Todd DJ, Heylings DJ, Allen GE, McMillin WP. Treatment of chronic varicose ulcers with pulsed electromagnetic fields: a controlled pilot study. *IR Med J.* 1991;84:54–55.

88. Kloth LC, Berman JE, Sutton CH, et al. Effect of pulsed radiofrequency stimulation on wound healing: a double-blind, pilot clinical study. In Bersani F, ed. *Electricity and Magnetism in Biology and Medicine.* New York, NY: Plenum; 1999:875–878.

89. Mayrovitz HN, Larsen PB. A preliminary study to evaluate the effect of pulsed radiofrequency field treatment on lower extremity peri-ulcer skin microvascularature of diabetic patients. *Wounds.* 1995;7:90–93.

90. Foley-Nolan D, Barry C, Coughlan RJ, et al. Pulsed high-frequency (27 MHz) electromagnetic therapy for persistent neck pain: a double-blind, placebo-controlled study of 20 patients. *Orthop.* 1990;13:445–451.

91. Foley-Nolan D, Moore K, Codd M, et al. Low-energy, high-frequency, pulsed electromagnetic therapy for acute whiplash injuries: a double-blind, randomized, control study. *Scan DJ Rehab Med.* 1992;24:51–59.

92. Weintraub, MI, Cole SP. Pulsed magnetic field therapy in refractory neuropathic pain secondary to peripheral neuropathy: electrodiagnostic parameters-pilot study. *Neuro Rehab, Neural Repair.* 2004;18:42–46.

93. Pickering SAW, Bayston R, Scammell BE. Electromagnetic Augmentation of antibiotic efficacy in infection of orthopaedic implants. *The J of Bone, Joint Surg.* 2003;85:588–593.

94. Weintraub MI, Cole SP. Novel device generating static and time-varying magnetic fields in refractory diabetic peripheral neuropathy: subset analysis of cohort with long-term exposure in nationwide, double-blind, placebo-controlled trial. *Diabetes.* 2007;(suppl):A-610.

95. Weintraub MI, Cole SP. A randomized, controlled trial of the effects of a combination of static and dynamic magnetic fields on carpal tunnel syndrome. *Neurol.* 2007; (supp1)68:A180.

96. Osenbach RK. Motor cortex stimulation for intractable pain. *Neuro Surg Focus.* 2006;21:1–17.

97. Cahn SD, Herzog AG, Pascual-Leone A. Paired-pulsed transcranial magnetic stimulation: effects of hemispheric laterality, gender and handedness in normal controls. *J Clin Neurophysiol.* 2003;20:371–374.

98. Pascual-Leon A, Wasserman EM, Davey NJ, eds. *Handbook of Transcranial Magnetic Stimulation.* London, England: Oxford University Press; 2002.

99. George MS, Lisanby SH, Sackeim HA. Transcranial magnetic stimulation: applications in neuropsychiatry. *Arc Gen Psychiatry.* 1999;56:300–311.

100. Wasserman EM. Risk and safety of repetitive transcranial magnetic stimulation: report and suggested guidelines from the International Workshop in the Safety of Repetitive Transcranial Magnetic Stimulation: June 5–7, 1996. *Electroencephalogr Clin Neurophysiol.* 1998;108:1–16.

101. Walsh V, Rushworth M. A primer of magnetic stimulation as a tool for neuropsychology. *Neuropsychologia.* 1999;37:125–135.

102. Terao Y, Ugawa Y. Basic mechanisms of TMS. *J Clin Neurophysiol.* 2002;19:322–343.

103. Lisamby, SH, Gutman D, Lubes B, et al. Intracerebral measurement of the induced electrical field and the induction of motor-evoked potentials. *Biol Psychiatry.* 2001a; 49:460–463.

104. Abbruzzese G, Trompetto C. Clinical and research methods for evaluating cortical excitability. *J Clin Neurophysiol.* 2002;19:307–321.

105. Amassian VE, Cracco RQ, Maccabee PJ. Focal stimulation of human cerebral cortex with the magnetic coil: a comparison with electrical stimulation. *Electroencephalograph Clin Neurophysiol.* 1989;74:401–416.
106. Chae JH, Nahas Z, Wasserman EM, et al. A pilot study using rtms to probe the functional neuroanatomy of tics in Tourette's syndrome. *Neuropsychiatry, Neuropsychol Behav Neurol.* In press.
107. Rollnik JD, Wusterfeld S, Dauper J, et al. Repetitive transcranial magnetic stimulation for the treatment of chronic pain: a pilot study. *Eur Neurol.* 2002;48:6–10.
108. Cantello R. Applications of transcranial magnetic stimulation in movement disorders. *J Clin Neurophysiol.* 2002;19:272–293.
109. Theodore WH. Transcranial magnetic stimulation in epilepsy. *Epilepsy Curr.* 2003; 3:191–197.
110. Orpin JA. False claims for magnetotherapy. *Can Med Assoc.* 1982;15:1375
111. DeRidder D, DeMulder G, Walsh W, et al. Magnetic and electrical stimulation of the auditory cortex for intractable tinnitus. *J Neuro Surg.* 2004;100:560–564.
112. George MS, Nahas Z, Kozel A, et al. Repetitive transcranial magnetic stimulation (rTMS) for depression and other indications. In: Rosch PJ, Markov MS, eds. *Bioelectromagnetic Medicine.* New York: Marcel Dekker; 2004:293–312.
113. Shellock FG. Biomedical implants and devices: assessment of magnetic field interactions with a 3.0T MR system. *J Magn Reson Imaging.* 2002;16:721–732.

FURTHER READING

Alfano AP, Taylor AG, Foresman PA, et al. Static magnetic fields for treatment of fibromyalgia: a randomized, controlled trial. *Alternative Comp Med.* 2001;7:53–64.

Bassett CA. Fundamental and practical aspects of therapeutic uses of pulsed electromagnetic fields (PEMFs). *Crit Rev Biomed Eng.* 1989;17:451–529.

Bassett CA. The development and application of pulsed electromagnetic fields (PEMFs) for ununited fracture and arthrodeses. *Orthop Clin North Am.* 1984;15:61–87.

Carter R, Aspy CB, Mold J. The effectiveness of magnetic therapy for treatment of wrist pain attributed to carpal tunnel syndrome. *J Fam Pract.* 2002;51:38–40.

Caselli MA, Clark N, Lazarus S, et al. Evaluation of magnetic foil and ppt insoles in the treatment of heel pain. *J Am Podiatry Med Assoc.* 1997;87:11–16.

Keck ME, Sillaber I, Ebner K, et al. Acute transcranial magnetic stimulation of frontal brain regions selectively modulates the release of vasopressin, biogenic amines and amino acids in the rat brain. *Eur J Neurosci.* 2000;12:3713–3720.

Leclaire R, Bourguin J. Electromagnetic treatment of shoulder periarthritis: a randomized, controlled trial of the efficacy and tolerance of magnetotherapy. *Arc Phys Med Rehab.* 1991;72:284–287.

McDonald F. Effect of static magnetic fields on osteoblasts and fibroblasts in-vitro. *Bioelectromagnetics.* 1993;14:187–196.

Rispoli FP, Corolla FM, Mussner R. The use of low frequency pulsing electromagnetic fields in patients with painful hip prostheses. *J Bioelectric.* 1988;7:181–187.

Ryaby JT. Electromagnetic stimulation in orthopedics: biochemical mechanisms to clinical applications. In: Rosch, PJ, Markov MS, eds. *Bioelectromagnetic Medicine.* New York: Marcel Dekker, Inc; 2004:411–422.

Segal NA, Toda Y, Huston J, et al. Two configurations of static magnetic fields for testing rheumatoid arthritis of the knee: a double-blind clinical trial. *Arch Phys Med Rehabil.* 2001;82:1453–1460.

Shellock FG, Crues JV. MR procedures: biological effects, safety and patient care. *Radiol.* 2004;232:635–652.

Thuile CH, Walzl M. Evaluation of electromagnetic fields in the treatment of pain in patients with lumbar radiculopathy or the whiplash syndrome. *Neuro Rehabil.* 2002;17:63–70.

Weintraub MI, Cole SP. Bi-axial rotating static magnetic fields in refractory carpal tunnel syndrome: a novel approach. (Under review).

CHAPTER 6

Animal-Assisted Therapy

Amy Tyberg and William H. Frishman

What is man without the beasts? If all the beasts were gone, man would die
from a great loneliness of the spirit. All things are connected.
—*Chief Seattle*

As it has become clear that psychosocial factors play an integral role
in health, particularly in influencing the progression and severity of
disease, scientists have begun to identify these factors with the goal
of uncovering methods to control them and thus affect the course of
an illness. Some of these studies have led to the hypothesis that the
presence of an animal companion is one such psychosocial factor. This
hypothesis is grounded in the significance of animals to people's lives.
The household pet plays such a large role in people's lives that 99% of
pet owners consider their pets to be part of the their families.[1] Pets are
present in 60% of households,[2] and a survey of 500 former pet-owners
now in a hospital setting showed that the "thing" they missed most was
their pets.[3] In the last half of the twentieth century, scientists began to
consider whether these animals have an actual physiologic effect on
people's health, and if so, whether they can be used as an integral part
of patient care.

This interest has spurred the emergence of animal-assisted therapy
(AAT) in hospitals and institutions across the country. In 1996 the Delta

Society, which is a leading international group that studies the human-animal bond, defined AAT as:

> a goal-directed intervention in which an animal meeting specific criteria is an integral part of the treatment process . . . AAT is designed to promote improvement in human physical, social, emotional, and/or cognitive functioning. AAT is provided in a variety of settings and may be group or individual in nature.[4]

GENERAL HISTORY OF ANIMAL-ASSISTED THERAPY

The earliest documented evidence of AAT dates back to the ninth century, when animals were used to help care for handicapped people in Belgium.[5] In 1792, physicians at a mental hospital in Great Britain used animals to help their patients learn to care for a living creature in a form of what we now call behavioral therapy and was then called moral therapy.[6] One hundred years ago, Florence Nightingale wrote that pets are perfect companions for patients that are confined to a hospital with a chronic illness.[7] More recently in the United States in 1940, hospitals established programs in which veterans interacted with animals in recovery units.[8] Presently, many health care establishments have programs with visiting and/or residential animals.

BENEFICIAL EFFECTS OF PETS

When used in the correct situation, AAT therapy is able to aid many aspects of a person's well-being. The participants of AAT should be carefully screened to ensure a positive interaction. The patient should not have a negative attitude towards animals and should be in a suitable medical condition in order to prevent any harm developing from the interaction. Katcher and Friedmann articulated nine beneficial conditions for humans that pets can help develop: "providing companionship, pleasurable activity, facilitating exercise, play and laughter, being something to care for and a source of consistency, allowing feelings of security, being a comfort to touch, and pleasurable to watch."[9] The presence of a pet provides a pleasant, nonevaluative external focus, promotes feelings of safety, and furnishes a source of comfort.[10]

AAT also improves physical health in several ways. A 10-month prospective study examined the changes induced by the acquisition of a pet in 71 subjects.[11] Dog owners were shown to have a highly significant reduction in minor health problems from the first month of ownership, with sustained effects up to the 10th month; cat owners initially reported these changes and returned to baseline after 6 months. Pet owners are shown to make fewer visits to the physician as well.[12]

ANIMAL-ASSISTED THERAPY IN CHRONIC NEUROLOGICAL AND PSYCHOLOGICAL DISEASES

The impact of AAT therapy on physical health has been studied more specifically in several areas of medicine. We have previously written on the influence of AAT in patients with cardiovascular disease.[13] This chapter considers the influence of AAT on patients with chronic, lifelong illnesses in the fields of neurology and psychiatry, specifically seizure disorders, dementia, and mental illness requiring chronic hospitalization.

Seizure Disorders

There have been several studies that have looked at the influence of AAT in patients with seizure disorders. Interest first arose in the this area in the 1980s when a women with a seizure disorder reported to the news media that her pet dog was able to predict when she was going to have an episode. A follow-up survey done in the 1990s showed that of 77 subjects with epilepsy, 10% felt their pet dog could predict when they were going to have a seizure, and 28% reported their dog stayed with them when they had a seizure and helped prevent them from injuring themselves.[14] A more recent survey conducted at the Alberta Children's Hospital in Canada examined this issue more specifically. The survey of 122 families with epileptic children found that 15% of those living with a pet dog reported their dogs were able to predict the children's seizures with a sensitivity of 80% and no false-positives.[15] It was also found that 40% of the dogs engaged in seizure specific behaviors, of which 50% were protective behaviors such as lying on top of the child and refusing to allow them to stand prior to a seizure or pushing the child away from the stairs prior to seizure onset. Additional studies performed in the United Kingdom confirmed the predictive ability of specially trained so-called seizure dogs to warn of impending seizures in their owners.[16] The studies found that the presence of seizure dogs also decreased the frequency of seizures in their owners. Of 10 subjects with epilepsy who were experiencing at least one tonic-clonic seizure per month, the frequency of tonic-clonic seizures decreased from baseline levels by 43% over 24 weeks (see Figure 6.1).[16,17]

The unpredictability of seizure occurrence remains the most difficult aspect of the disease for patients with epilepsy, according to patients in one large survey.[18] Thus, the existence of seizure dogs that could help predict seizure occurrence and decrease the frequency of seizures in patients with epilepsy is an exciting potential adjuvant to drug therapy. The previously mentioned study from the Alberta Children's Hospital found that quality of life was significantly improved for those families whose pet dogs were able to predict seizure onset and engage in protective behavior towards the epileptic children;[15] however, the effectiveness of seizure dogs remains ambiguous, as more recent studies have found seizure dogs to be less effective than originally suggested. Two studies done at Johns Hopkins University and the Swedish Epilepsy Center in Seattle monitored seven individuals who had been using seizure dogs via video electroencephalogram. The studies found that seizure dogs were actually predicting psychosocial seizures rather than epileptic seizures.[19,20] Additionally, the studies from the United Kingdom mentioned above used specially trained seizure dogs in their studies.[16] In a comparative study using untrained dogs, it was found that almost 50% of the dogs died or engaged in aggressive behavior towards humans when their owners had seizures.[21] While AAT shows some promise in patients with seizure disorders, the current research remains inconclusive (see Figure 6.1).

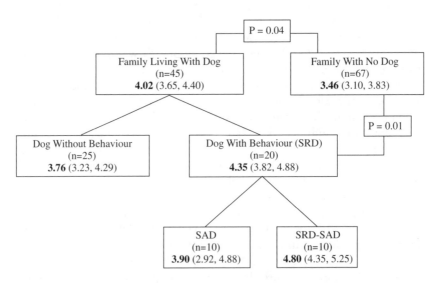

FIGURE 6.1   Overall quality of life in pediatric epilepsy as assessed by the Impact of Pediatric Epilepsy Scale (IPES) is higher in families living with a dog, particularly if that dog demonstrates seizure-related behaviors (SRD).[15] SAD, seizure-alerting dogs. From Kirton A, Krauss GL, Lesser RP. Pseudoseizure dogs. *Neurology.* 2004;62(23):2303–2305.

Dementia

There is undisputed evidence that AAT has a positive impact on individuals with degenerative cognitive illnesses. Studies show that both behavioral and psychological aspects of dementia can be improved with the implementation of AAT. By interacting with an animal, calling it by name, and asking for behavior from the animal, patients can improve short-term memory and communication. Similarly, seeing an animal can often trigger long-term memory in demented patients.[22] In a literature review from the University of Sydney, it was found that several small studies together showed that the presence of a pet-therapy dog decreased aggression and agitation and increased social behaviors among patients with dementia.[23] In another study it was shown that residents in several chronic care facilities were "coming alive" in the presence of pets; residents who were previously unable to be engaged began to speak and interact with residents and staff in the presence of canine visitors.[24] One study done at the University of Nebraska College of Nursing looked specifically at the effect of AAT on problem behaviors in patients with dementia. Using the Nursing Home Behavior Problem Scale, residents were studied over 4 weeks before and after the placement of a dog in the facility and were found to show significantly fewer problem behaviors in the presence of the dog.[25]

In addition to improving behavioral and psychological aspects of dementia, AAT has also been shown to improve physical health in patients with dementia. A study from the Purdue University School of Nursing of 62 individuals with Alzheimer's disease in chronic care facilities found that the presence of fish aquariums was associated with the improved nutritional status of patients. Both the nutritional intake and the weights of the patients increased, and the amount of nutritional supplementation required decreased during the 8 weeks of the study.[26] AAT provides clear benefit to patients with dementia; however, the mechanism behind these improvements, as well as the exact frequency and duration of AAT required to elicit maximum improvement remains to be discovered.

Mental Illness Requiring Long-Term Hospitalization

Several studies have been done looking at the effects of AAT in chronically mentally ill patients on psychiatric wards. Hospitalized psychiatric patients often have severe impairments in social functioning, with little chance for improvement due to the limited social interaction available on psychiatric inpatient wards. AAT provides a potential social outlet for these patients. This was first investigated in the 1960s, when studies showed that pet dogs helped schizophrenic patients remain more "grounded in reality."[27] A more recent study looked at the effects of AAT in 20 elderly schizophrenic patients in a hospital in Israel. The results showed that patients exposed to AAT had more positive scores on the Scale for Social Adaptive Functioning Evaluation compared to their own baseline levels, as well as compared to the patients not exposed to AAT. These patients also showed improvements in interpersonal contact, communication, and various activities of daily living such as personal hygiene.[28]

AAT has also been shown to help psychiatric inpatients in other areas besides social improvement. A study of 230 hospitalized psychiatric patients from the Medical College of Virginia showed that AAT sessions significantly decreased anxiety levels in patients with psychotic disorders, mood disorders, and other psychiatric conditions.[29] Additional studies have demonstrated that chronically hospitalized patients were found to have a lower incidence of depression after AAT than those who did not participate in AAT.[27] The benefits of AAT in psychiatric inpatients is evident; however, as in the dementia studies, the mechanism behind these improvements and the frequency and duration of AAT required to inspire maximum improvement remains to be seen.

SIDE EFFECTS OF ANIMAL-ASSISTED THERAPY

Although AAT has been shown to provide many benefits to a variety of patients with various medical conditions, adverse effects of AAT programs must also be considered. Animals carry a variety of zoonotic diseases that could potentially be transmitted to the patients they are in contact with, including rabies, ringworm, external parasitism, internal parasitism, and intestinal infections (see Table 6.1).[29] Animals can also induce allergies in patients, as well as bite or scratch the patients they interact with.[29] Additionally, animals interacting with multiple patients could serve as a vector for disease transmission. Yet, despite these potential risks, AAT therapy appears to be relatively safe. In 1993, David Walter-Toews surveyed 124 animal care agencies in the United States and Canada to determine the types of measures used to prevent disease transmission, as well as the prevalence of disease transmission among animal care agencies.[29] The responses indicated that less than 50% of community-based animal care programs consulted a physician or veterinarian about disease transmission, and less than 10% had printed guidelines about controlling zoonotic diseases. Hospital-based programs fared better, with 95% having consulted a health professional about disease transmission, and 70% having printed guidelines for controlling a disease outbreak.[29] Yet despite these results, transmission of zoonotic diseases remains uncommon. A study by Stryler-Gordon et al. of 284 Minnesotan nursing homes with

TABLE 6.1 Zoonotic Disease Concerns in Animal Visitation and Animal-Assisted Therapy Programs in Canada and the United States

Disease	Program		Hospitals[a]	Total
	Canada	United States		
Rabies	14 (29%)[b]	12 (17%)	1 (5%)	27 (20%)
Ringworm	5 (10%)	10 (15%)	1 (5%)	16 (12%)
External parasitism	5 (10%)	5 (7%)	—	10 (7%)
Allergies	1 (2%)	4 (6%)	1 (5%)	6 (4%)
Internal parasitism	3 (6%)	3 (4%)	—	6 (4%)
Intestinal infections	1 (2%)	2 (3%)	3 (16%)	6 (4%)
Bites and scratches	3 (6%)	3 (4%)	—	6 (4%)

[a]Hospitals with animal-assisted programs listed by the Delta Society
[b]Number of programs reporting concern (% of programs in that country/category). Categories are not mutually exclusive
From: Walter-Toews D. Zoonotic disease concerns in animal-assisted therapy and animal visitation programs. *Can Vet J.* 1993;34(9):549–551.

live-in dogs over a 1-year period found a 0% transmission rate of zoonotic diseases.[30] Thus, while the potential for adverse effects exists, so far AAT seems to be a relatively safe treatment approach; however, as AAT programs gain popularity and expand in size and number, standardized methods to prevent infection transmission should be implemented.

CONCLUSION

Neurology and psychiatry are areas of medicine in which current medical treatment options often fall short. Patients with chronic conditions in these fields, such as seizure disorders, dementia, or mental illnesses, often start out or become refractory to traditional pharmacotherapy throughout the course of their illnesses. It is increasingly recognized that pharmacotherapy for these illnesses has inherent limitations, as well as carrying significant, and in some cases unacceptable, risks of it own. Additionally, many patients with these conditions have cognitive impairments and impairments in social functioning that cannot be easily treated with medications. AAT can be a useful adjuvant treatment for these patients. AAT therapy has been shown to increase social interaction and to decrease problem behaviors in patients with dementia, as well as to improve the nutritional status of such patients. Patients with schizophrenia show not only improvements in social functioning but also a decreased incidence of anxiety and depression in the presence of AAT. Although the role of AAT in patients with seizure disorders remains less concrete, it shows the potential to both decrease the frequency of seizures and relieve some of the uncertainty of seizure occurrence by helping predict when they will occur; however, the mechanisms of these improvements, as well as the ideal duration and frequency of AAT, is yet to be determined.

Overall, AAT has been shown to have beneficial effects on many chronic, potentially treatment-refractory conditions in the fields of neurology and psychiatry. With the implementation of better mechanisms to prevent and control the spread of zoonotic disease, AAT has the potential to be an extremely useful complementary therapy that could improve the quality of life of many chronically ill patients.

REFERENCES

1. Voith V. Attachment of people to companion animals. *Vet Clin North Amer: Small Animal Practice*. 1985;15:289–295.
2. Marx MB, Stallones TF, Garrity JR, Johnson TP. Demographics of pet ownership among US adults 21–64 years of age. *Anthrozoos*. 1988;2(1):33–37.
3. Francis GM. Loneliness: measuring the abstract. *Intl J Nurs Studies*. 1976;13:153–160.
4. Delta Society. Standard of practice for animal assisted activities and therapy. Renton, WA. 1996.
5. Bustad LK, Hines L. Historical perspectives of the human-animal bond. In: Bustad, LK, Hines, L, eds. *The Pet Connection: Its Influence on our Health and Quality of Life*. Minneapolis, MN: University of Minnesota Press; 1984.
6. Jones B. *The Psychology of the Human/Companion Animal Bond: An Annotated Bibliography*. Philadelphia, PA: University of Pennsylvania Press; 1985.
7. Nightingale F. *Notes on Nursing*. New York, NY: Dover Publications; 1969 (originally published in 1859).
8. Kear L. Pet-facilitated therapy and the elderly. *Dog World*. 1990;75: 25–27
9. Katcher A, Friedmann E. Potential health value of pet ownership. *Compendium of Continuing Education Prac Vet*. 1980;2(2):117–121.
10. Odendaal JSJ. Animal-assisted therapy: magic or medicine? *J Psychosom Res*. 2000; 49:275–280.
11. Serpell J. Beneficial effects of pet ownership on some aspects of human health and behavior. *J R Soc Med*. 1991;84(12):717–720.
12. Siegel JM. Companion animals: in sickness and in health. *J Social Issues*. 1993;9:157–167.
13. Wolff AI, Frishman WH. Animal-assisted therapy and cardiovascular disease. In: Frishman WH, Weintraub MI, Micozzi MS, eds. *Complementary and Integrative Therapies for Cardiovascular Disease*. Philadelphia, PA: Elsevier/Mosby; 2005:362–368.
14. What about seizure dogs? Epilepsy Association of Central Florida Web site. http://www.epilepsycf.org/seizure_dogs.htm. Accesed February 29, 2004.
15. Kirton A, Wirrell E, Zhang J, Hamiwka L. Seizure alerting and response behaviors in dogs living with epileptic children. *Neurol*. 2004;62(12):2303–2305.

16. Strong V, Brown SW, Walker R. Seizure-alert dogs—fact or fiction? *Seizure.* 1999;8: 62–65.
17. Strong V, Brown S, Huyton M, Coyle H. Effect of trained seizure alert dogs on frequency of tonic–clonic seizures. *Seizure.* 2002;11:402–405.
18. Fisher RS, Vickrey BG, Gibson P, et al. The impact of epilepsy from the patient's perspective: descriptions and subjective perceptions. *Epilepsy Res.* 2001;41:39–45.
19. Krauss GL, Choi JS, Lesser RP. Pseudoseizure dogs. *Neurol.* 2007;68(4):308–309.
20. Doherty MJ, Haltiner AM. Wag the dog. skepticism on seizure alert canines. *Neurol.* 2007;68:309.
21. Strong V, Brown SW. Should people with epilepsy have untrained dogs as pets? *Seizure.* 2000;9(6):427–430.
22. Laun L. Benefits of pet therapy in dementia. *Home Healthcare Nurse.* 2003;21(1): 49–52.
23. Filan SL. Llewellyn-Jones RH. Animal-assisted therapy for dementia: a review of the literature. *Intelligence Psychogeriatr.* 2006;18(4):597–611.
24. Shaw G. Dementia therapy goes to the dogs. *Neurology Now.* March/April 2007.
25. McCabe BW, Baun MM, Speich D, Agrawal S. Resident dog in the Alzheimer's special care unit. *West J Nurs Res.* 2002;24(6):684–696.
26. Edwards NE, Beck AM. Animal assisted therapy and nutrition in Alzheimer's disease. *West J Nurs Res.* 2002;24(6):697–712.
27. Barker S, Dawson K. The effects of animal-assisted therapy on anxiety ratings of hospitalized psychiatric patients. *Psychiatric Serv.* 1998;49:797–801.
28. Barak Y, Savorai O, Mavashev S, Beni A. Animal-assisted therapy for elderly schizophrenic patients: a one-year controlled trial. *Am J Geriatr Psychiatry.* 2001;9(4): 439–442.
29. Walter-Toews D. Zoonotic disease concerns in animal-assisted therapy and animal visitation programs. *Can Vet J.* 1993;34(9):549–551.
30. Stryler-Gordon R, Beall N, Anderson RK. Facts and fiction: health risks associated with pets in nursing homes. *J Delta Soc.* 1985;2(1):73–74.

CHAPTER 7

Headache: An Intraoral Etiology and Noninvasive Treatment

Mark Friedman

Primary headache is the most common neurologic problem presenting to family physicians and neurologists, with migraine and tension-type headache (TTH) comprising the vast majority of these cases.[1] This most prevalent problem worldwide is responsible annually for 156.9 million lost workdays in the United States alone.[2] When one includes headaches in homemakers, students, children, and the elderly, epidemic proportions are suggested. Because those afflicted are basically healthy, the pervasive nature of this disorder is generally not appreciated. Because the response and side effect profile of traditional medication is often unsatisfactory, more than 200 different medications have been prescribed, chiefly for migraine, and extreme measures are often considered, such as Botox or surgical implants of antimigraine devices. Nearly 12 million Americans take prescription drugs for migraines. Few medications have been produced specifically for TTH (the most common headache)[3] or posttraumatic headache.

The pathophysiology of migraine is controversial, but the prevailing theory describes a persistent neurogenic dural inflammation with plasma extravasation (swelling).[4,5] Our research suggests that this neurogenic inflammation may also occur locally, closely adjacent to a relatively accessible maxillary nerve segment.[6]

Demonstrating the uncertainty also associated with migraine etiology is the continual emergence of new models, such as vascular theory, continuum theory, central sensitization, and convergence hypothesis. The etiology of TTH remains unresolved, and knowledge about key pathophysiological factors is limited. In the *Handbook of Headache Management,* Saper and Silberstein state "Because of the significant uncertainty regarding TTH, we have decided against a detailed review of this entity."[7]

Our treatment is based on the discovery of a distinct area of maxillary intraoral tenderness (MIT), which can be palpated consistently in patients with migraine, TTH, and posttraumatic headache, even in the headache-free state. Absent or inconsistent in pain free individuals, or in those with temporomandibular joint disorders, it is also noted in patients with atypical facial pain[8,9] and cervical muscle spasm.[10] This marker is located adjacent to the maxillary second and third molar root apices, even if the area is edentulous, and is closely related to the laterality and severity of symptoms.[6] This zonal tenderness approximates the plexus formed by the posterior superior alveolar branch of the maxillary nerve. A multihospital study has demonstrated that the tenderness is caused by a local inflammation.[11] The resultant edema (swelling) exerts pressure on the maxillary nerve, causing the headache. *Because the etiology is local, safer and more effective localized antiinflammatory treatment can be used.* The extraordinary results obtained for both headache prevention and elimination tends to validate this localized headache etiology theory.

BACKGROUND RESEARCH

Palpation Studies

In preliminary data analysis, this tenderness was palpated in 1,026 out of 1,100 (93.2%) mostly asymptomatic migraine and TTH patients, with laterality and degree of tenderness closely related to laterality and severity of reported symptoms.[12]

To identify the maxillary alveolar tenderness (MAT), the examiner's index finger is pressed upward and backward as far as possible along the vestibule forming the roof of the cheek pouch when the mouth is partially opened—when opened fully, muscular contraction reduces space for the examination. If necessary for clearance, individuals are instructed to move the mandible laterally to the side being examined. Palpation is performed from the apical area of the maxillary third molar (whether the tooth is present or not) forward as far as the cuspid region. The MAT does not extend this far anteriorly, but tenderness can be better appreciated when compared with the adjacent nonsensitive gingiva.[10]

The MAT is described by some dentists and chiropractors as lateral pterygoid muscle hyperactivity (spasm). However, this main jaw opening muscle lies far from the surface and therefore is not accessible to palpation.[13,14] It can, however, be assessed indirectly; isometric force application to this muscle elicits pain if spasm is present; the patient resists a strong closing (upward) force applied to the chin.[15] On over 2,500 patients examined in this manner, no relationship was observed between lateral pterygoid muscle spasm and MAT. Chiropractors occasionally report relief from MAT palpation—local edema is dispersed, reducing pressure against the maxillary nerve.

Temperature Studies

On 40 patients during unilateral migraine or TTH, the posterior maxillary molar apical areas were palpated bilaterally, and their temperatures recorded with a long stem laboratory thermometer (covered with a disposable plastic sheath for sterility). The temperature was consistently higher (37 of 40) and the area more tender (39 of 40) on the ipsilateral side.[11] *Tenderness and elevated temperature are signs of inflammation.*

The study was performed in the Departments of Neurology and Medicine at New York Medical College, the Department of Emergency Medicine at Westchester Medical Center, Our Lady of Mercy and St. Agnes Hospitals, and the principal investigator's office.

Medical Device for Intraoral Chilling

An apparatus was developed by the author to resolve edema by *local* vasoconstriction. Chilling of the edematous MAT area decreases intracapillary pressure by reducing local blood flow; edema (excessive interstitial fluid) is encouraged to return to the micro circulation via the capillary wall, reducing pressure against the maxillary nerve. The device consists of hollow metal tubes shaped to fit over the MAT. The metal is covered by a disposable plastic sheath. The tubes are connected to an ice water source by rubber tubing. The ice water, driven by a small pump, passes through and chills the metal, then flows to an identical arrangement on the opposite side, and back to its source.[10]

Even if symptoms are unilateral, the device is applied bilaterally because unilateral application occasionally caused a symptom (and MAT) side-shift. In all applications, the device is held by the patient—usually for 37 minutes—based on extensive symptomatic patient applications using varying times.

In over 4,000 applications in two private clinics, a tertiary medical center emergency department, and a department of medicine out-patient controlled study, side effects have not been observed. The device has received FDA approval for migraine and muscle spasm, and has been declared a nonsignificant risk by the New York Medical College and the Westchester Medical Center Institutional Review Boards (IRBs).[12] Because the procedure involves *local* intraoral vasoconstriction, it is referred to as IVC, and the device is called the IVC device.

Emergency Department Acute Migraine and TTH Study

Of 25 patients presenting to a tertiary medical center emergency department with *severe* migraine or TTH (average pretreatment headache duration over 30 hours), 20 were relieved of symptoms within 40 minutes, solely by IVC. The mean migraine score (0–10 scale) went from 7.74 to 3.7 and the mean TTH score from 7.8 to 2.7, with no rebound effect 24 hours later. In this nonfunded study, the eight treating emergency medicine physicians used no medication.[16]

The study was unusual: (a) pregnant women were included, (b) no side effects were reported, (c) moderate headaches were not included, (d) profound effects were tabulated immediately, and (e) pretreatment headache duration was recorded.

Acute Migraine Study

Thirty-five patients were treated in the out patient department of the New York Medical College Department of Medicine and a faculty practice at St. Agnes Hospital, during severe migraine (average pretreatment duration 17+ hours). In randomized fashion, the patients were treated by 40 minutes of IVC, as in the above study, 50 mg of oral sumatriptan, or (placebo) tongue chilling (40 minutes), using the same device.

Results. Significant mean headache relief was obtained by IVC and sumatriptan at 1, 2, 4, and 24 hours after the initiation of treatment, with poor relief obtained by placebo (0–10 scale). IVC was more effective than sumatriptan at all four time intervals. Significant nausea relief was obtained by IVC and sumatriptan at the same posttreatment time intervals. At 24 hours, some headache and nausea recurrence was noted with sumatriptan but not with IVC.[17]

In the above studies, a 10-point scale was used, as opposed to the usual 4-point scale: headache free, mild, moderate, and severe. This four-point scale, used in standard headache studies, assigns equal success to a symptomatic decrease from one category on the scale to four categories, that is, a decrease from severe to headache-free is equal to a decrease from moderate to mild.

Evoked Potentials

Cryotherapy (IVC) accesses the trigeminal system intraorally, where it is unprotected by skin or bone, which may be a factor in the dramatic results obtained. Evoked potentials (EPs), the electric responses of the nervous system to various stimuli, induce a cortical response, the amplitude of which increases linearly with pain intensity and decreases when pain is attenuated.[18] In pharmaceutical research, EP amplitudes are commonly used to evaluate drugs because the placebo effect is eliminated.

Low-level (noncutting) lasers also produce a local anti-inflammatory effect. In this trigeminal somatosensory (as opposed to visual or auditory), placebo-controlled EP study, the infraorbital foramen was used as the electrical input. The author was the first of 12 pain-free patients used to evaluate the relevance of a proposed placebo-controlled EP study.

After electrical input at the left infraorbital foramen, on 24 experimentally blinded pain-free subjects, Helium Neon laser irradiation (1.mW, 632.5nm, 50 Hz) was performed for 2 minutes on 12 of these subjects, and sham irradiation on the other 12, at the left maxillary third molar apical area. Four far field step latencies and amplitudes were recorded at base line, immediately after intervention, and 10 and 20 minutes after intervention. Laser irradiation was performed on the same intraoral area used for headache treatment.

Results. In the irradiated group, an immediate (average) somatosensory trigeminal evoked potential (STEP) amplitude decrease from baseline of 60% occurred, with further reduction to 65% and 72%, at the 10- and 20-minute intervals. No significant change occurred in the sham irradiation group.[19]

Intraoral Application of Topical, Nonsteroidal Antiinflammatory Medication

If secondary edema from a local inflammation causes migraine and TTH, and responds to local anti-inflammatory treatment (chilling), topical NSAID application to the same area should also aid in treatment of these headaches. The following experiment was designed to further test the above theory and also to develop effective headache prevention therapy.

A *topical* anti-inflammatory gel (Ketoprofen) was designed to adhere to the oral mucosa. It was applied by the patients to the same intraoral area for headache prevention. Twenty episodic migraine, TTH, and posttraumatic headache patients were enrolled in an open-label headache prevention study.[20]

Patients kept a headache diary for 60 days, recording headache type, frequency, severity (1–10 scale), duration (total monthly headache hours), headache medications analgesics taken, and side effects. During the second 30 days, medication was applied. Ketoprofen was compounded with organogel, serving as the vehicle to deliver the drug to the tissue. Patients placed a disposable cheek shield between the molar teeth and the cheek; patients then applied the gel to the tissue bilaterally, using a cotton applicator. This procedure was followed once daily. If symptoms were exclusively unilateral, the medication was applied to the symptomatic side only.

Results. Headache burden was defined as the average intensity of each headache (0–10 scale) multiplied by its duration in hours. The average monthly headache burden score for the 20 patients enrolled in the study went from 454.8 (30-day baseline) to 86.5 p<0.001 during the 30-day treatment phase. Additionally, analgesic and headache medication intake was significantly reduced from baseline during the treatment phase, and side effects were minimal. Usually, migraine preventive medications must be taken for at least a few months before effectiveness can be determined and are rarely prescribed for TTH.[21] In practice, because the gel is now more adhesive, the cheek shield is rarely used.

PHYSIOLOGY

The movement of fluid in and out of the microcirculation—arterioles, capillaries, and venules—is regulated by the balance between intravascular hydrostatic pressure, forcing fluid out of the vessels, and the opposing effects of osmotic pressure, exerted by the plasma proteins, which tend to retain fluids within the vessels (Starling's Law).

To inflame literally means to "set afire." In addition to heat, redness, and tenderness, swelling is also produced.[22] The inflammatory process is controlled by a group of vasoactive neuropeptides within the body. When unknown triggers liberate these chemicals, they relax the smooth muscle layer of small blood vessels (arterioles) and the precapillary sphincters. *Vasodilatation* (expansion) of capillaries and opening of previously inactive capillaries can result in as much as a tenfold increase in local blood flow, increasing local temperature and hydrostatic pressure.

In addition to vasodilalation, these chemicals increase vascular permeability, by shrinking endothelial cells surrounding the blood vessels. The end result—*edema*—is caused by increased blood flow and "leaky" blood vessels due to vascular permeability from the intracellular gaps. This combination of factors makes it easier for fluid and large molecular plasma proteins to leave the blood vessels and enter the extravascular space. These proteins increase the tissue osmotic pressure, further attracting fluid from the blood vessels. In the intraoral tender (headache marker) area, this local swelling exerts constant pressure on an accessible maxillary nerve segment, for conduction of head and facial pain. Application of anti-inflammatory medication or cold reverses the above effect; in other words, *local* antiinflammatory treatment reduces edema (swelling).

Most of the antimigraine drugs—the ergots, Imitrex, Midrin, Sansert, and so forth—are *systemic* vasoconstrictors. Common examples include chest tightness after taking a triptan, resulting from cardiac smooth muscle constriction, and uterine muscle contraction from dyhydroergotamine (DHE).

THE CERVICAL CONNECTION

Persistent neurogenic inflammation in the maxillary nerve area appears to mediate not only headache but cervical muscle spasm as well. This observation is not surprising as the head and neck operate as a single functional unit.[10,23] This connection can easily be demonstrated to the reader—place your left hand lightly over the left sternomastoid (SCM) muscle while applying a strong lateral force to the right side of your chin with your right hand (resist mandibular movement to the left). A distinct SCM (cervical) reaction to the lateral force can be felt immediately. In addition to affecting function, joints and muscles often refer symptoms to adjacent areas. Referred head and neck pain may be confusing because referred pain does not travel down specific neural pathways rather the pain may occur from an error in cortical perception. Areas A, B, C, D, and F are innervated by cervical nerves, respectively.

Over 100 years ago, Sherrington reported that in the decerebrate cat, excitation of a portion of the trigeminal nerve is enough to cause relaxation of the rigid neck muscles.[24]

Since then, experiments have confirmed a close trigemino-cervical relationship.[25,26] Because the head and neck are one functional unit, cervical musculoskeletal disorders can refer as headache, jaw, or facial pain.[27] Correction of only one area—headache, with existing cervical muscle spasm—is much less satisfactory. Similarly, a knee rehabilitation in a patient with an incorrect gait caused by an ankle problem on the same side is problematic. In examining a symptomatic headache patient, an important question to ask "Does your neck bother you—*between* headaches?" If the answer is yes, cervical physical therapy is indicated.

Occipital headaches are often described as a type of TTH, but we believe that this occipital or suboccipital condition is cervicogenic, that is, referred pain from a cervical disorder.[28–30] In almost every individual with significant cervical muscle spasm, the author has noted the same MAT. Again, the severity and laterality of the MAT is closely related to the severity and laterality of the cervical problem. In a study of patients with cervical muscle spasm and pain, MAT was palpated in 623 out of 663 cases (93.9%).[10] It was also noted that in severe trauma cases with major cervical injury, MAT is severe and cannot be eliminated, even by instillation of local anesthetic to the area.

A nonblinded study was performed on 12 subjects with clinically determined cervical muscle spasm (hyperactivity). All subjects reported neck pain at rest and during cervical range of motion (ROM), and six reported headache. MAT was present in all cases. Upper trapezius surface electromyography (EMG) was performed before and after relatively brief IVC. Following treatment, 9 out of 12 subjects demonstrated a reduction of EMG activity. In these same nine subjects, there was a mean increase of 10.58° plus or minus 6.95° of motion in the single most painful cervical cervical spine movement. Resting neck pain was relieved or eliminated in 8 out of 12 subjects, and four out of six accompanying headaches were also relieved, from only 15 minutes of IVC.[10] Since that time, we have extended IVC to 37 minutes. On over 4,000 applications, we have recorded an 80% success rate (significant improvement immediately after treatment), with no side effects.[10] In headache, MAT may well be the origin of the problem. In cervical muscle spasm, the dysfunction appears to create the MAT, further perpetuating cervical muscle spasm. This type of loop is not unique. For example, lactic acid is created from muscle contraction and further exacerbates the muscle pain and soreness. IVC interrupts the loop. In some cases, this treatment replaces cervical physical therapy or chiropractic. More often, we use it as an adjunct to ongoing cervical treatment. It works especially well in headaches coexisting with cervical muscle spasm.

Posttraumatic Headache

In addition to the immediate pain following a head injury, posttraumatic headache (PTH), a more prolonged and enduring headache, may develop. This condition often resembles migraine or TTH, and may last for weeks, months, or years. We have treated large numbers of these patients, usually resulting from motor vehicle accidents. The vast majority also suffer from cervical problems, which partially explains why local antiinflammatory treatment (NSAID gel) works exceptionally well for this condition; the cervical muscle spasm is treated simultaneously.

CONCLUSION

In practice, IVC is used once or twice on new headache patients, and then the topical gel is prescribed—for daily home use (initially). Most successful patients can soon reduce the daily application. Patients return for IVC in case of a headache flare-up. This technique has considerable advantages over standard migraine treatment: (a) it is effective, not only for migraine but for TTH and PTH as well; and (b) it is significantly more effective than standard migraine medications, which demonstrate minimal effectiveness. For example, five migraine preventive studies published in the journal *Headache* report 0.8, 0.5, 0.7, 0.6, and 1.7 migraine/month less than placebo![31-35] Treatment is often effective for chronic daily (constant) headache; because TTH is a large component of this condition, migraine medications are ineffective.

Another benefit of this treatment is the *minimal side effects,* as opposed to numerous (and often serious) side effects produced by the migraine preventive drugs. We often use the topical gel for medically compromised patients.[36] Unlike typical migraine medications, IVC and the topical NSAID gel do not affect the coronary vessels.

Based on our research (palpation and temperature studies, laser-evoked potential results, IVC response in open-label and controlled studies, IVC results in more than 7,000 in-office headache treatments and home application of the NSAID topical gel), I conclude that these primary headaches are mediated by a persistent neurogenic maxillary alveolar mucosal inflammation and that they respond exceptionally well to local anti-inflammatory treatment.

REFERENCES

1. Rasmussen BK, Jensen R, Schroll M, Olesen J. Epidemiology of headache in a general population—a prevalence study. *J Clin Epidemiology.* 1991;44:1147–1157.
2. The Nuprin Pain Report. *Newsweek.* January 11, 1999.
3. Jensen J, Olesen J. Tension-type headache: an update on mechanism and treatment. *Curr Opin Neurol.* 2000;13:285–289.
4. Goadsby PJ, Edvinsson L, Eckman R. Vasoactive peptide release in the extracerebral circulation of humans during migraine headache. *Ann Neurol.* 1990;28:183–187.
5. Moskowitz MA. Interpreting vessel diameter changes in vascular headache. *Cephalalgia.* 1992;12:5–7.
6. Friedman MH. Local inflammation as a mediator of migraine and tension-type headache. *Headache.* 2004;44:767,771.
7. Saper JR, Silberstein S, Gordon CD, Hamel RI. Episodic tension-type headache. In: Saper, JR, Silberstein, S, David, C, et al., eds., *Handbook of Headache Management.* 2nd ed. Philadelphia, PA: Lippincott Williams & Wilkins; 1999:192.
8. Friedman MH. Atypical facial pain: the consistency of ipsilateral maxillary area tenderness and elevated temperature. *JADA.* 1995;126:855–860.
9. Friedman MH, Weintraub MI, Forman S. Atypical facial pain: a localized maxillary nerve disorder? *Am J Pain Man.* 1994;4:149–152.
10. Friedman MH, Nelson AJ. Head and neck pain review: traditional and new perspectives. *J Orthop Sports Phys Ther.* 1996;24:268–278.

11. Friedman MH, Luque AF, Larsen EA. Ipsilateral intraoral tenderness and elevated temperature during unilateral migraine and tension-type headache. *Headache Quart.* 1997;8(4):341–344.

12. These findings were submitted to the New York Medical College and Westchester Medical Center Institutional Review Boards, in our successful application for research classification as a "non-significant risk."

13. Johnstone DR, Templeton M. The feasibility of palpating the lateral pterygoid muscle. *J Prosthet Dent.* 1980;44:318–323.

14. Friedman MH, Agus B, Weisberg J. Neglected conditions producing preauricular and referred pain. *J Neurol Neurosurg Psychiatry.* 1983;46:1067.1072.

15. Friedman MH, Weisberg J. Screening procedures for temporomandibular joint dysfunction. *Am Fam Physician.* 1982;25:157.160.

16. Friedman MH, Nehrbauer NJ, Larsen EA. An alternative approach to acute headache treatment: an emergency department pilot study. *Headache Quart.* 1999;10: 131–134.

17. Friedman MH, Peterson SJ, Behar CF, Zaidi Z. Intraoral chilling vs. oral sumatriptan for acute migraine. *Heart Dis.* 2001;3:357.361.

18. Chen ACN, Chapman CR, Harkins SW. Brain evoked potentials are functional correlates of induced pain in man. *Pain.* 1979;6:365–374.

19. Nelson AJ, Friedman MH. Somatosensory trigeminal evoked potential amplitudes following low level and sham irradiation over time. *Laser Ther.* 2001;14:60–64.

20. Friedman MH, Peterson SJ, Frishman WH, Behar CF. Intraoral topical nonsteroidal antiinflammatory drug application for headache prevention. *Heart Dis.* 2002;4:212–215.

21. Noble SL, Moore KL. Drug treatment of migraine: part II. Preventive therapy. *Am Fam Physician.* 1997;56(9):2279–2286.

22. Trowbridge HO, Emling RC. *Inflammation: A Review of the Process.* 5th ed. Chicago, IL: Quintessence Publishing Co Inc; 1997:9–14.

23. Friedman MH, Weisberg J. The craniocervical connection: a retrospective analysis of 300 whiplash patients with temporomandibular disorders. *J Craniomandib Pract.* 2000;18(3):163–167.

24. Sherrington CS. Decerebrate rigidity and reflex coordination of movement. *J Physiol (London).* 1898;22:319–332.

25. Abrahams VC, Richmond FJR, Rose PK. Absence of monosynaptic reflex in dorsal neck muscle of the cat. *Brain Res.* 1975;92:130–131.

26. Kerr FWL, Olafsson RA. Trigeminal cervical volleys: convergence on single units in the spinal gray at C1 and C2. *Arch Neurol.* 1961;5:171–178.

27. Friedman MH, Weisberg J. Application of orthopedic principles in evaluation of the temporomandibular joint. *Phys Ther.* 1982;62(5);597.603.

28. Fredricksen TA, Hovdal H, Sjaastad O. Cervicogenic headache: clinical manifestation. *Cephalalgia.* 1987;7147.7160.

29. Hunter CR, Mayfield FH. Role of the upper cervical roots in the production of pain in the head. *Am J Surg.* 1949;48:743–751.

30. Wilson PR. Chronic neck pain and cervicogenic headache. *Clin J Pain.* 1991;7:5–11.

31. Becker WJ, Christie SN, Ledoux S, Bind C. Topiramate prophylaxis and response to triptan treatment for acute migraine. *Headache.* 2006;46:1424–1430.

32. Rapoport A, Mauskop A, Diener H-C, et al. Long-term migraine prevention with topiramate: open-label extension of pivotal trials. *Headache.* 2006; 46: 1151–1160.

33. Storey JR, Calder CS, Hart DE, Potter DL. Topiramate in migraine prevention: a double-blind placebo-controlled study. *Headache.* 2001;41:968–975.

34. Winner P, Pearlman EM, Linder SL, Jordan DM, et al. Topiramate for migraine prevention in children: a randomized double-blind, placebo-controlled trial. *Headache.* 2005;45:1304–1312.

35. Limmroth V, Biondi D, Pfeil J, Schwalen S. Topiramate in patients with episodic migraine: reducing the risk for chronic forms of headache. *Headache.* 2007;47:13–21.
36. Friedman MH, Peterson SJ. Intraoral migraine treatment in a medically compromised patient: a case report. *Conn Med.* 2001;65:707,709.

PART II

Manual and Hand-Mediated Modalities

CHAPTER 8

Therapeutic Massage

Elaine Calenda and Sharon Weinstein

Every civilization has used touch as a form of healing. The Egyptians, Greeks, and Romans developed forms of massage similar to techniques used today, including traction, rubbing the muscles, and passively moving joints. Well-documented accounts of massage as therapy are also common in Chinese medical history. The words *Tui-na* and *Anma*, meaning "to rub" and "to press," are found in Chinese literature dating back to 2000 B.C. *Romi-romi* is the term used by the Polynesians to describe their method of manual healing, and Hawaiians use the term *Lomi-lomi*. Although many names have been used to denote massage, the translation generally produces similar meanings, such as rubbing, pressing, lifting, beating, and stretching.

Modern methods of massage and bodywork also are known by many names. The European styles are credited to the work of Per Henrik Ling of Sweden and Dr. Johan Georg Mezger of Holland. The Swedish system developed by Ling is still the most recognized by the Western world. Ling attempted to scientifically systematize massage as a medical therapy. He organized exercises and the basic elements of traditional massage technique according to the principles of anatomy and physiology as they were understood at the time. Thus the system became known as *Swedish massage and remedial gymnastics*.[1]

Although Ling is no longer credited with introducing the French names of massage techniques, he did popularize massage and particularly passive movements. Mezger of Amsterdam, and his followers, organized massage into a form and gave the techniques their French names. Massage combined with heat and exercise was a fundamental technique used by physical therapists during polio epidemics. From 1920 to 1950 numerous works on the effects of massage were published, including Harvey Kellogg's *Art of Massage,*[3] which is still in publication.

As the field of physiotherapy, or physical therapy, made advances in the treatment of neurologic diseases, higher education became necessary. However, when physical therapists were required to learn neuroanatomy, neurophysiology, and kinesiology, the practice of massage decreased. During the 1950s, modern modalities, such as galvanic stimulation, automated traction, and other treatments performed by machinery emerged in physical medicine, leading to a further decline in the use of massage. Although these devices proved effective and saved time, a vital personal element of health care was lost.

In the years that followed, the practice of massage was confined to health clubs and spas, and its practitioners were referred to as *masseuses* and *masseurs.* Training, offered by only a handful of schools, fell under the auspices of vocational education along with ophthalmic dispensers and bartenders. During the physical fitness and holistic health movements of the 1970s, massage regained its status as an effective health care modality. Today, there are hundreds of schools, some that offer Associate of Occupational Studies (A.O.S.) degree programs. Schools throughout America are developing similar programs in higher education. These progressive schools are laying the groundwork for the resurgence of a profession that was once nearly extinct. Despite widespread use of massage and some scientific progress in demonstrating its physiologic effects, there are few studies of its clinical application. In the 1950 American Medical Association's *Handbook of Physical Medicine and Rehabilitation,* Pemberton stated, with regard to massage, "there is probably no other measure of equal known value in the entire armamentarium of medicine which is so inadequately understood and utilized by the profession as a whole."[4] Currently massage therapy remains largely outside the realm of standard medical practice; it is considered "unconventional" or "alternative" care. The extent to which the American public seeks such care is remarkable as evidenced by out-of-pocket expenditures.[5]

STATUS OF THE PROFESSION

Statistics

According to the AMTA data collection base, there are between 250,000 and 300,000 massage practitioners in the United States providing some

230 million sessions per year. These calculations suggest that the massage therapy profession generates over \$11 billion annually.[2] Other surveys report more Americans than ever are seeking and utilizing massage therapy and 85% of those report a favorable response. Over 90% paid out-of-pocket for massage therapy suggesting that the American public places a high value on its benefits.[3] Hospital-based massage is on the rise as well, and according to the bi-annual survey conducted by the Health Forum in 2004, the number of hospitals offering massage therapy has increased by more than one third in 2 years. The breakdown of massage service utilization in hospital settings is as follows:

Indications for Massage[4]

Medical conditions

Stress management and comfort (71%)
Pain management (67%)
Improving mobility and movement (52%)
Part of physical therapy regimen (50%)
Edema (33%)
Postoperative care (25%)
Preoperative care (17%).

Patient population

Cancer patients (52%)
Staff for stress management (67%)
Pregnant women (51%)
Hospice or end-of-life care (37%)
Infants (24%)

Multiple indications for massage in the same person are represented.

According to AMTA's 2005 Consumer Survey, 21% of American adults indicated that they discussed massage therapy with their doctor or other health care provider, up from 14% in 2002. More health care providers advised massage therapy than in years past. Sixty percent of adult Americans were referred by their physicians, 50% by a physical therapist, and 38% by a chiropractor. Seventy percent of the massage therapists surveyed indicated that they receive referrals from health care providers, averaging two per month. The National Survey conducted by the Health Forum/American Hospital Association in 2003 showed that 82% of hospitals offering complementary and alternative medicine (CAM) therapies include massage therapy among their health care offerings and of those, 70% use massage therapy for pain management and pain relief.[5]

Education

While licensure is a step in the right direction for the profession, a credential is only as good as the education behind it. The national educational standard for massage therapy education remains at 500 hours; however, as with the value of the credential, there is a trend toward increasing this number. The number of massage and shiatsu training programs has grown exponentially in the last two decades in part because of an increasing public demand for more natural approaches to health care. A number of regulating bodies govern the practice of massage and bodywork. In the last decade programs providing 1,000 to 1,200 hours of training and associate degree programs (equivalent to 2-year college programs) have become more common. A series of school surveys collected by the Associated Bodywork and Massage Professionals (ABMP) showed a continuous and rapid increase in the number of new massage training programs, particularly within the career college arena. ABMP followed the trend which seemed to correspond to the tremendous number of massage school enrollees and graduates from 1998 to 2004. The ABMP recently revealed their 2007 analysis and the first slight decline in these numbers, showing enrollment decreased by 9.8% from 73,933 entrants in 2004 to 66,653 in 2006. Massage therapy program graduates declined from 71,272 in 2004 to 62,784 in 2006.[6]

Massage therapy and bodywork schools have a fairly standardized curriculum base, which includes communication skills, Eastern and Western bodywork modalities and philosophies, anatomy, physiology, pathology, kinesiology, business practices, ethics, and first aid/CPR. In addition to the classroom studies, students gain experiential knowledge by participating in supervised clinical internships. Some schools and colleges require externships as well, which generally take place in hospitals, hospices, assisted care facilities, athletic departments, and corporations. Massage therapy had become a part of mainstream America and can be obtained in full view at airports, events, fairs, and shopping malls. It seems the more technology creates a virtual world, the more we seek out human touch to maintain a healthy balance.

Credentialing

States that regulate massage therapy increased from 14 in 1989 to 38 in 2007, and many of the remaining states have introduced legislation. The surge in regulation of the profession began in the 1990s, when the American Massage Therapy Association, set on establishing a national minimum standard in education, formed the National Certification Board for Therapeutic Massage and Bodywork (NCBTMB).[1] The board's mission was to foster high standards of ethical and professional practice. Support for regulation swelled as more practitioners viewed licensing as a way to further legitimize a profession that had separated from the medical model of physical therapy in the 1950s and become enmeshed in out-dated entanglements with prostitution. Many of the states had and continue to have ordinances that require massage therapists be tested for AIDS and other sexually transmitted diseases and receive regular physicals. This antiquated system, which attempted to curtail and control prostitution, is vanishing as the massage therapy profession asserts ownership and protection of the massage therapy title.

There are a number of professional massage and bodywork organizations and associations in the United States and Canada. The American Massage Therapy Association (AMTA), founded in 1943, now has more than 56,000 members. The AMTA supports its members by providing continuing education through regional and national conferences and conventions and by offering liability insurance. The National Certification Board for Therapeutic Massage and Bodywork (NCBTMB) developed the first national examination in therapeutic massage and bodywork. As of 2007, 38 states and the District of Columbia, utilize or recognize the national certification board's examination as their credentialing requirement. Some massage and bodywork schools are accredited by organizations like the Accrediting Commission of Career Schools and Colleges of Technology (ACCSCT), the Accrediting Council for Continuing Education and Training (ACCET), the Council on Occupational Education (COE), and the Commission on Massage Therapy Accreditation (COMTA). The majority of schools however are not accredited by these organizations.

Research

Until the 1990s, research in the field had been isolated to animal experimentation, cardiac massage, and other postoperative procedures. One of the pioneers of modern massage therapy research is Tiffany Field, PhD, from the Touch Research Institute (TRI), University of Miami School of Medicine, Florida.[7] To date, the TRI is credited with publishing over 30 research articles on the efficacy of massage on a variety of conditions. Several massage programs have begun to conduct pilot and case studies. The number of studies in massage therapy has increased in the last 20 years from a few dozen to a few thousand. While this is not a large number, it reflects a maturing of the industry. The Massage Therapy Foundation was established by the American Massage Therapy Association (AMTA) in 1990. In addition to funding research, the foundation hopes to contribute to changing the perception of touch. The National Center for

Complementary and Alternative Medicine (NCCAM) has joined in the investigation of massage therapy and its role in integrated health care. They have funded research on the effects of massage for chronic neck and back pain, for cancer patients at the end of life, depression, and sickle cell anemia pain. Other studies have explored how massage therapy helps healthy people and quality of life.

DEFINITIONS

Massage

From the Latin word *massa,* meaning "to knead," massage describes a means of touch that manipulates the skin and muscle against the bones with a kneading action. Massage therapy, or therapeutic massage, is described as the practice of skilled touch for the purposes of reducing pain brought about by injury, disease, or prolonged stress. It includes muscular rehabilitation and preventive care.

Myofascial Release

Myofascial release is a technique that works on the principle of thixotropy (from the Greek words *thingein* [stem: thix-], meaning "to touch," and *tropy,* meaning "a turn or change") and the sol to gel principles. *Sol* is a term used to describe the warm fluid environment of the body during activity, and *gel* denotes the negative solidifying effects of disuse. The heat generated by the hands of the practitioner during manipulation of the muscles and fascia promotes the gel to sol reaction. The technique is divided into three components: broad-base approach, general approach, and specific approach. The system is designed to release the skin from the fascia and the fascia from the muscle to establish the optimal cellular environment and increase joint range of motion.[1]

Muscle Energy Techniques

Muscle energy techniques fall into the category of neuromuscular therapy. These techniques are similar to Ling's Swedish gymnastics in that they require the patient's active participation through a series of controlled muscle contractions. The techniques include proprioceptive neuromuscular facilitation, pandiculation, and active isolated stretching. Other techniques are based on Sherrington's law of reciprocal inhibition and use postisometric relaxation and reciprocal inhibition.

Hydrotherapy and Cryotherapy

Hydrotherapy is a term used to describe the therapeutic use of water in the form of hot or cold applications or emersions. *Cryotherapy* refers to the use of ice or ice massage.

Zen Shiatsu

Developed by Shizuto Masunaga, zen shiatsu is one of several forms of Asian and Oriental bodywork. Shiatsu (Japanese for "finger pressure") is a Japanese bodywork modality that approaches the human form in both health and disease according to ancient Asian and Oriental beliefs and methodologies. Shiatsu directly affects the meridian systems that govern the organs of the body. The manipulation of Qi (life force) by skillful and intuitive contact of the *tsubos* (points) along meridians is the basis of treatment. The needs of the patient are assessed by an evaluation of the Hara before, during, and after the session. Shiatsu is mentioned throughout this chapter when a more energetic approach may be indicated, particularly if the patient cannot tolerate much movement against the body.

Physiologic and Psychological Effects

Massage may be studied in terms of the physiologic basis of its effects (the psychological effects; the effects of different techniques; and the effects on tissue, organ, or system) or its application as a treatment for a specific condition. Mennell categorized the mechanisms of the effects of massage as mechanical, chemical, reflex, and psychological.[7] Pemberton and Scull summarized the physiologic effects of massage in 1944.[8] Beard reviewed the scientific literature over the 10 years before 1972.[9] What follows is a summary of the relevant findings as documented in the medical literature over the last few decades:

- Massage improves the circulation of blood and lymph.[10–17]
- Massage effectively reduces lymphedema in cancer patients.[18]
- Massage speeds recovery of fatigued muscles,[19–21] may improve joint range of motion,[22,23] induces muscle relaxation,[24–27] may be used to break down joint adhesions,[28] and improves neuromuscular function after spinal cord injury.[29]
- Serum myoglobin levels rise after massage in patients diagnosed with fibrositis.[30]
- Massage improves ventilation.[31,32]
- Massage may result in a transient increase in sympathetic nervous tone in healthy and critically ill patients.[33–35]

- Changes in skin temperature and function are observed after massage.[36,37]
- Changes in serum enzymes, urinary hormones, and cerebrospinal fluid enzymes have been noted as a result of massage.[38–40]
- Serum endorphins may transiently rise in humans after massage.[41,42]
- The neuroendocrine effects of touching the skin have been investigated in nonhuman primates and human infants; it has been demonstrated that touch is vital to growth and development.[43,44]
- Rats handled early in infancy show better responses to stress and fewer aging changes in the brain.[45]
- Lowered glucocorticoid levels have been demonstrated in preterm infants after massage.[46,47]

Skin is the primary organ through which psychological nurturing occurs.[48] A person receiving massage may enter a hypnagogic state of deep relaxation resembling sleep. The psychological accompaniment of this effect may be the release of psychological defenses, allowing the individual to feel cared for and nurtured. Massage reduces anxiety.[49,50] Physiological changes accompanying relief of anxiety also have been shown.[51–58] Massage has been used as an adjunctive treatment for chemical dependency.[59]

Providers with other credentials also may offer massage. Soft tissue manipulation may be included in chiropractic care. Osteopathic physicians, once uniformly trained in soft tissue manipulation, may or may not incorporate this therapy into their medical practices. Swedish massage technique is used in the standard "back rub" taught in nursing schools. Physical therapists employ Swedish massage, trigger point stimulation, and myofascial manipulation. Podiatrists may provide foot massage. Cosmetologists give facial, scalp, and neck massages. Many other bodywork techniques that may properly fall under the category of soft tissue manipulation, such as reflexology, Feldenkrais, Rolfing, and shiatsu (acupressure), are practiced without regulation. Mechanical massage devices are used routinely for specific medical indications, such as to prevent thrombosis of the veins of the lower extremities during convalescent care and to reduce postmastectomy lymphedema.

TREATMENT

Pain

Pain is a function of the nervous system. Nociceptive (pain) signals are transduced in specialized neural receptors, transmitted along neurons, modulated at all levels of the nervous system, and finally processed in the higher cortical centers. Pain is defined as a complex perceptual phenomenon, a dynamic product of multiple neural circuits. There is no known pain center in the brain.

Acute pain is the result of active tissue damage and the release of inflammatory and algesic (pain) mediators. Nociception may arise in any pain-sensitive tissue (somatic, visceral, or connective). Chronic pain states may result from a number of different processes occurring in the peripheral and central nervous tissues. Chronic pain may result from an abnormal peripheral or central pain generator. This type of pain is generally termed *neuropathic*.

Somatic back pain syndromes may derive from musculoskeletal tissues of the spine, such as ligaments, facets, and intrinsic muscles. All of these structures, including the intervertebral disks, are considered pain sensitive. Pain arising from these areas does not appear to be caused by neurologic compromise or nerve root compression but rather by inflammatory or degenerative processes resulting from injury, disease, or normal wear and tear. Orthopedic assessment tests assist the practitioner in the formulation of a treatment plan for the individual and as a means of noting progress.

Preliminary data on the use of massage therapy in the treatment of cancer-related pain are limited.[60] Small studies of patients with nonmalignant pain have demonstrated that massage results in lowered pain intensity scores and reduced analgesic consumption.[61-65]

The term *myofascial pain syndrome* refers to that type of pain induced when muscle and soft tissue are inflamed and pressure is applied. Pressure applied directly on an active trigger point in the levator scapulae muscle often elicits pain in the midback and along the spine of the scapula. Postural and mechanical problems contribute to the formation of trigger points, which are nodules of fibrous tissue that have become ischemic. Trigger points also are related to holding patterns and the pain/spasm/pain cycle. Treatment of trigger points is most successful when a combination of direct digital pressure followed by thorough passive stretching is used.

Posttraumatic pain may have several sources. Examples include pain that follows physical injury resulting from an accident, assault, poisoning, near-drowning, and recovery from surgery. Psychological trauma also must be addressed in these patients because some degree of mental anguish coincides with the cause of their pain. For treatment to be fully successful, therefore, the individual must pursue help on all levels by participating in physical therapy that includes massage and psychological, emotional, or spiritual counseling.

Headache and Migraine

A comfortable, quiet, and dimly lit environment is helpful during massage treatments, particularly when trying to combat a headache. If a migraine is already in progress, even the most gentle massage may be too disturbing. Most headaches, including migraines, are relieved or greatly reduced by massage of the cranium, cervical region, and facial structures. Shiatsu point pressure on the cranium can quell even the worst pounding headache in minutes. The relief from pain may last for hours or days, depending on the causative factors. One study of patients with chronic headache showed that massage produces analgesia accompanied by improvement in mood.[66] Massage may abort migraine headache,[67] and patients may readily accept massage therapy.[68]

There are nine studies of the efficacy of massage for pain relief, representing more than 500 patients. These studies are best described as well-designed quasiexperimental studies, well-designed nonexperimental studies, and case series. The limitations of these studies include lack of specificity of the condition treated, limited details of the treatment applied, and lack of standardized pain assessments. As judged by the general outcome criteria of self-reported reduced pain, reduced analgesic requirement, and improved physical functioning, these studies provide weak evidence to suggest massage may be beneficial for some chronic pain conditions, including tension headache, migraine with aura, postconcussive headache, nonspecific low back pain, nonspecific neck pain, inflammatory joint pain, and regional muscle pain.

A parasympathetic response is achieved by gently stroking in rhythmic patterns. The patient can participate by breathing slowly and deeply during the session. Guided imagery is helpful for patients who find it difficult to release muscle tension. Lymphatic drainage, traction of the cervical vertebrae, and friction at the temporal and occipital regions are extremely beneficial for the reduction of muscle tension and fluid retention. Gentle vibratory percussions promote drainage of the sinuses and thus reduce pain. Massage of the abdomen, the lower extremities, and reflex points on the feet also has been effective as part of a more complete approach to the treatment of headache.

MOTOR SYMPTOMS

Weakness/Spastic Paralysis

The primary goals when treating paralysis are to enhance the patient's comfort, to assist venous return, and to inhibit spasticity through the application of rhythmic kneading, compression, and percussion.

Increased Tone

One of the symptoms of subacute paralysis is increased muscle tone. The violent muscle contraction and severe pain are controlled by muscle relaxants. Massage can be beneficial as a means of promoting circulation, but care must be taken not to disrupt brittle fibers. Medium pressure should be used to prevent a hyperreflexive reaction.

Decreased Tone

One of the symptoms of long-term paralysis is decreased muscle tone. The limbs lay flaccid, and tissue wasting is evident. Gentle massage that includes skin rolling and lifting can promote hydration of the tissues.

Weakness

Massage combined with muscle energy techniques can retard the progression of atrophy and improve function at the neuromuscular junction.

Loss of Coordination

Lack of coordination is a common symptom of nervous system disorders, especially those that affect the cerebellum or the inner ear. A systematic massage of the entire body that includes passive movements like those used in patients recovering from stroke is similarly beneficial for patients with muscular disorders.

MUSCULAR DISORDERS AND PAIN

Cramps

A muscle cramp is a type of sustained muscle contraction caused in part by a disturbance in blood and lymph flow. Cramps tend to occur during periods of rest. Dehydration, faulty alignment, microscopic tears, and poor walking or running habits contribute to the incidence of cramps. Fibrous formations resulting from previous injuries can interfere with normal activity and circulation.

During a severe cramp, reciprocal inhibition and intermittent percussions are generally successful as first aid pain relief. When the cramp subsides, muscular kneading promotes better circulation. As soon as it can be tolerated, friction should be applied to disrupt excessive collagen formation. Passive stretching is used to stretch the muscles, nerves, and fascia in the affected area. The stretching facilitates the optimal flow of lymph and blood through the tissues.

Multiple Sclerosis

The etiology of multiple sclerosis is unknown, but viral infection is suspected. Symptoms vary from mild loss of motor function to severe dysfunction of the lung or bladder. Complications in these organs can cause death. Symptoms arise in individuals between the ages of 20 and 40 years, and episodes may last only a few years and then spontaneously subside. For others the disease is more progressive and completely debilitating. Insults to the nervous system caused by multiple spinal traumas (i.e., whiplash) may exacerbate symptoms. Muscular symptoms include a feeling of weakness in the extremities, especially in the lower limbs; cramping at the proximal hamstring; and ataxia.

Common symptoms of the nervous system include numbness and neuralgia, which may be severe or mild. In mild cases massage treatment can be administered for up to 1 hour and should include passive range of motion, as tolerated, to relieve stiffness. The fingertips can be used to rake the muscles from the proximal to the distal attachments and stimulate motor excitement. In addition, general massage that lifts the muscle from the bone or rolls muscle onto bone effectively improves circulation, sensation, and strength. Very light massage may frustrate patients and leave them feeling restless. The massage therapist must explore different pressures and track how much time is spent on each area to determine the best therapy for each patient. The beneficial effects of massage may last for several hours or days, depending on the stage of disease.

MOVEMENT DISORDERS

Rigidity

Lymphatic drainage therapy is beneficial for decreasing edema. Myofascial release and cross-fiber friction of the ligaments facilitate increased movement and diminish stiffness of the tissues.

Tremor

Massage and muscle energy techniques have been successful in decreasing the fatigue factor associated with tremors.

Parkinson's Disease

Parkinson's disease begins as a slow degeneration of the central nervous system, initially destroying the substania nigra neurons that produce the neurotransmitter dopamine. In primary Parkinsonism the pigmented cells of the substania nigra that are dispersed along the putamen and caudate nucleus die off. These cells are important structures in the basal ganglia that control muscle coordination. Once these cells die, balance and muscular control diminish. The disease generally presents between the ages of 40 and 60 years, but juvenile Parkinsonism can occur in younger persons. Although the exact cause is unknown, drugs that block dopamine receptors or cause metallic toxicity are contributing factors.

Treatment is directed toward decreasing rigidity. Rigidity is present whenever tremor is not. As the disease progresses, fine tremors of the head, hand, or foot develop. General massage and muscle energy techniques are beneficial.

Amyotrophic Lateral Sclerosis

Massage is indicated for relief of muscle spasms and fatigue. Gentle kneading, jostling, and stretching temporarily relieve symptoms and promote a feeling of increased strength. Shorter treatments several times per week are most productive.

CEREBROVASCULAR DISEASE

Cerebrovascular accidents (or strokes) affect hundreds of thousands of people each year. Stroke is related to cardiovascular disease, as in cerebral insufficiency, or results from hypertension or atherosclerosis. Massage therapists must have medical clearance before working with individuals who have had strokes.

Massage therapy can be extremely helpful in assisting patients with deficient circulation and can restore a sense of calm after such an episode. However, the practitioner must be aware of any blood clot or emboli before undertaking the case. Knowledge of the side effects of the patient's medications is also an important consideration, especially if analgesics are being administered. The massage therapist must take care not to apply pressure too vigorously or deeply. The primary goals are to provide comfort, assist venous return, and reduce stress.

PERIPHERAL NEUROPATHY AND NEURALGIA

The nerves most commonly affected by neuralgia are the trigeminal (third cranial), sciatic, and brachial nerves. Myofascial release and nerve release techniques effectively alleviate pain but only temporarily in some cases.

Neuralgia is often a symptom of muscular atrophy or hypertrophy, which may be further aggravated by unhealthy blood chemistry. Viral infection also can produce neuralgic pain, and in these cases many nerves may be affected. Myofascial release and percussion along the course of the nerve are extremely helpful. The underlying cause, however, should determine the treatment. Patients in the acute phase react differently to direct pressure. Some patients respond positively to direct pressure, but for others the effect is quite adverse and may exacerbate symptoms. This extreme difference in reaction may be a result of the individual's pain tolerance and how the nerve is situated in the soft tissues.

NERVE ENTRAPMENT

Carpal Tunnel Syndrome

Carpal tunnel syndrome is described as a compression of the median nerve where it passes through the carpal tunnel at the wrist and through the volar surface of the hand. Causative factors include narrowing of the space between the carpal bones and the transverse carpal ligament (flexor retinaculum) and laxity of the carpal ligaments resulting from repetitive motion, strain, the intrusion of certain hormones, and maintaining static wrist positions. Differential diagnostic testing is essential to rule out other causes and syndromes. To date, Tinel's and Phalen's tests continue to be reliable and widely used.

Impingement of the median nerve causes a sharp shooting pain that starts at the proximal wrist flexors and extends into the wrist. Pain often begins after activity and can disturb sleep. Chronic impingement causes atrophy of the thenar muscle. Practitioners must conduct physical assessment tests to determine whether other impingements exist. Some of the commonly associated areas of neurovascular compression, such as the cervical, interscalene, subclavicular, pectoral, cubital, and Guyon's canal (ulnar nerve), should be explored. These areas must be investigated in treatment because they are factors in most cases. To be successful, treatment also must address the holding patterns that can develop. The shrug mechanism is the most common type of muscular contracture and can limit recovery if not treated. The other holding pattern is the tendency to splint the arm, which impedes axillary circulation and interferes with the healing process.

Treatment should include general massage and lymphatic drainage techniques to prepare the patient for deeper pressure. Myofascial release and specific nerve release techniques are used in areas where nerves are compromised or compressed. Squeezing the ulna and radius at the wrist during passive movement improves ligamental tone and helps restore the carpal arch. Passive mobilization of the neck, shoulder, elbow, and wrist ensures complete coverage of related areas.

Cubital Tunnel Syndrome (Ulnar Neuropathy)

Cubital tunnel syndrome responds to the treatment outlined for carpal tunnel syndrome, but the ulnar nerve release technique must be added to the regimen. This technique involves thrusting with a "plucking" motion the flexor carpi ulnaris muscle from the medial surface of the ulna, from just below the elbow, through Guyon's Canal and the hypothenar muscle.

Radial Tunnel Syndrome (Posterior Interosseous Nerve Syndrome)

Techniques that thrust the extensor carpi radialis longus and extensor carpi radialis brevis muscles medially from the posterior surface of the radius should be performed from the proximal to the distal portions of the bone. Vigorous friction along the interosseus membrane is also helpful.

Thoracic Outlet Compression Syndrome

Thoracic outlet compression syndrome involves an interference of proper pulsation and blood flow through the subclavian artery as it passes through the interscalene triangle. This condition can result from a variety of mechanical impingements and osseous compressions. Myofascial release of neurovascular compression at the interscalene triangle, subclavicular area, and pectoralis minor muscle has been quite successful in conservative and postsurgical care.

CONVULSION/SEIZURE DISORDER

When working with seizure patients, massage therapists should be prepared to move the patient to a safe place if he or she has a seizure during a session. The patient should be helped from the massage table onto the floor, all objects should be removed from the area, and an ambulance should be called if the seizure does not subside quickly. General massage is indicated to relax muscles and decrease anxiety.

PANIC ATTACK

Panic attacks are common, but most people recover without medication or physical treatment. If panic attacks occur frequently and appear to worsen over time, additional medical attention should be sought. The panic reaction to stress usually begins at an early age and may disappear in adulthood, only to return during periods of great stress. During a panic attack the individual experiences both psychological terror and physical discomfort.

A variety of symptoms are associated with a panic attack, but a true panic attack must include several of the following symptoms: increased perspiration, feeling of terror, difficulty breathing or shortness of breath, uncontrollable yelling or screaming, tightness in the chest, dizziness, uncontrollable muscle trembling or contraction, fear of dying, fear of losing control, thoughts of going insane, out of body experience, and other similar sensations related to the flight or fight response of the autonomic nervous system.

Persons pursuing massage therapy for panic attacks can benefit from the soothing effect massage has on the nervous system. The treatment should consist of gentle strokes performed in rhythmic, predictable patterns. Deep and continuous breathing should be encouraged and monitored throughout the session.

SLEEP DISORDERS (INSOMNIA)

Sleep disorders, including difficulty sleeping and insufficient sleep, are often associated with chronic pain, anxiety, and dietary factors. Ideally the treatment should be given late in the day or even just before the patient's usual bedtime. Gentle, predictable, and repetitive strokes can induce sleep. Massage of the face, spine, and feet has a particularly hypnotic effect on the CNS.

HICCOUGH (SINGULTUS)

Hiccoughs are involuntary repetitive spasmodic contractions of the diaphragm, followed by a sudden closure of the glottis. Low levels of carbon dioxide (CO_2) increase the incidence of hiccoughs, whereas high blood levels of CO_2 inhibit it. Deep tissue massage temporarily increases the release of CO_2 from the body tissues, often causing patients to hold their breath. Although breath holding is strongly discouraged during massage, it is the body's instinctive attempt to balance the blood gases.[2] Thus the therapist may try using flushing strokes during consistent breathing patterns and sustained pressures and squeezing techniques during breath holding.

Several other massage techniques can be used to treat hiccoughs; however, specialized training is mandatory before performing any of the following techniques:

Squeezing the cervical musculature to increase vagal stimulation.

Applying judicious pressure to the phrenic nerves behind the sterno-clavicular joints.

Applying intermittent and sustained carotid sinus pressure.

Slowly, steadily compressing the sternum as many as 12 times.

Massaging the diaphragm just below the xiphoid process and continuing to just above the umbilicus in four to six passes, with each pass gradually becoming deeper.

Using intermittent flipping frictions up from under the costal arch to achieve myofascial release.

DYSPHAGIA

Before undertaking any of the suggested treatments for dysphasia, the practitioner should complete specialized training beyond the standard 500 hours. General massage for relaxation should precede the medical portion of the treatment for dysphagia and should be used throughout the session to reduce anxiety. Placing the hand on the forehead as a method of distraction and tapping lightly on the sternum after a challenging technique calms patients. Facial and cranial massage is useful to reduce rigidity of the muscles. A tongue depressor is used to urge the tongue to elongate; the patient is instructed to push the tongue up against the depressor for 8 to 10 seconds and then slowly relax. This technique is beneficial for those who habitually press the tongue to the roof of the mouth, sometimes throughout the night, which eventually weakens the tongue muscle and may cause the gums to recede. The patient is then asked to protrude the tongue from the mouth as far as possible and is taught techniques for self-massage of the interoral structures. Massage may continue, using myofascial techniques that elongate the platysma. Direct digital pressure is placed against the myohyoid beneath the mandible until relaxation is perceived. The same procedure may be used to achieve a similar effect on the genio-hyoid and digastric muscles. The subhyoidal structures also must be treated, but direct pressure should be applied with great caution. Using the tips of the thumb and first and second digits, the practitioner pulls and collects small portions of the skin covering the trachea as a way of gently massaging the trachea. This technique is followed with transverse mobilization of the trachea from the thyroid cartilage to just above the sternum. Slow, firm pressures on the sternum are followed through to the epigastric region, elongating the stomach and duodenum. The practitioner frequently returns to the submandibular, sublingual, and parotid glands, applying upward and circular massage to stimulate salivary secretions. This procedure facilitates swallowing as well.

URINARY INCONTINENCE

The bladder is situated just behind the pubic bone in the pelvis. Undue direct digital pressure on the bladder should be avoided.

The patient is in the supine position with the bolster under the knees so the abdominal muscles relax. General myofascial lifting, with the whole surfaces of the hands placed at the lower *abdomen*, should be performed during the patient's full inhalation and exhalation. Massage of the lower extremities and systemic circulatory massage indirectly stimulates urine production and urgency. When massaging a patient with bladder dysfunction (incontinence), the practitioner must place a special mattress pad under the treatment sheet on the bed or massage table. Use of this pad protects the treatment surfaces, puts the patient at ease, and helps avoid unnecessary embarrassment. If the patient has increased urinary urgency and frequency, the practitioner must ensure that a restroom or other accommodation is nearby. Because massage stimulates urine output, the therapist may choose to limit the session to 30 minutes.

ANOSMIA

Gentle massage of the head and neck initially stimulates the flow of saliva. If there has been physical damage to the olfactory bulbs, the senses of smell and taste are not likely to return. The mood-enhancing effect of massage may relieve some of the anger and frustration related to this sensory loss. It also facilitates the body's attempt to heal the damaged tissue by containing edema. Before any work is done inside the mouth or the nostrils, the procedure and its beneficial outcomes must be fully explained to and understood by the patient. Use of a skull to demonstrate the technique is helpful. After the procedure has been explained, the patient must be allowed to choose whether to submit to the treatment. Vinyl or powder-free latex gloves must always be worn by the practitioner performing oral and nasal massage.

Massage of the platysma, sternocleidomastoid, and scalene muscles and the submandibular area should precede interoral work. Gentle facial massage is relaxing and can be repeated throughout the session to reduce the patient's anxiety.

Patients who have had extensive plastic surgery may require special consideration because of scarring, altered sensitivity and tolerance, and surgical implants (plastic or dental). Open communication with the patient is essential. Describing the procedure and the expected beneficial effect is strongly advised.

Interoral procedures can be accomplished by using a tongue depressor and the digits. The tongue depressor can be inserted horizontally and turned to a vertical position as it is pressed against the inner wall of the cheek. The tissue is gently stretched laterally, with upward and downward movements. Techniques are executed on both sides, and vibration is used to finish the area before the tongue depressor or the practitioner's fingers are removed from the oral cavity. Digital palpation and pressure should be used to explore areas of muscle tension and to reduce the rigidity of the temporomandibular joints. Other structures involved in the restriction of movement include the pterygoid, digastric, and superior and inferior hyoid muscles. Extreme caution should be exercised at all times, and stimulation of the gag reflex should be avoided as much as possible.

NASAL AND ORAL HYGIENE

The treatment generally consists of inserting a fingertip into one of the nostrils and sustaining digital pressure against the maxilla for several seconds, then repeating in the other nostril. Not all patients consent to nasal massage even though massage therapists do not penetrate past the nasal bone. In these instances an attempt is made to teach patients to perform self-massage using a cotton-tipped swab to apply gentle pressure in a circular movement just inside the nostrils. The same is true of interoral massage. It should be encouraged as part of an oral hygiene program.

PSYCHIATRIC SYMPTOMS

Massage therapists lack the education to treat patients with severe neurosis; however, practitioners who have pursued degrees in psychology may be better equipped to handle such cases. Massage therapists are trained to recognize common neuroses, such as dissociation, the physical symptoms of eating disorder, hypochondriasis, and the like. Such patients are then referred for psychological counseling. Some massage therapists work in psychiatric facilities where they serve as apprentices acting under direct supervision.

SAFETY

When performed by a trained professional, massage therapy is safe. Isolated case reports of complications of massage include sigmoid perforation, aggravation of thyrotoxicosis, communication of herpes-zoster virus, and arterial dissection. The general contraindications to massage are an open skin lesion, bleeding diathesis, fever, and hemodynamic instability; the sites of tumors and fractures should not be massaged.

REFERENCES

1. Travell J. *Myofascial Pain and Dysfunction: The Trigger Point Manual, Upper Half of the Body.* vol. 1. Baltimore, MD: Williams & Wilkins; 1983.
2. Kellogg J. *The Art of Massage.* Brushton, NY: TEACH Services; 1999.
3. American Massage Therapy Association (AMTA) Houston Unit Newsletter [newsletter]. Houston, TX: The Association; May 1993:4.
4. Pemberton R. The physiology of massage. In: *American Medical Association Handbook of Physical Medicine and Rehabilitation.* Philadelphia, PA: American Medical Association; 1950.
5. Barnes PM, Powell-Griner E, McFann K, Nahini RL. Comlementary and Alternative Medicine Use Among Adults: United States, 2002. *Seminars in Integrative Medicine.* 2004;2:54–71.
6. Matsumoto K, Birch S. *Hara Diagnosis: Reflections on the Sea.* Brookline, MA: Paradigm; 1988.
7. Mennell JB. *Physical Treatment.* 5th ed. Philadelphia, PA: 1945.
8. Pemberton R, Scull CW. Massage. In Glasser O, ed. *Medical Physics.* Chicago, IL: Yearbook; 1944.
9. Wood C. *Beard's Massage Principles and Techniques.* 2nd ed. Philadelphia, PA: WB Saunders; 1974.
10. Hovind N, Nielsen SL. Effect of massage on blood flow in skeletal muscle. *Scand J Rehabil Med.* 1974;6(2):74–77.
11. Hansen TI, Kristensen JH. Effect of massage, shortwave diathermy and ultrasound upon 133Xe disappearance rate from muscle and subcutaneous tissue in the human calf. *Scand J Rehabil Med.* 1973;5(4):179–182.
12. Ek AC, Gustavsson G, Lewis DH. The local skin blood flow in areas at risk for pressure sores treated with massage. *Scand J Rehabil Med.* 1985;17(2):81–86.
13. Wyper DJ, McNiven DR. Effects of some physiotherapeutic agents on skeletal muscle blood flow. *Phys Ther.* 1976;62(3):83–85.
14. Severini V, Venerando A. The physiological effects of massage on the cardiovascular system. *Europa Medicophys.* 1967;3:165–183.
15. Severini V. Venerando A. Effect on the peripheral circulation of substances producing hyperemia in combination with massage. *Europa Medicophys.* 1967;3:184–198.
16. Mortimer PS et al. The measurement of skin lymph flow by isotope clearance—reliability, reproducibility, injection dynamics, and the effect of massage. *J Invest Dermatol.* 1990;95(6):677–682.
17. Xujain S. Effect of massage and temperature on the permeability of initial lymphatics. *Lymphol.* 1990;23(1):48–50.
18. Gray B. Management of limb oedema. *Nurs Times.* 1987;83(49):39–41.
19. Cafarelli E et al. Vibratory massage and short-term recovery from muscular fatigue. *Int J Sports Med.* 1990;11(6):474–478.
20. Rodenburg JB et al. Warm-up, stretching and massage diminish harmful effects of eccentric exercise. *Int J Sports Med.* 1994;15:414–419.

21. Smith LL et al. The effects of athletic massage on delayed onset muscle soreness. creatine kinase, and neutrophil count: a preliminary report. *J Orthop Sports Phys Ther.* 1994;19(2):93–99.

22. Crosman LJ, Chateauvert SR, Weisberg J. The effects of massage to the hamstring muscle group on range of motion. *J Orthop Sports Phys Ther.* 1984;6(3):168–172.

23. Wiktorsson-Meller et al. Effects of warming up, massage and stretching on range of motion and muscle strength in the lower extremity. *Am J Sports Med.* 1983;11(4): 249–252.

24. Goldberg J, Sullivan SJ, Seaborne DE. The effect of two intensities of massage on H-reflex amplitude. *Phys Ther.* 1992;72(6):449–457.

25. Morelli M, Seaborne DE, Sullivan SJ. H-reflex modulation during manual muscle massage of human triceps surae. *Arch Phys Med Rehabil.* 1991;72(11):915–919.

26. Sullivan SJ et al. Effects of massage on alpha motoneuron excitability. *Phys Ther.* 1991;71(8):555–560.

27. Matheson DW et al. Relaxation measured by EMG as a function of vibrotactile stimulation. *Biofeedback Self Regul.* 1976;3:285.

28. Hammer WI. The use of transverse friction massage in the management of chronic bursitis of the hip or shoulder. *J Manipulative Physiol Ther.* 1993;16:107–111.

29. Goldberg J et al. The effect of therapeutic massage on H-reflex amplitude in persons with a spinal cord injury. *Phys Ther.* 1994;74(8):728–737.

30. Danneskold-Samse B et al. Regional muscle tension and pain ("fibrositis"): effect on massage on myoglobin in plasma. *Scand J Rehabil Med.* 1983;15(1):17–20.

31. Chopra SK et al. Effects of hydration and physical therapy on tracheal transport velocity. *Ann Rev Resp Dis.* 1977;115(6):1009–1014.

32. Petersen LN et al. Foot zone therapy and bronchial asthma—a controlled clinical trial. *Clin Trial.* 1992;154(30):2065–2068.

33. Naliboff BD, Tachiki KH. Autonomic and skeletal muscle responses to nonelectrical cutaneous stimulation. *Percept Mot Skills.* 1991;72(2):575–584.

34. Tyler DO et al. Effects of a 1-minute back rub on mixed venous oxygen saturation and heart rate in critically ill patients. *Heart Lung.* 1990;19(5Pt2):562–565.

35. Barr JS, Taslitz N. The influence of back massage on autonomic functions. *Phys Ther.* 1970;50(12):1679–1691.

36. Olson B. Effects of massage for prevention of pressure ulcers. *Decubious.* 1989;(4):32–37.

37. Bogdan FL et al. Epithelial mesenchymal interrelations at the skin level. *Morphol Embryol.* 1982;28(1):3–9.

38. Jian H, Yang Z. Influence of finger pressing massage on cAMP and cGMP in the cerebrospinal fluid in prolapsed intervertebral disc. *Chin J Mod Dev Tradit Med.* 1990;10(1):27–29.

39. Arkko P, Pakarinen AJ, Kari-Koskinen O. Effects of whole body massage on serum protein, electrolyte and hormone concentrations, enzyme activities and hematologic parameters. *Int J Sports Med.* 1983;4(4):265–267.

40. Bork K, Karling GW, Faust G. Serum enzyme levels after "whole body massage." *Arch Dermatol Forsch.* 1971;240:342–348.

41. Kaada B, Tosteinbo O. Increase of plasma beta- endorphins in connective tissue massage. *Gen Pharmacol.* 1989;20(4):487–489.

42. Day JA, Mason RR, Chesrown SE. Effect of massage on serum level of *b*-endorphin and *B*-lipotropin in healthy adults. *Phys Ther.* 1987;67(67):926–930.

43. Wheeden A et al. Massage effects on cocaine-exposed preterm neonates. *Dev Behav Pediatr.* 1993;14(5):318–322.

44. Scafidi F et al. Factors that predict which preterm infants benefit most from massage therapy. *Dev Behav Pediatr.* 1993;14(3):176–180.

45. Meaney MJ et al. Effect of neonatal handling on age- related impairments associated with the hippocampus. *Science.* 1987;239:766–768.

46. Acolet D et al. Changes in plasma cortisol and catecholamine concentrations in response to massage in preterm infants. *Arch Dis Child.* 1993;68(Suppl 1):29–31.

47. Rice RD. Premature infants respond to sensory stimulation. *APA Monitor.* 1975; 6(11):8–9.

48. Montagu A. *Touching: The Human Significance of the Skin.* New York, NY: Harper & Row; 1978.

49. Fraser J, Kerr JR. Psychophysiological effects of back massage on elderly institutionalized patients. *J Adv Nurs.* 1993;18(2):238–245.

50. McKechnie AA et al. Anxiety states: a preliminary report on the value of connective tissue massage. *J Psychosom Res.* 1983;27(2):125.

51. Longworth JC. Psychophysiological effects of slow stroke back massage in normotensive females. *ANS.* 1982;4(4):44–61.

52. Ho KH et al. Reduction of post-operative swelling by a placebo effect. *J Psychosom Res.* 1988;32(2):197–205.

53. Zanolla R et al. Evaluation of the results of three different methods of postmastectomy lymphedema treatment. *J Surg Oncol.* 1984;26:210–213.

54. Meek SS. Effects of slow stroke back massage on relaxation. *Image J Nurs Sch.* 1993; 25(1):17–21.

55. Platania SA et al. Relaxation therapy reduces anxiety in child and adolescent psychiatric patients. *Acta Paedopsychiatr.* 1992;55(2):115–120.

56. Field T et al. Massage reduces anxiety in child and adolescent psychiatric patients. *J Am Acad Child Adolesc Psychiatry.* 1992;31(1):125–131.

57. Bumpus S et al. The effect of caring touch on the psychological well-being of selected residents of a long-term care facility. *SC Nurs.* 1993;8(1):26–27.

58. Groer M et al. Measures of salivary secretory immunoglobulin A and state anxiety after a nursing back rub. *Appl Nurs Res.* 1994;7(1):2–6.

59. Milkman H, Metcalf D, Reed P. An innovative approach to methadone detoxification. *Int J Addict.* [[year]];15(8): 1199–1211.

60. Weinrich SP, Weinrich MC. The effect of massage on pain in cancer patients. *Appl Nurs Res.* 1990;3(4):140–145.

61. Konrad K et al. Controlled trial of balneotherapy in treatment of low back pain. *Ann Rheum Dis.* 1992;51(6):820–822.

62. Koes BW et al. Randomised clinical trial of manipulative therapy and physiotherapy for persistent back and neck complaints. results of one year follow up. *Br Med J.* 1992;304(6827):601–605.

63. Koes BW et al. The effectiveness of manual therapy, physiotherapy, and treatment by the general practitioner for nonspecific back and neck complaints. *Spine.* 1992;17(1): 28–35.

64. Marin I et al. Postoperative pain after thoracotomy: a study of 116 patients. *Rev Mal Respir.* 1991;8(2):213–218.

65. Jensen OK, Nielsen FF, Vosmar L. An open study comparing manual therapy with the use of cold packs in the treatment of post-traumatic headache. *Cephalalgia.* 1990; 10(5):2241–2250.

66. Puustjarvi K, Airaksinen O, Pontmen PJ. The effects of massage in patients with chronic tension headache. *Acupunct Electrother Res.* 1990;15(2):159–162.

67. Lipton SA. Prevention of classic migraine headache by digra massage of the superficial temporal arteries during visual aura. *Ann Neurol.* 1986;19(5):515–516.

68. Engel JM et al. Value of physical therapy from the viewpoint of the patient: results of a questionnaire. *Z Rheumatol.* 1987;46(5):250–255.

FURTHER READING

American Massage Therapy Association, compiled data, 2005.

American Massage Therapy Association, consumer survey, 2004.

American Massage Therapy Association, industry survey, 2005.

American Massage Therapy Association Press Release, 2003.

Associated Bodywork and Massage Professionals, survey analysis, 2007.

National Certification Board for Therapeutic Massage and Bodywork, press release.

Touch Research Institute, University of Miami School of Medicine, research to date, 2007.

CHAPTER 9

Therapeutic Touch

Eric Leskowitz

It is always a good idea to get a map before setting out for new territory. So before discussing this chapter's specific topic—the use of therapeutic touch (TT) in pain management—a brief overview of the field of complementary and alternative medicine (CAM) is in order. This overview is designed to emphasize the multidimensional nature of human beings and the importance of having a full spectrum of therapeutic approaches to deal with illness and health. This perspective is particularly important in considering therapies that may at first appear to have no basis in scientific fact, according to the Western medical model.

THE MULTIDIMENSIONAL MODEL
OF HUMAN FUNCTION

It is helpful to think of human beings as having four main levels of function and structure. The most concrete level is physiology, once a major focus of medical school training and modern medical and surgical therapies. In the biomedical model, which focuses on this level, the human body is seen as a complex mechanism that is the source of illness and the target for treatments. The biomedical model focuses all its treatments, whether pharmaceuticals, surgery, radiation, or genetic manipulation, on this concrete level.

Emotions and thoughts constitute the next important levels. In some traditions, such as yoga and Theosophy, these are believed to be two distinct levels; however, for the purposes of this chapter, the realm of thoughts, beliefs, attitudes, and emotions are considered as one level. This dimension is addressed by psychotherapy and other mind-body techniques. A large body of knowledge in the field of psychoneuroimmunology has demonstrated that psychologic and emotional events can influence the onset and course of most important medical syndromes. A whole range of mind-body techniques that are discussed elsewhere in this book addresses this area. For example, hypnosis, biofeedback, meditation, imagery, and specific psychotherapies all fit into this second paradigm. (see Figure 9.1).

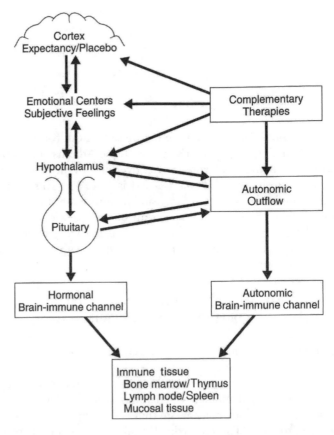

FIGURE 9.1   Psychoneuroimmunological pathways of mind-body medicine.

The last dimension is the spiritual. The most lasting value of holistic medicine may be that it finally bridges the long-standing gap between religion and science. We now have scientific data validating the clinical efficacy of interventions like prayer[1] and the laying on of hands,[2] two approaches that were formerly taboo for medical researchers to investigate, let alone prescribe. What these and other spiritually based therapies have in common is an insistence that human beings are animated by a special type of vital energy. This vital energy fills individuals up with health when they are inspired and is drained when they are ill. Many cultures speak of the phenomenon in their own language. In China, the energy is called *qi;* in India, yogis call it *prana;* in Hebrew mysticism, it is called *ruach;* but in Western medicine there is no word or concept for this vital energy. The end result is called *homeostatic balance,* but there is no knowledge as to how it comes about.

A wide range of alternative medicine therapies deal with this dimension of subtle energy. These therapies tend to be the ones that are most controversial and the most difficult for mainstream science to make sense of. Some of the most prominent energy-based therapies are addressed elsewhere in this book, including acupuncture, qigong, homeopathy, shiatsu, and tai chi. The focus for this chapter is on one of the few Western-based techniques that acknowledges and harnesses this so-called subtle energy, therapeutic touch (TT).

HISTORIC PRECURSORS OF THERAPEUTIC TOUCH

To be fair, some of the medical renegades of the Western medical tradition did try to characterize this subtle life energy. Sigmund Freud talked of libido, Wilhelm Reich researched orgone, Henri Bergson wrote of élan vital, and most importantly for this chapter, Franz Mesmer tried to harness "animal magnetism." Although widespread opinion holds that Mesmer's work was that of a charlatan, his technique was actually a precursor of TT and was more valid than he was ever given credit for. In addition, the reception he was given by the medical establishment of his time has interesting overtones considering the American Medical Association's (AMA) once hostile reaction to CAM and the recent controversy over a widely publicized attempt to debunk TT.

Austrian physician Franz Anton Mesmer participated in the intellectual ferment that swept Europe in the late 1700s, in particular the interest in the newly discovered forces of electricity and magnetism.[3] He developed a wildly popular form of magnetic therapy that used magnetic stones and his own personal store of so-called animal magnetism to heal his wealthy aristocratic patients. The wide range of disorders that he healed would probably be labeled as conversion symptoms today. However, because the medical establishment was threatened by his runaway success, both medical and financial, King Louis XVI asked the Royal Society to investigate the claims of Mesmerism. These eminent scientists, including Antione Lavoisier, Joseph Guillotine, and Benjamin Franklin, found that his patients did, in fact, get better, but only through the powers of imagination and suggestion. They discounted the magnetic "fluidium" that Mesmer claimed to transmit to his patient by making his famous Mesmeric passes. These passes consisted of stroking the air several inches from the patient's body in repeated downward movements. The fact that a commission completely vindicated Mesmer after his death was no solace, as he had effectively been run out of town, never again to recover his reputation or influence.

Two hundred years later, the twentieth century having drawn to a close, the tide has turned. Modern biomagnetism has documented that there is an energy field surrounding the human body.[4] The process has shown that purported energy healers emit measurable negative body potential surges of up to 90 volts under experimental conditions.[5] In the early 1970s, a team consisting of nurse Delores Krieger and medical intuitive Dora Kunz developed a standardized treatment known as Therapeutic Touch.[6] The purpose of TT was to allow medical professionals, particularly nurses, to harness some of the same subtle energies that saints and mystics and healers had been working with for centuries.

THE TECHNIQUE OF THERAPEUTIC TOUCH

The standardized TT treatment protocol involves five steps.[7] The first and most important step is centering, in which the nurse healer takes a moment to quiet the mind and focus on a heart-centered wish to be of service to the patient. The second step is known as the assessment, in which the nurse scans the patient's external energy field by placing the palms of her hands several inches away from each part of the patient's body. The nurse tries to sense alterations in the subtle perceptions of tingling or temperature that are typically experienced in this process. These alterations are thought to reflect underlying physiologic problems and indicate the regions to be addressed in step three.

In the third treatment step, the nurse tries to unruffle and clear these apparent energy blocks with a series of slow, stroking movements down the patient's energy field. The nurse does not actually make any physical contact. These movements are identical in form to the Mesmeric passes. In the next step, the nurse focuses his or her hands on one particular region and directs and modulates the flow of energy there. This balancing phase may also involve direct physical contact with the patient's body. In the final phase, the nurse evaluates the changes in the patient's energy field hoping to detect the symmetric and open flow that marks a successful treatment.

SCIENTIFIC STUDIES

In the past 20 years, a large amount of clinical literature has built up around TT. There are 129 references listed at the end of the Rosa article cited later, and Medline gave 317 TT citations as of October 2000. The technique has been applied to a wide range of conditions, not only measuring subjective variables, such as pain, anxiety, and self-esteem, but also objectively measuring physiologic processes, including immune function, wound healing, and general medical conditions. Experimental rigor, as usually defined by clinical medicine, is hard to come by, in part due to the nature of TT itself. A sham TT technique has been developed in which patients can be blinded to TT. In this technique, nurses move their hands in the typical downward strokes of TT, but occupy their minds with mental arithmetic rather than the attitude of compassionate caring that marks true TT. Unfortunately, the nurse cannot be blinded to the treatment being given because, by definition, he or she is aware of which of these two states of mind is being used. Hence, TT research can at best be only single blind.

Two key physiologic studies follow as well as some case vignettes that illustrate how TT has been integrated into the Pain Management Program at Spaulding Rehabilitation Hospital (SRH) in Boston.

Stress is known to inhibit numerous physiologic processes. One such process that is susceptible to objective monitoring is wound healing, that is, the rate of repair of damaged skin. For example, the skin of people under high stress, in this case caregivers of Alzheimer's patients, heals much more slowly from punch biopsies than does the skin of matched controls.[8] In contrast, TT has been shown to accelerate the rate of wound healing in healthy volunteers. In an elegant study, Daniel Wirth[2] controlled for placebo and expectancy effects when he demonstrated that after 15 days, none of the 50 mm^2 biopsy wounds in the untreated control group had completely healed. However, 50% of the TT recipients had healed. The level of statistical significance was $p < 0.0001$. Although this crucial study has never been replicated by independent researchers, it provides a tantalizing clue as to how clinicians might be able to enhance the body's healing response after surgery or injury.

Another important study[9] showed that stress-induced immunosuppression could be reversed by TT, as measured by serum levels of immunoglobulins A and M in medical students during final exam time. Again, a clinically important physiologic variable was effected in a positive manner by a relatively brief course of TT. The potential clinical applications are intriguing, especially given the wide range of medical conditions that are characterized by immune dysfunction.

THERAPEUTIC TOUCH IN PAIN MANAGEMENT

It is possible to pick out important nuggets from the medical literature and some intriguing research data suggesting that TT can influence mind and body. But what about pain management? The next section focuses on several specific neurologic conditions and highlights some relevant research and clinical findings.

Peripheral Neuropathy

Two clinical case studies from SRH highlight potential applications of TT to peripheral neuropathy; however, no formal research studies have yet been done with this specific syndrome.

Case 1: Dan was a 39-year-old man with AIDS-related peripheral neuropathy. His bilateral foot pain had not responded to opiates, tricyclics, or anticonvulsants. His primary nurse attempted to alleviate his attendant anxiety with a course of TT and found, much to her surprise, that not only did Dan's anxiety level decrease with TT, but his pain level went from a self-rating of "very bad" to "not much." Unfortunately, his pain returned the next day. He continued to respond favorably to each TT session, although his carryover only lasted several hours. He was lost to follow up after discharge.

Case 2: Lillian was a 68-year-old woman who had developed neuropathic pain in the distribution of her femoral nerve, which had been accidentally injured during vascular surgery several years earlier. She was able to obtain only slight relief with standard medications for neuropathic pain. In addition, her allodynia was so severe that she could not participate in any form of rehab that involved direct physical contact, including physical therapy (PT) manipulation and tactile thermal desensitization; however, during the course of a TT treatment she felt the sensitivity decrease to such an extent that she allowed the TT practitioner to physically touch her leg. This was the first time she had allowed another person to touch her. This decreased sensitivity opened the door to a range of other standard pain management approaches, which were able to significantly decrease her discomfort. Interestingly, the other intervention that lessened her pain level was psychotherapy, during which she was able to express for the first time her rage and disappointment at the trusted surgeon who had damaged her nerve.

Phantom Pain

The SRH clinic has recently reported on the successful use of TT in treating cases of phantom limb pain.[10,11] A fascinating aspect of this work, which merits further study, is the finding that the TT therapist can perceive the energetic outlines of the phantom limb in what appears to be empty space. The patient is also able to detect when the therapist's hands make contact with his phantom limb. These findings suggest validity to the notion that a subtle energetic anatomy exists independent of our physiology. The TT process, when successful, creates a feeling that has been described as draining the pain out of the affected limb. Benefits last from hours to days, and patients have been taught to administer this treatment to themselves for sustained long-term benefits.

Case 3: Mary was a 73-year-old woman who had a below-the-knee amputation of her left leg to prevent the worsening of peripheral-vascular-disease-induced gangrene. She had expected to lose only a toe, not a limb, and from the moment she awoke from surgery she experienced severe phantom pain in the toe that was gangrenous. No standard medications such as opiates, anticonvulsants, or antidepressants were helpful, but she responded almost immediately to TT. She felt the pain drain out of the bottom of her phantom foot and became pain free for the first time in more than a year. She could amplify the effects of this treatment by visualizing a soothing blue light coating her painful limb. She eventually learned to perform TT on herself and reported that she could start each day with a TT session and remain quite comfortable throughout the day, unless her stress level rose above a certain threshold.

Multiple Sclerosis

Several reports in the nursing literature describe the use of TT in the care of multiple sclerosis (MS) patients. One case study[12] highlights the adjunctive role of TT in MS care, noting in particular its benefits for such subjective symptoms as mood and comfort. Another paper[13] emphasizes the high rate of use of various alternative therapies by MS patients and indicates that TT is one of the most popular. Results are reported in terms of quality of life but are not quantified by using, for example, the Schatsky functional rating scale or the Functional Improvement Measure (FIM). These simple steps could greatly strengthen the TT literature on MS. In addition, given the current conceptualization of MS as an autoimmune disorder, the previously mentioned demonstration of enhanced immune functioning following TT takes on added significance.

Dementia

No studies exist concerning the use of TT to reverse the degenerative process, but several papers describe its use in bringing about behavioral changes in Alzheimer's patients. In one naturalistic study,[14] TT was introduced as a stress-management technique. It was found to induce a relaxation response in demented patients who had a history of agitated behavior, but it was not effective in decreasing the actual levels of these behaviors. Direct physical contact, as in hand massage, proved more effective than TT in reducing agitation in these patients suggesting that with a certain degree of brain damage, the effects of TT may be too subtle to translate into overt behavioral changes.

Headache

One of the best-designed TT studies ever performed looked at the effects of TT on tension headache pain.[15] By using the sham TT intervention mentioned earlier, expectancy and placebo factors could be taken into consideration. A matched group of 60 headache patients was studied, all of whom were naive to prior TT treatments. Ninety percent of the members of the active treatment group experienced improvements in symptoms following TT, averaging a 70% decrease in degree of symptom intensity. Of the control patients, 80% reported pain reduction that averaged only 37% in degree. It should be noted that both groups practiced deep breathing. Therefore the placebo group was actually receiving a treatment known to be somewhat helpful in itself for mild headache symptoms, and the treatment group actually received two treatments, TT plus breathing. Furthermore, this differential benefit was even more pronounced 4 hours after the initial treatment, again favoring TT over sham TT controls.

Postoperative Pain

In a single-blind clinical trial that measured postoperative pain in 108 patients, Meehan found[16] that a single TT treatment reduced the patients' need for analgesic medication, although reported pain levels were similar between patients who received genuine TT and those who received the sham TT control intervention. Presumably, the untreated patients used additional analgesics to make up for the differential impact of TT. An extension of this work should look at the role of regular TT applications.

Presumably there would be a sort of dosage effect, with greater impact coming from more regular application of the modality. The author cautiously notes that TT may be best conceptualized as an adjunctive pain therapy, rather than as a primary treatment modality.

Burn Pain

Pain, anxiety, and impaired immune function are all known to follow significant burns to the body surface. One study[17] measured the impact of regular TT treatments on these three variables on patients in a hospital burn unit. Again using sham TT control intervention, this single-blinded randomized clinical trial determined that 5 days of regular TT caused statistically significant reductions on self-reported pain (the McGill Pain Questionnaire Rating Index) and anxiety (the Visual Analogue Scale). Immune function was also altered, as reflected by a 13% decrease in CD8+ cell concentration, although the clinical significance of this cellular change was not clear. Again, the authors call for more studies to look at the long-term effects of ongoing TT and to control more tightly for behavioral variables that might influence outcome.

TWO RECENT CONTROVERSIES

Despite this promising list of neurologic and other medical/physiologic processes that have been proven to be affected by TT, the general populace's view of this technique has become one of extreme skepticism. This stems in part from a lack of awareness of the body of research data cited previously. However, it stems more directly from the massive publicity given to a unique report—the *Journal of the American Medical Association's (JAMA)* publication of an 11-year-old schoolgirl's science fair project, titled "A Closer Look at Therapeutic Touch."[18] This study is important on so many levels that it is worth discussing in some detail.

A Unique Study of Therapeutic Touch in the *Journal of the American Medical Association*

At the level of basic science, this study is noteworthy for using an elegantly simple research protocol to test whether nurse practitioners of TT could in fact reliably detect the presence of the so-called energy field of their client. In this protocol, the nurses were effectively blindfolded and then asked to guess over which of their outstretched hands the researcher was placing her own hand. In other words, they were asked to sense the energy field emanating from the experimenter's hand. Interestingly enough, the nurses were only accurate 40% of the time in their guesses, indicating that they performed even more poorly in their energy assessments than would be expected with random guessing. The authors then concluded that because there was no experimental validation of the energy fields that purportedly underlie TT therapy, there could be no clinical effectiveness to TT as a treatment intervention. The *JAMA* editors joined in, urging patients to refuse to pay for such treatments until scientific evidence of its efficacy could be produced.

As a tide of rebuttal letters to *JAMA*[19] and editorial commentaries elsewhere[20,21] pointed out, there were numerous crucial methodologic flaws in the study. There were also logical fallacies in the conclusions reached by the authors and the editor. Of note, the degree of expertise of the TT volunteers was not reported, and they did not in fact enter into the true TT process outlined previously because they were never asked to elicit their inner intent to heal. This omission raises questions about what technique was actually being assessed. Many of the sessions were videotaped in a television studio, which could easily have generated performance anxiety. More importantly, there was no control for experimenter bias, a significant possibility given that the girl's parents, the article's coauthors, were members of Quackwatch Inc., a now discredited organization devoted to debunking alternative therapies.

Regardless, it is a basic tenet of energy-based therapies that the frame of mind of the healer influences the degree of energy effect he or she creates.[22] If the girl had been a master healer emitting huge bursts of energy, it would be striking that the success rates were so low; however, if she had at some unconscious or conscious level wanted negative results, she might have literally shut down her own energy field, making it even harder than normal to detect its presence. Perhaps this is the true significance of the low detection scores—the nurses may have been accurately responding to a negative alteration in the test energy field. Contrast these apparently negative data with results from an earlier study[23] that reported a successful detection rate of more than 65% using a similar protocol. Interestingly, this study was not referenced in the otherwise exhaustive TT bibliography cited in the *JAMA* paper. *JAMA* authors summarily dismissed this research literature as being without significant scientific merit.

Even more striking than these methodologic problems is the authors' unwarranted conclusion that TT is clinically useless. No clinical outcomes were assessed in this study, so no conclusions could logically be made in the domain of clinical efficacy. One wonders what led the usually judicious editorial staff of *JAMA* to make such an uncalled-for statement decrying the use of a therapeutic intervention other than to conduct another of *JAMA*'s periodic publicity stunts. The resemblance to Mesmer's run-in with the Royal Society is striking: an attempt by political influence to destroy work that threatens the dominant medical paradigm.

Another controversy concerns a body of research that had generally been accepted within the energy medicine community as strongly validating the efficacy of TT in enhancing the normal physiologic process of wound healing. A study by Daniel Wirth, published in 1990, purported to show that even in double blind conditions, TT could dramatically speed up the rate at which standardized punch biopsies of the skin could heal in normal healthy subjects.[2] Due to the tightly controlled conditions and strikingly positive statistics, this study (and several other subsequent ones by the same author) have been regarded as providing the foundation for energy medicine research.

However, in recent years, several researchers (including Wirth's former supervisor, and the author of this chapter) became troubled by their inability to obtain any information about the research protocol from Wirth directly, and they began to investigate his research methods more fully.[24] They found that no documentation could prove that the study was performed as described; the coauthors believe that some, if not all, of Wirth's primary data was fabricated; however, they point out that sufficient subsequent research has established the validity of energy medicine, and of TT, to such an extent that even absent the entire body of Wirth's work, the field of energy medicine has a strong research foundation.

CONCLUSION

Certainly there has been a good measure of deserved resistance by the medical establishment to novel energy-based therapies like TT, but the tide is turning. The field of biomagnetics is documenting the existence of human subtle-energy fields. A rapidly growing body of evidence is proving that TT and its relatives can be effective in a wide range of clinical situations. This includes most prominently a variety of pain conditions, as research on TT in other neurologic conditions is still in its infancy. Further research is needed to move beyond the reporting of subjective variables into the realm of functional measurements and biological parameters. The current situation is full of promise for future discoveries in the application of energy-based therapies to the problems of medicine, in general, and pain medicine in particular.

REFERENCES

1. Byrd R. The effects of intercessory prayer on patients in a coronary care unit. *South Med J.* 1988;81(7):826–829.
2. Wirth D. The effect of noncontact therapeutic touch on the rate of healing of full thickness dermal wounds. *Subtle Energies.* 1990;1(1):1–21.

3. Ellenberger H. *The Discovery of the Unconscious.* New York, NY: Basic Books; 1970.

4. Becker R. *Crosscurrents: The Promise of Electromedicine, the Perils of Electropollution.* Los Angeles, CA: J Tarcher; 1990.

5. Green E et al. Anomalous electrostatic phenomena in exceptional subjects. *Subtle Energies.* 1991;2(3):69–81.

6. Wager S. *A Doctor's Guide to Therapeutic Touch.* New York, NY: Perigee Books; 1996.

7. Mulloney S, Wells-Federman C. Therapeutic touch: a healing modality. *Cardiovasc Nurs.* 1998;(28):117–125.

8. Kiecolt-Glaser J et al. Slowing of wound healing by psychological stress. *Lancet.* 1995; (346):1194–1196.

9. Olson M et al. Stress-induced immunosuppression and therapeutic touch. *Altern Ther.* 1997;3:68–74.

10. Leskowitz E. Phantom limb pain: subtle energy perspectives. *Subtle Energy Energy Med.* 1999;8(2):125–152.

11. Leskowitz E. Phantom limb pain and complementary medicine: a case report. *Arch Phys Med Rehab.* 2000;81:522–524.

12. Payne M. The use of therapeutic touch with rehabilitation clients. *Rehab Nurs.* 1989;14(2):69–72.

13. Fawcett J et al. Use of alternative health therapies by people with multiple sclerosis: an exploratory study. *Holist Nurs Pract.* 1994;8(2):36–42.

14. Snyder M, Egan E, Burns K. Interventions for decreasing agitation behaviors in persons with dementia. *J Gerontol Nurs.* 1995;21(7):34–40.

15. Keller E, Bzdek V. Effects of therapeutic touch on tension headache pain. *Nurs Res.* 1986;35(2):101–106.

16. Meehan T. Therapeutic touch and postoperative pain: a Rogerian research study. *Nurs Sci Q.* 1993;6(12):69–78.

17. Turner J et al. The effect of therapeutic touch on pain and anxiety in burn patients. *J Adv Nurs.* 1998;28(1):10–20.

18. Rosa L et al. A close look at therapeutic touch. *JAMA.* 1998;279:1005–1010.

19. Freinkel A et al. An even closer look at therapeutic touch. *JAMA.* 1999;280(22):1905–1908.

20. Achterberg J. Clearing the air in the therapeutic touch controversy. *Alt Ther.* 1999; 4(4):100–101.

21. Leskowitz E. Un-debunking therapeutic touch. *Alt Ther.* 1999;4(4):101–102.

22. Brennan B. *Hands of Light.* New York, NY: Bantam New Age; 1992.

23. Schwartz G, Russek L, Beltran J. Interpersonal hand- energy registration: evidence for implicit performance and perception. *Subtle Energies.* 1995;6:183–200.

24. Solfvin J, Leskowitz E, Benor D. Questions concerning the work of Daniel P Wirth [letter]. *J Alt Comp Med.* 2005;11(6):949–950. http://www.wholistichealingresearch. com/WirthQ.html. Accessed September 11, 2007.

CHAPTER 10

Chiropractic

Daniel Redwood

Over 90% of patients seen by chiropractors seek care for musculoskeletal pain, primarily back pain, neck pain, and headaches.[1] Chiropractors also treat painful extremity disorders including sprain and strain injuries and carpal tunnel syndrome, as well as a smaller number of patients with visceral pain disorders including infantile colic, dysmenorrhea, and otitis media.

Following a 1975 conference sponsored by the United States federal government that found a paucity of research on the subject of spinal manipulation,[2] there has been a substantial increase in both basic science research and clinical trials related to this signature chiropractic method. Over 40 randomized controlled trials (RCTs) have evaluated spinal manipulation (also called spinal adjustment) for lower back pain, and more than 20 RCTs have studied its effects for upper spine conditions including neck pain and headaches. Together, these three conditions comprise the vast majority of chiropractic cases.[3]

A special panel commissioned by the U.S. Health Resources and Services Administration recently reviewed over 700 published research studies and determined that spinal manual therapy is an effective treatment for both acute and chronic back pain.[4]

Aside from back pain, neck pain, and headaches, the number of RCTs on spinal manipulation is small, with no other condition having been the focus of more than a few. It is noteworthy that across the broad sweep of several dozen chiropractic-related RCTs, spinal manipulation has never performed more poorly than a comparison treatment or placebo, and no significant injuries have been reported. Summaries and examples of this research will be presented in this chapter.

THE CHIROPRACTIC PROFESSION

The United States is home to approximately 65,000 of the world's 90,000 chiropractors.[5] Chiropractors are licensed throughout the English-speaking world and in an increasing number of other nations. Rigorous educational standards are supervised by government-recognized accrediting agencies, including the Council on Chiropractic Education (CCE) in the United States. After fulfilling college science prerequisites analogous to those required for admission to medical or osteopathic schools, chiropractic students must complete a 4-year chiropractic school program, which includes a wide range of courses in anatomy, physiology, pathology, and diagnosis, as well as spinal adjusting, physical therapy, rehabilitation, and nutrition.

As noted by Meeker and Haldeman,[3] utilization of chiropractic in the United States tripled over 17 years, from about 3.6%[6] to an estimated 11%, according to a 1997 national random telephone survey.[7] American chiropractors log approximately 190 million patient visits per year, or about 30% of visits to all complementary practitioners.

In recent years, the mainstreaming of chiropractic has taken many forms. Low back guidelines from government agencies in the United States,[8] Great Britain,[9] Sweden,[10] Denmark,[11] Australia,[12] and New Zealand[13] have recognized spinal manipulation as one of a very small number of effective treatment methods for lower back pain, the condition most often treated by chiropractors. The U.S. guidelines found that only two categories of professionally administered procedures (spinal manipulation and anti-inflammatory or analgesic medications) had proven efficacy and that only manipulation provided both pain relief and functional improvement.

Chiropractic care is included in the U.S. Medicare system that serves the elderly and disabled. The majority of private health insurance plans in the United States, including a majority of HMOs, include coverage for chiropractic services. Chiropractors serve on the U.S. Olympic medical staff, and professional sports teams across the country make chiropractic care available to their athletes.. In the past decade, chiropractors have been hired as staff members for Veterans Administration (VA) hospitals and Department of Defense (DOD) bases of all branches of the U.S.

armed services, in a gradual phase-in leading toward eventual system-
wide access to chiropractic care throughout the VA and DOD health
systems. At the same time, chiropractors have attained staff privileges
at hundreds of civilian hospitals, and there has been significant growth
in the number of interdisciplinary and integrative clinics where chiropractors work alongside medical physicians and other conventional or
complementary health practitioners. These and other ongoing changes
reflect an evolution of the profession from alternative to mainstream
status.

THE CHIROPRACTIC PARADIGM

Definitions of Chiropractic, Role of the Chiropractor

Though the vast majority of chiropractic patients present with pain as
the primary symptom, national and international definitions of chiropractic omit any mention of pain. The World Federation of Chiropractic,
which represents all major national chiropractic organizations, defines
chiropractic as follows:

> A health profession concerned with the diagnosis, treatment and pre-
> vention of mechanical disorders of the musculoskeletal system, and the
> effects of these disorders on the functions of the nervous system and
> general health. There is an emphasis on manual treatments including
> spinal adjustment and other joint and soft-tissue manipulation.[14]

The Association of Chiropractic Colleges definition of chiropractic
reflects a consensus of all chiropractic college presidents in North
America:

> Chiropractic is a healthcare discipline that emphasizes the inherent re-
> cuperative power of the body to heal itself without the use of drugs or
> surgery. The practice of chiropractic focuses on the relationship be-
> tween structure (primarily the spine) and function (as coordinated by
> the nervous system) and how that relationship affects the preservation
> and restoration of health. In addition, doctors of chiropractic recog-
> nize the value and responsibility of working in cooperation with other
> health care practitioners when in the best interest of the patient.[15]

Chiropractors have historically emphasized the intimate relations
between structure and function, the preeminent mediating role of the
nervous system, and the need for restoration and maintenance of structural and functional balance of the spine and musculoskeletal system.
From this perspective, balance is the key and the presence or absence of
pain is incidental.

For patients, however, pain is almost always the primary concern. The public identifies chiropractors as musculoskeletal specialists and the profession's reputation is largely based on chiropractors' ability to help people with physical pain. The differences between the public's perception of chiropractic and the self-perception and self-definition of chiropractors are a source of ongoing discussion within the profession. A brief review of the fundamentals of the chiropractic worldview can offer helpful context for understanding the ways chiropractors define their role.

Common Domain Principles

Chiropractors trace their philosophical roots to principles shared with other natural healing arts. Basic principles of natural healing, which have been part of chiropractic from the beginning and are incorporated into the curricula at chiropractic training institutions, include the following:

1. Humans possess an innate healing potential, an inner wisdom of the body.
2. Maximally accessing this healing system is the goal of the healing arts.
3. Addressing the cause of an illness should take precedence over suppressing its surface manifestations in most cases.
4. Pharmaceutical suppression of symptoms can sometimes compromise and diminish the body's ability to heal itself.
5. Natural, nonpharmaceutical measures (including chiropractic spinal adjustments) should generally be an approach of first resort, not last.
6. A balanced, natural diet is crucial to good health.
7. Regular exercise is essential to proper bodily function.[16]

These principles, endorsed and elucidated by chiropractors for more than a century, are currently recognizable as the foundation of the contemporary wellness paradigm.

Core Chiropractic Principles

In addition to precepts shared with other natural healing arts, the following core theoretical constructs form the underpinning of chiropractic principles:

1. Structure and function exist in intimate relation with one another.
2. Structural distortions can cause functional abnormalities.

3. Vertebral subluxation (spinal joint motion restriction or misalignment causing aberrant nerve signaling) is a significant form of structural distortion and dysfunction and leads to a variety of functional abnormalities.
4. The nervous system occupies a preeminent role in the restoration and maintenance of proper bodily function.
5. Subluxation influences bodily function primarily through neurologic means.
6. The chiropractic adjustment is a specific and definitive method for the correction of the vertebral subluxation.[16]

Chiropractic and Medical Approaches to Pain

In my experience, conventional medical physicians engage in symptom suppression much more than chiropractors and also more frequently assume that the site of a pain is the site of its cause. Thus, knee pain is generally assumed to be a knee problem, shoulder pain is assumed to be a shoulder problem, and so forth. This pain-centered diagnostic logic frequently leads to increasingly sophisticated and invasive diagnostic and therapeutic procedures. For example, if physical examination of the knee fails to define the problem clearly, the knee is radiographed. If the X-ray film fails to offer adequate clarification, magnetic resonance imaging (MRI) of the knee is performed, and in some cases a surgical procedure follows.

As with their allopathic colleagues, chiropractors use diagnostic tools such as radiography and MRI. The point here is not to criticize these useful technologies but to present an alternative diagnostic model. Chiropractors are familiar with patients in whom this entire high-tech diagnostic scenario, as in the previous knee example, is played out, after which the knee problem is discovered to be a compensation for a mechanical disorder in the lower back, a common condition that too often remains outside the medical diagnostic loop.

If the lower back is mechanically dysfunctional and in need of spinal adjustment, this can often place unusual stress on one or both knees. In these patients, medical physicians can and often do spend months or years medicating the knee symptoms or performing surgery, often failing to address the source of the problem.

Regional and Whole-Body Context: Neurology and Biomechanics

The chiropractic approach to musculoskeletal pain involves evaluating the site of pain in a regional and whole-body context. Although shoulder, elbow, and wrist problems can be caused by injuries or pathologies in these areas, pain in and around each of the shoulder, elbow, and wrist joints can also have as its source segmental dysfunction (subluxation) in the cervical spine. Similarly, symptoms in the hip, knee, and ankle can also originate at the site of the pain, but in many cases the source lies in the lumbar spine or sacroiliac joints. Besides pain, other neurologically mediated symptoms (e.g., paresthesia) can have a similar etiology. The need to consider this chain of causation is built into the core of chiropractic training.

Chiropractors intentionally refrain from assuming that the site of a symptom is the site of its cause. They assume instead that *the source of the pain should be sought along the path of the nerves leading to and from the site of the symptoms, or in a kinematic chain of which the symptomatic structures are a part.* Thus, pain in the knee might come from the knee itself, but tracing the nerve pathways between the knee and the spine reveals possible areas of causation in and around the hip, in the deep muscles of the buttocks or pelvis, in the sacroiliac joints, or in the lumbar spine.

Furthermore, if joint dysfunction does exist, for example, at the fourth and fifth lumbar levels, it might have its primary source at L4–L5, or it might represent a compensation for another subluxation elsewhere in the spine, perhaps in the lower or middle thoracic vertebrae or in a mechanical dysfunction of the muscles and joints of the feet. Such an integrative, whole-body approach to structure and function is of great value.

For patients whose presentation includes visceral organ symptoms, chiropractic diagnostic logic includes (once so-called red flag contraindications to manipulation have been ruled out) evaluation of the spine, with particular attention to spinal levels providing autonomic nerve supply to the involved area, as well as consideration of possible nutritional, environmental, and psychological factors.

RESEARCH AND CLINICAL DECISION MAKING

Low Back Pain

Low back pain (LBP) constitutes the majority of chiropractic practice. Accordingly, it has also been the primary focus of chiropractic research, with dozens of clinical trials on manual manipulation. Generally, LBP is divided into acute, subacute, and chronic types. While definitions vary, acute pain is commonly defined as having been present 3 weeks or less; subacute pain, between 3 weeks and 3 months; and chronic pain, longer than 3 months, or more than six episodes in 12 months.

Avoiding chronicity has increasingly emerged as a central focus for chiropractic and all other health disciplines dealing with LBP, leading to a substantially increased focus on reactivation and rehabilitation, with a commensurate decrease in long-term intensive treatment programs relying mainly upon doctor-administered passive care (e.g., manual adjustments and physical therapy). This is a major paradigm shift that now appears well-rooted enough to endure. It is driven in part by research supporting exercise-driven active care for subacute and chronic cases, and in part by diminished willingness on the part of third party payers to reimburse long-term passive care.

Central to this active care model is its requirement for active participation by patients in their own healing and its implicit recognition that too much passive care leads to patient dependency. Some chiropractic practitioners and educators, most notably Craig Liebenson, are recognized as world leaders in this interdisciplinary rehabilitation movement.[17]

Spinal adjustment or manipulation is widely recognized as a valuable therapy for acute LBP. As summarized by Meeker and Haldeman,[3] 43 randomized trials of spinal manipulation for treatment of acute, subacute, and chronic LBP have been published. Thirty favored manipulation over the comparison treatments in at least a subgroup of patients, and the other 13 found no significant differences. None of these LBP studies has shown manipulation to be less effective than a comparison approach, control group or placebo. As noted earlier, consensus panels evaluating the data have consistently placed spinal manipulation on the short list of recommended procedures for acute LBP.

Key Clinical Trials. In an influential trial with more than 700 patients, British orthopedic surgeon T. W. Meade compared chiropractic manipulation with standard hospital outpatient treatment for LBP, which consisted of physical therapy and wearing a corset.[18,19] Patients with low-back pain in whom manipulation is not contraindicated, had long-term benefit from chiropractic in comparison to hospital outpatient management.[18,19] He described the applicability of these findings for primary care physicians as follows:

> Our trial showed that chiropractic is a very effective treatment, more effective than conventional hospital out-patient treatment for low-back pain, particularly in patients who had back pain in the past and who [developed] severe problems. So, in other words, it is most effective in precisely the group of patients that you would like to be able to treat. . . . One of the unexpected findings was that the treatment difference—the benefit of chiropractic over hospital treatment—actually persists for the whole of that three-year period [of the study]. . . . the treatment that the chiropractors give does something that results in a very long-term benefit.[20]

Meade's study was the first large randomized clinical trial to demonstrate substantial short-term and long-term benefits from chiropractic care. Because it dealt with both acute LBP patients and chronic LBP patients, Meade's data support the use of chiropractic care for both populations.

Acute vs. Chronic Low Back Pain. Consensus panels and meta-analyses have not fully resolved the question of whether the literature supports recommending spinal manipulation for both chronic and acute LBP patients. In general, as reflected in the various guidelines cited earlier, strong agreement exists that the literature supports the appropriateness of manipulation for many acute LBP cases, but debate still surrounds chronic LBP. The perceived current insufficiency of data favoring manipulation for chronic LBP has led some reviewers to rate it as "inappropriate" for chronic LBP,[21] although other analysts have found the literature to support the efficacy of manipulation for chronic LBP.[22]

When Shekelle and colleagues[21] rated the "appropriateness" of decisions to initiate manipulative therapy, they deemed manipulation "inappropriate" for all cases of chronic lower back pain. Although this lowered the percentage of cases in which chiropractic was considered appropriate, both Shekelle's group and Micozzi[23] aptly noted that the study offered solid justification for primary care physicians to refer many more of their LBP patients to chiropractors.

Evidence for Manual Methods in Chronic Cases. Seeing that manipulation may be considered "inappropriate" for chronic LBP, physicians and other health practitioners might logically conclude that until further convincing evidence emerges, they should not refer patients with chronic LBP to chiropractors. However, physicians frequently refer chronic LBP patients for physical therapy, based on perceptions that its effectiveness and appropriateness significantly exceed its research documentation.[24] Because a primary care physician's decision about whether and where to refer LBP patients hinges on which treatments are expected to yield the most satisfactory outcomes, a summary of studies on spinal manipulation for chronic LBP may aid the decision-making process.

Besides Meade's work,[18,19] an impressive prospective study of LBP was performed at the University of Saskatchewan hospital orthopedics department by Kirkaldy-Willis, a world-renowned orthopedic surgeon, and Cassidy, a chiropractor who later became the department's research director.[25] The approximately 300 subjects in this study were "totally disabled" by LBP, with pain present for an average of 7 years. All had gone through extensive, unsuccessful medical treatment before participating as research subjects. After 2 to 3 weeks of daily chiropractic adjustments, more than 80% of the patients without spinal stenosis had good to excellent results, reporting substantially decreased pain and increased mobility. After chiropractic treatment, more than 70% were improved to the point of having no work restrictions. Follow-up a year later demonstrated that the changes were long-lasting. Even those with a narrowed spinal canal, a particularly difficult subset, showed a notable response. More than half the patients improved, and about one in five were pain free and on the job 7 months after treatment.

In a randomized trial of 209 patients, Triano and colleagues[26] compared manipulation to education programs for chronic LBP, which they defined as pain lasting 7 weeks or longer, or more than six episodes in 12 months. These investigators found greater improvement in pain and activity tolerance in the manipulation group, noting that immediate benefits from pain relief continued after manipulation, including for the last encounter at the end of the 2-week treatment interval."[26] there appeared to be clinical value to treatment according to a defined plan using manipulation even in LBP exceeding 7 weeks duration. Koes and colleagues[27] compared manipulation to physiotherapy (PT) and treatment by a general practitioner (GP) in a randomized trial of 256 chronic cases that included back and neck pain. Physiotherapy included exercises, massage, heat, electrotherapy, ultrasound, and short-wave diathermy. General practitioner care included medication (analgesics, nonsteroidal anti-inflammatory drugs [NSAIDs]), and advice about posture, rest, and activity. Data indicated that both manipulation and PT were much more effective than GP treatment, with manipulation marginally surpassing PT. This advantage was sustained at 12-month follow-up.

Another randomized trial compared the effects of chiropractic and NSAID treatments, each combined with supervised trunk exercise for 174 chronic LBP patients.[28] Both regimens were found to produce similar and clinically important improvement over time that was considered superior to the expected natural history of long-standing chronic LBP. The manipulation plus trunk-strengthening exercise group showed a sustained reduction in medication use at 1-year follow-up. Also, continuation of exercise during the follow-up year was associated with better outcomes for both groups.

In a study of 115 patients with chronic spinal pain, Giles and Muller[29] compared the effects of medication (NSAID or analgesic not previously ineffective for the individual patient), spinal manipulation, and acupuncture. Treating practitioners were told to follow their normal office procedures to determine whether manipulation or acupuncture was appropriate, as well as which manipulative procedures or acupuncture points should be used. Electrical stimulation was not applied to the acupuncture needles. The highest proportion of early recovery (asymptomatic status) was found for manipulation (27.3%), followed by acupuncture (9.4%) and medication (5%). Manipulation also outperformed the other interventions on a variety of other measures, with one notable exception: acupuncture achieved the best results on the visual analog scale measurement for neck pain improvement (50% for acupuncture vs. 42% for manipulation).

A recent systematic review on manual therapies for low back and neck pain by Bronfort et al[30] concluded that spinal manipulation has demonstrated effectiveness for patients with LBP categorized as acute, chronic, and combined acute/chronic.

Preventing Acute Cases From Becoming Chronic. Because the prognosis for patients with acute LBP is better than for those with chronic pain, high priority must be accorded to preventing acute cases from becoming chronic. However, a key factor leads physicians to minimize this concern: conventional wisdom that 90% of LBP resolves on its own within a short time. Findings published in the *British Medical Journal* call for urgent reassessment of the assumption that most LBP patients seen by primary care physicians attain resolution of their complaints. Contrary to prevailing assumptions, Croft and colleagues[31] found that *at 3-month and 12-month follow-up, only 21% and 25%, respectively, had completely recovered in terms of pain and disability.* However, only 8% continued to consult their physician for longer than 3 months. In other words, the oft-quoted 90% figure actually applied to the number of patients who stopped seeing their physicians, not the number who recovered from their back pain. Their dissatisfaction with conventional medical care was also reminiscent of earlier studies.[32,33] Croft stated the following:

> We should stop characterizing low-back pain in terms of a multiplicity of acute problems, most of which get better, and a small number of chronic long-term problems. Low back pain should be viewed as a chronic problem with an untidy pattern of grumbling symptoms and periods of relative freedom from pain and disability interspersed with acute episodes, exacerbations and recurrences. This takes account of two consistent observations about low-back pain: firstly, a previous episode of low-back pain is the strongest risk factor for a new episode, and, secondly, by the age of 30 years almost half the population will have experienced a substantial episode of low-back pain. These figures simply do not fit with claims that 90 percent of episodes of low-back pain end in complete recovery.[32(p33)]

The patients in Croft's study were not referred for manual manipulation, and most developed chronic LBP. Based on the Agency for Healthcare Policy and Research (AHCPR) guidelines,[8] which emphasize the functionally restorative qualities of manipulation, it seems reasonable to expect that early chiropractic adjustments could have prevented this progression in many patients. Recall that follow-up in both the Meade (1 year and 3 year) and the Kirkaldy-Willis (1 year) studies showed that the beneficial effect of manipulation was sustained for extended periods.[18,19,25] The decision not to refer patients to chiropractors may mean that many LBP patients will develop long-standing problems that could have been avoided.

Low Back Pain Patients With Leg Pain. Differential diagnosis is crucial for cases in which LBP radiates into the leg. Specifically, motor, sensory, and reflex testing should be used to screen for signs of radicular syndromes and cauda equina syndrome. However, a British study of primary care practitioners found that a majority of these physicians do not routinely examine for muscle weakness or sensation, and 27% do not regularly check reflexes.[34] Such factors play a central role in determining which patients should be referred directly for surgical consultation and which should be referred for manual manipulation. Chiropractic training places strong emphasis on conducting a proper neurologic examination on each patient's first visit, with appropriate follow-up evaluations throughout the course of care.

The AHCPR guidelines state that manipulation is appropriate for acute LBP cases that include nonradicular pain radiating into the lower extremity.[34] in cases where radicular signs such as muscle weakness or decreased reflex response are present, however, some evidence suggests that chiropractic can yield beneficial results. In a series of 424 consecutive cases, Cox and Feller[35] reported that 83% of 331 lumbar disc syndrome patients completing care (13% of whom had previous low back surgeries) had good to excellent results. ("Excellent" was defined as >90% relief of pain and return to work with no further care required, and "good" as 75% relief of pain, return to work, with periodic manipulation or analgesia required). There was a median of 11 treatments and 27 days to attain maximal improvement.

BenEliyahu[36] followed 27 patients receiving chiropractic care for cervical and lumbar disc herniations, the majority being lumbar cases. Pretreatment and posttreatment MRI studies were performed; 80% of the patients had a good clinical outcome, and 63% of the post-MRI studies showed herniations either reduced in size or completely resorbed.

In a study of 14 patients with lumbar disc herniation, Cassidy and colleagues[37] reported that all but one obtained significant clinical improvement and relief of pain after a 2- to 3-week regimen of daily side-posture manipulation of the lumbar spine, directed toward improving spinal mobility. All patients received computed tomography (CT) scans before and 3 months after treatment. In most patients the CT appearance of the disc herniation remained unchanged after successful treatment, although five showed a small decrease in the size of the herniation, and one patient showed a large decrease.

Neck Pain

Chiropractors have treated chronic and acute neck pain and related upper extremity symptoms since the profession's beginnings, but research specifically addressing this subject is far less extensive than for LBP. This is also the case for nonmanual methods of treating neck pain (e.g., medications). Meeker and Haldeman[3] found that of the 11 randomized controlled trials of spinal manipulation for neck pain conducted, four demonstrated positive findings, seven equivocal findings, and none negative.

A more recent review of the literature on manual methods for chronic neck pain[38] analyzed 16 trials on manual therapies for chronic neck pain not due to whiplash (9 for manipulation, 5 for mobilization, and 2 for other manual methods). The investigators found moderate- to high-quality evidence that subjects with chronic neck pain not due to whiplash and without arm pain and headaches show clinically important improvements from a course of spinal manipulation or mobilization at 6, 12, and up to 104 weeks posttreatment. They also found that current evidence does not support a similar level of benefit from massage.

An earlier review by Vernon et al on acute neck pain not due to whiplash[39] found only three relevant clinical trials in the literature. There was limited evidence of the benefit of spinal manipulation and transcutaneous electrical nerve stimulation. The authors remarked on the lack of adequate research in this area.

Studies on spinal manipulation and manual therapies for whiplash are few and far between. Again, it is worth noting that the same holds true for nonmanual methods. A recent review[40] found only two primary studies and concluded that there is insufficient evidence at this time to support the efficacy of manipulation for whiplash.

Application in Clinical Practice. All practitioners who treat musculoskeletal conditions function within empirical traditions that preceded by many years the development of RCT-based clinical research. Recognizing that patients in pain cannot wait years or decades for definitive conclusions to be reached by researchers, and that the development of best practices recommendations requires thoughtful, integrative evaluation of available research and clinical experience, an increasingly well-accepted approach is to form consensus panels of recognized experts in the field to develop guidelines.

RAND released such a report on manipulation and mobilization of the cervical spine, involving a literature review and a multi-disciplinary panel appropriateness study for cervical spine, headache, and upper extremity disorders.[41] RAND's cervical spine literature review suggested that short-term pain relief and enhancement of the range of motion might be accomplished by manipulation or mobilization in the treatment of subacute or chronic neck pain; acute neck pain was deemed to have too little literature to reach any recommendation.

Headache

While chiropractors' treatment of headaches is less well known than their work on back and neck pain, headache is a condition for which manual adjustment (usually of the cervical spine) has been studied and found to be effective.

The International Headache Society (IHS) classifies benign headaches into three major groups—tension-type, cervicogenic, and migraine. While a headache from any category can be quite painful, migraines are generally the most severe and disabling while tension-type headaches are the mildest.

Tension-Type Headache. Among the most noteworthy chiropractic research to emerge from the United States is the work on headaches conducted in the 1990s by Boline and colleagues at Northwestern College of Chiropractic in Minnesota.[42] These investigators found chiropractic to be more effective than the prescription medication amitriptyline for long-term relief of tension-type headache pain.

During the treatment phase of the trial, pain relief among those treated with medication was comparable to the chiropractic group. revealingly, however, the chiropractic patients maintained their levels of improvement after treatment was discontinued, whereas those taking medication returned to pretreatment status in an average of 4 weeks after its discontinuation.[22,43,44] This strongly implies that while medication suppressed the symptoms, chiropractic addressed the problem at a more causal level.

It is noteworthy that the Boline et al study was rated the highest in quality of all trials compared in three independent systematic literature reviews.

Chiropractic treatment of tension headaches is supported by two other randomized controlled trials.[45,46] High-velocity thrusting did not seem to confer additional benefits upon patients given massage and trigger-point (TP) therapy, as shown in a trial by Bove and Nilsson.[47] Proper interpretation of this study requires consideration of the fact that *chiropractors typically utilize both interventions* (manipulative thrust and massage/TP therapy) in treating headache patients. Both groups of patients showed significant improvements over baseline values in all the outcome measures observed, but because the outcomes for the two groups did not differ significantly from each other, physicians perusing the literature might inaccurately conclude that no benefit was conferred. The danger of misinterpretation arises when chiropractic care is equated with only one of its elements, high-velocity manipulation.

Cervicogenic Headache. The research literature on manipulation for cervicogenic headache is supportive. In comparing patient groups given either high-velocity cervical spinal adjustments or low-level laser treatments as a nontherapeutic control, Nilsson[48] observed improvements of the manipulated group in terms of pain experienced, headache hours per day, and need for less analgesic medication to alleviate discomfort. Both the control and experimental groups had also received massage. Nilsson's investigation demonstrates the importance of employing large enough groups to achieve statistical significance, since his own earlier report had shown a statistically insignificant tendency toward improvement because the number of subjects was too small.[49]

Migraines and Unclassified Headaches

Using a very similar design to that utilized in investigations of chiropractic treatment of tension headache,[50] Nelson's group at Northwestern College of Chiropractic observed comparable results in his clinical trial involving patients with migraine headache. There was no advantage to combining amitriptyline and spinal adjustment for treatment. As was the case in the Boline et al tension headache study, clinically important improvements were observed in all three study groups, but significant differences emerged during the follow-up period—with reductions of the headache index amounting to 24% for the amitriptyline group, 42% for chiropractic adjustments, and 25% for the combined group. In a later study comparing manipulation to detuned ultrasound for treating migraine patients, Tuchin et al reported statistically significant improvements from manipulation in headache frequency, duration, disability, and level of medication use.[51]

Some headache research involves unclassified headache (headaches other than tension, migraine, and cervicogenic). In an examination of 100 patients with chronic headaches treated by manipulation, Turk and Ratkolb[52] demonstrated an absence of headaches in 25% and an improvement in 40% of the patients 6 months after completing treatment. The remaining 35% reported improvement that lasted for approximately 1 month. Comparing cold pack treatment with mobilization, Jensen showed a reduction of posttraumatic headache pain by 43% in the manual therapy population compared to the cold therapy group at 2 weeks following treatment.[53]

The Duke Headache Evidence Report. The Agency for Health Research and Quality began in 1994 a process of systematic review of the literature on headaches as part of its ongoing process of guidelines development, which had included the low back guidelines mentioned earlier. However, funding cuts to the agency eliminated all future guidelines development and stopped work on all pending guidelines. The work of the AHCPR multidisciplinary committee charged with performing the literature evaluation and developing ratings of the evidence was ultimately sent to the Duke Center for Health Policy Research and Education, which later produced a report[54] based on the work begun by AHCPR.

Among the physical interventions reviewed in this report were cervical spine manipulation; low-force manual techniques such as cranial sacral therapy, massage (including trigger point release); mobilization; stretching; heat therapy; ultrasound; transcutaneous electrical nerve stimulation (TENS); surgery; and exercise. Among the behavioral interventions reviewed were relaxation, biofeedback, cognitive-behavioral (stress management) therapy, and hypnosis.

The final report concluded that nonpharmacological treatments (including manual manipulation) are of growing importance and, that if they are effective and available, they may be the first choice for most patients.[54]

Extremity Pain

Repetitive Stress Disorders Research. Manipulation of the musculoskeletal system for treatment of pain and reduced motion is not limited to the back or neck. Over the past decade, the extremities have become increasingly recognized as an area responsive to manual therapy. Compression of the median nerve at the wrist may lead carpal tunnel syndrome (CTS), involving unilateral or bilateral paresthesia in the fingers, with or without pain in the wrist, palm, and/or forearm proximal to the area of compression. One of its major causes is protracted strain on an extended or flexed wrist caused by repetitive stress, often found in the workplace. The rationale for manipulation is to take pressure off the transverse carpal ligament and add carpal adjustments to help decompress the tunnel.

Randomized clinical trials addressing the extremities are few in number but offer some preliminary indications of benefit from manipulation and other manual methods.[55-57] Improvements are comparable to those achieved by the other interventions; manipulation can yield improvement in certain groups of patients,[55] although corticosteroid injections produced more rapid improvements in patients with disorders of the shoulder girdle.

Case control studies supporting chiropractic intervention in the management of CTS suggest that, in 38 subjects, a broad array of dietary, exercise, and manipulative interventions result in statistically significant improvements in several strength measures of up to 25% over pretreatment values;[58] improved objective pain and distress levels were observed in 22 returning subjects to persist for at least 6 months posttreatment.[59]

Manipulation has also been shown to be effective in two case series studies by Benjamin Sucher. The first, involving four patients with CTS, showed both clinical improvement and changes in MRI imaging that revealed that the anteroposterior and transverse dimensions of the carpal canal increased significantly after treatment. Electrical improvement consistent with the clinical recovery was documented by EMG/NCS measurements.[60] Both clinical and electrical improvement were subsequently observed in a larger group of 16 patients with CTS.[61]

Visceral Pain

Although the bulk of recent and current chiropractic research still focuses on musculoskeletal disorders, research on somatovisceral disorders is also underway.

Infantile Colic. In 1999 a breakthrough study in visceral disorders was published in *Journal of Manipulative and Physiological Therapeutics.* This randomized controlled trial by chiropractic and medical investigators at Odense University in Denmark showed chiropractic spinal manipulation to be effective for treating infantile colic.[62] An estimated 22.5% of newborns suffer from colic, a condition marked by prolonged, intense, high-pitched crying. Numerous studies have explored a possible gastrointestinal (GI) etiology, but the cause of colic has long remained a mystery.

Health visitor nurses from the National Health Service recruited 50 participants for this study, whose parents consented to a 2-week trial of either dimethicone or spinal manipulation by a chiropractor. Dimethicone, which decreases foam in the GI tract, is prescribed for colic, even though several controlled studies have shown it to be no better than placebo.[63,64]

The infants in the Wiberg study were 2 to 10 weeks of age and had no symptoms of diseases other than colic. Inclusion criteria included at least one violent crying spell lasting 3 hours or more for at least 5 of the previous 7 days. Mothers of infants in both groups also received counseling and advice on breast-feeding technique, mother's diet, air swallowing, feeding by bottle, burp technique, and other advice normally given to parents by health visitor nurses. The main outcome measure was the percentage of change in the number of hours of infantile colic behavior per day as registered in the parental diary, an instrument with validated reliability.

The 25 infants randomized to the chiropractic group were given a routine case history and a physical examination that included motion palpation of the spinal vertebrae and pelvis. The articulations restricted in movement were manipulated (mobilized) with specific light pressure with the fingertips for up to 2 weeks (three to five sessions) until normal mobility was found in the involved segments.[62] The areas treated were primarily in the upper and middle thoracic regions, the source of sympathetic nerve input to the digestive tract.

The mean daily hours of colic in the chiropractic group were reduced by 66% on day 12, which is virtually identical to the 67% reduction in a previous prospective trial. In contrast, the dimethicone group showed a 38% reduction.

The Wiberg study on infantile colic was the first randomized controlled trial to demonstrate effectiveness of chiropractic manipulation for a disorder generally considered nonmusculoskeletal. Addressing this issue, the authors conclude that their data lead to two possible interpretations; (1) either spinal manipulation is effective in the treatment of the visceral disorder infantile colic or, (2) infantile colic is, in fact a musculoskeletal disorder."[62]

A contrasting view is provided by a study performed under the auspices of a university pediatrics department in Norway.[65] In this study, 86 infants were randomly assigned to chiropractic care or placebo (held for 10 minutes by nurse, rather than given 10-minute visit with chiropractor). In the chiropractic group, adjustments were administered by light fingertip pressure. The methods used to identify involved segments were not described, and no mention was made of which regions were most frequently involved. Both groups experienced substantial decreases in crying, the primary outcome measure; 70% of the chiropractic group improved versus 60% of those held by nurses. However, no statistically significant differences were found between the two groups in terms of the number of hours of crying, or as measured on a five-point improvement scale (from "getting worse" to "completely well"). The researchers concluded that spinal manipulation is no more effective than is placebo in the treatment of infantile colic.

Otitis Media. A pilot study by Fallon, a New York pediatric chiropractor, evaluating chiropractic treatment for children with otitis media demonstrated improved outcomes compared to the natural course of the illness. Using both parental reports and tympanography with a cohort of more than 400 patients, data suggest a positive role for spinal and cranial manipulation in the management of this challenging condition.[66,67]

Dysmenorrhea. Two small controlled clinical trials evaluating the effects of chiropractic adjustment/manipulation for primary dysmenorrhea showed encouraging results, with both pain relief and changes in certain prostaglandin levels noted.[68,69] However, a larger randomized controlled trial failed to demonstrate significant benefits from adjustment/manipulation.[70] Dysmenorrhea may be a condition for which manipulation helps certain individuals but not the majority of patients necessary to attain a statistically significant result.

DIVERSITY OF CHIROPRACTIC STYLES

Among the defining characteristics of chiropractic and other manual healing arts is their diversity of technique.[71] Chiropractic training institutions teach a variety of adjustive approaches for every joint, on the assumption that in healing, one size does not fit all. These methods include the classical thrust maneuvers for which chiropractors are best known, but also a broad spectrum of gentler adjustments, some of which utilize specialized tables or adjusting instruments. For example, the widely utilized flexion-distraction technique utilizes a form of angled traction for lumbar disc syndrome and other low back conditions that has its origins in early 20th-century osteopathy and the similarly popular Activator™ approach utilizes a low-force, spring-loaded adjusting instrument. In general, these alternative approaches were developed by practitioners who found certain patients unresponsive to standard methods, were unwilling to accept failure, and applied their manual or engineering skills to the problem at hand. Other such methods widely utilized by chiropractors today are the Thompson technique that utilizes mechanical "drop pieces" to provide a biomechanical assist and the Graston technique that employs stainless steel instruments for soft tissue therapy.

CHIROPRACTOR'S ROLE BEFORE AND AFTER SURGERY

Chiropractic scope of practice includes neither pharmaceuticals nor surgery. However, many patients who are possible surgical candidates consult chiropractors as their initial point of contact with the health care system. Thus, an important aspect of the chiropractor's role is to evaluate painful conditions that may require surgery.

To properly serve their patients, most chiropractors develop collegial relations with neurosurgeons and orthopedic surgeons in their communities. In a small percentage of cases, if the chiropractic intake examination reveals major abnormalities of motor, reflex, or sensory function indicative of cauda equina syndrome or severe nerve root compression, referral may be immediate. More often, in less severe cases a trial of chiropractic care is attempted for up to a month. If this fails to result in significant improvement, surgical referral follows.

Chiropractors not only play a first-contact triage role in potential surgical cases but also sometimes serve in a treatment capacity in cases where surgery has not helped or has not helped enough. While the specific site of a surgical procedure (e.g., the L5-S1 motor unit) should not be directly thrust upon, it is not uncommon for adjacent areas (e.g., the sacroiliac joints) to require adjustment after a surgical site has healed. Such manual manipulation often provides significant pain relief.

Back and neck pain are not the only conditions to potentially benefit from postsurgical chiropractic intervention. A case report by Browning,[72] though hardly typical, provides a powerful example of chiropractic's potential. This case involved a woman who had undergone an appendectomy, left oophrectomy and partial hysterectomy, three bowel surgeries, and four bladder surgeries over a period of 18 years. These procedures failed to resolve her many complaints related to pelvic organic dysfunction, and she presented to Browning with pelvic pain, rectal bleeding, diarrhea, bladder discomfort, pain on intercourse, and anorgasmy. Browning used flexion-distraction adjustments as his primary treatment. Within 4 weeks, her symptoms had noticeably improved, and there was complete resolution at 30 weeks. Particularly noteworthy in this case was the conspicuous absence of one symptom in particular—LBP.

SAFETY

All health care interventions entail risk, which is best evaluated in relation to other common treatments for similar conditions (i.e., manipulation vs. anti-inflammatory medications for neck pain). Medications with a safety profiles comparable to that of spinal manipulation are considered quite safe. Although minor, temporary soreness after a chiropractic treatment is not unusual, major adverse events resulting from chiropractic treatment are few and infrequent. As a result, chiropractic malpractice insurance premiums are substantially lower than those for medical and osteopathic physicians.

The potential reaction to chiropractic treatment that has raised the greatest concern is cerebrovascular accident, or stroke, following cervical spine manipulation. This occurs so rarely that it is virtually impossible to study other than on a retrospective basis, because the cohort necessary for a prospective study would involve hundreds of thousands of patients.

Lauretti[73] provides an excellent summary of chiropractic safety issues and makes the following key points:

- Every reliable published study estimating the incidence of stroke from cervical adjustment/manipulation agrees that the risk is less than 1 to 3 incidents per 1 million treatments and approximately 1 incident per 100,000 patients.
- Haldeman and colleagues[74] found the rate of stroke to be 1 in 8.06 million office visits, 1 in 5.85 million cervical adjustments, 1 in 1,430 chiropractic practice years, and 1 in 48 chiropractic practice careers.
- NSAIDs, the medications most widely utilized for neck pain and headaches, have an unenviable safety profile[75] that should be considered when evaluating the risks and benefits of potential treatments for these conditions.

Chiropractors' extensive diagnostic training prepares them to identify the signs and symptoms of impending stroke and to recognize their significance. However, some cases of vascular compromise provide no advance warning signs. In situations where a patient on the verge of having a stroke presents to a chiropractor's office (or a beauty parlor, or an athletic event, or any other situation where neck rotation and/or extension is likely to occur), some strokes will occur. Whether causation may accurately be ascribed to chiropractic cervical adjustments has been an area of controversy for many years.

However, a major step toward the resolution of this controversy emerged in a 2008 article by Cassidy and colleagues,[76] in which a team of Canadian investigators performed a population-based, case control and case-crossover study reviewing Ontario health records from 1993 to 2002 (848 strokes in 100 million person years) to determine whether there was any correlation between vertebrobasilar accidents (VBA) and recent visits to a chiropractor.

A previous review of Ontario records by Rothwell and colleagues[77] had found such a correlation, but only for those under age 45. Though Rothwell and colleagues cautioned against attributing causation based on their findings, their 2001 article led to widespread media headlines connecting chiropractic to stroke causation. The new review by Cassidy and colleagues found that the correlation between chiropractic visits and stroke was no larger (it was actually marginally smaller) than the correlation between medical visits and stroke. The authors concluded VBA stroke is a very rare event, that people on the verge of strokes may experience headaches and neck pain, and that there is no evidence of excess risk of VBA stroke associated with chiropractic care compared to primary care.

FUTURE TRENDS IN CHIROPRACTIC AND PAIN MANAGEMENT

The vast majority of chiropractic practice involves treating patients with neuromusculoskeletal pain and treatment of such pain is central to the public's perception of the chiropractor's role in the health care system. It is therefore not surprising that the most significant steps toward chiropractic integration into health care groups and systems have involved becoming joining pain management teams.

The health systems of the United States Department of Defense and Department of Veterans Affairs have developed integrative models over the past decade that may serve as a template for future efforts at integration. Despite initial concerns by some chiropractors that requiring referral from a gatekeeper medical physician would sharply limit the number of patients able to access chiropractic services, the DOD and VA chiropractic programs have generally proved a resounding success. Making chiropractors an integral part of the health care team has in many cases resulted in advances in interprofessional understanding and cooperation, with patients as the prime beneficiaries.

Transplanting this success from the single payer model of military health care to America's far more eclectic private health care system is a significant challenge. The answers will probably take a variety of forms incorporating joint medical-chiropractic teams operating under one roof along with more fully developed referral arrangements among private practitioners of both professions. To the extent that chiropractors become full partners in the health care system, patients will be the ultimate beneficiaries.

REFERENCES

1. Plamondon R. Summary of 1994 ACA annual statistical study. *J Am Chiropr Assoc.* 1995;32(1):57–63.
2. Goldstein M. *The Research Status of Spinal Manipulative Therapy.* Washington, DC: U.S. Government Printing Office; 1975.
3. Meeker WC, Haldeman S. Chiropractic: a profession at the crossroads of mainstream and alternative medicine. *Ann Intern Med.* 2002;136(3):216–227.
4. Meeker W, Lawrence D, Micozzi MS et al. Consensus development on treatment of lower back pain. American Public Health Association, Washington, DC; 2007.
5. Chapman-Smith DA. *The Chiropractic Profession.* Des Moines, IA: NCMIC Group; 2000.
6. Von Kuster T. *Chiropractic health care: a national study of cost of education, service, utilization, number of practicing doctors of chiropractic and other key policy issues.* Washington, DC: Foundation for the Advancement of Chiropractic Tenets and Science; 1980.

7. Eisenberg DM, Davis RB, et al. Trends in alternative medicine use in the United States, 1990–1997: results of a follow-up national survey. *JAMA*. 1998;280(18):1569–1575.

8. Bigos S, Bowyer O, et al. *Acute Lower Back Pain in Adults. Clinical Practice Guideline, Quick Reference Guide Number 14.* Rockville, MD: U.S. Department of Health and Human Services, Public Health Service, Agency for Health Care Policy and Research; 1994.

9. Rosen M. *Back Pain: Report of a Clinical Standards Advisory Group Committee on Back Pain.* London, England; HMSO; 1994.

10. Commission on Alternative Medicine. *Social Departementete: Legitimization for vissa kiropraktorer.* Stockholm, Sweden. 1987;12:13–16.

11. Danish Institute for Health Technology Assessment 1999.

12. Thompson CJ. *Second Report, Medicare Benefits Review Committee.* Canberra, Australia: Commonwealth Government Printer; 1986.

13. Hasselberg PD. *Chiropractic in New Zealand: Report of a Commission of Inquiry.* Wellington, New Zealand:, Government Printer; 1979.

14. Definition of chiropractic. World Federation of Chiropractic; 2001.

15. Association of Chiropractic Colleges, 1996

16. Redwood D. Chiropractic. In: Micozzi MS, ed. *Fundamentals of Complementary and Integrative Medicine.* 3rd ed. New York, NY: Elsevier; 2006:139–163.

17. Liebenson C. *Rehabilitation of the Spine: A Practitioner's Manual.* Baltimore, MD: Lippincott, Williams and Wilkins; 2007.

18. Meade TW, Dyer S, et al. Low back pain of mechanical origin: randomised comparison of chiropractic and hospital outpatient treatment [see comments]. *BMJ*. 1990; 300(6737):1431–1417.

19. Meade TW, Dyer S, et al. Randomised comparison of chiropractic and hospital outpatient management for low back pain: results from extended follow up [see comments]. *BMJ*. 1995;311(7001):349–351.

20. Meade TW. Interview on Canadian Broadcast Corporation. *Chiropractic: A Review of Current Research.* Arlington VA: Foundation for Chiropractic Education and Research; 1992.

21. Shekelle PG, Coulter I, et al. Congruence between decisions to initiate chiropractic spinal manipulation for low back pain and appropriateness criteria in North America [see comments]. *Ann Intern Med.* 1998;129(1):9–17.

22. Bronfort G, Assendelft WJ, et al. Efficacy of spinal manipulation for chronic headache: a systematic review. *J Manipulative Physiol Ther.* 2001;24(7):457–466.

23. Micozzi MS. Complementary care: When is it appropriate? Who will provide it? *Ann Intern Med.* 1998;129:65–66.

24. Cherkin DC, Deyo RA, et al. Physician views about treating low back pain. The results of a national survey. *Spine*. 1995;20(1):1–10.

25. Kirkaldy-Willis W, Cassidy J. Spinal manipulation in the treatment of low back pain. *Can Fam Phys.* 1985;31:535–540.

26. Triano JJ, McGregor M, et al. Manipulative therapy versus education programs in chronic low back pain. *Spine*. 1995;20:948–955.

27. Koes BW, Bouter LM, et al. A blinded randomized clinical trial of manual therapy and physiotherapy for chronic back and neck complaints: physical outcome measures. *J Manipulative Physiol Ther.* 1992;15(1):16–23.

28. Bronfort G, Goldsmith CH, et al. Trunk exercise combined with spinal manipulative or NSAID therapy for chronic low back pain: a randomized, observer-blinded clinical trial. *J Manipulative Physiol Ther.* 1996;19(9):570–582.

29. Giles LG, Muller R. Chronic Spinal Pain: A randomized clinical trial comparing medication, acupuncture, and spinal manipulation. *Spine*. 2003;28(14):1490–1502.

30. Bronfort G, Haas M, et al. Efficacy of spinal manipulation and mobilization for low back pain and neck pain: a systematic review and best evidence synthesis. *Spine J.* 2004;4(3):335–356.

31. Croft PR, Macfarlane GJ, et al. Outcome of low back pain in general practice: a prospective study [see comments]. *BMJ.* 1998;316(7141):1356–1359.

32. Cherkin D, Deyo A, et al. Evaluation of a physician education intervention to improve primary care for low back pain I: impact on physicians. *Spine.* 1991;16(10):1168–1172.

33. Cherkin D, MacCornack FA, et al. Family physicians' views of chiropractors: hostile or hospitable? [see comments]. *Am J Public Health.* 1989;79(5):636–637.

34. Little P, Smith L, et al. General practitioners' management of acute back pain: a survey of reported practice compared with clinical guidelines. *BMJ.* 1996;312:485–488.

35. Cox JM, Feller JA. Chiropractic treatment of low back pain: a multicenter descriptive analysis of presentation and outcome in 424 consecutive cases. *JNMS: Journal of the Neuromusculoskeletal System.* 1994;2:178–190.

36. BenEliyahu DJ Magnetic resonance imaging and clinical follow-up: study of 27 patients receiving chiropractic care for cervical and lumbar disc herniations [see comments]. *J Manipulative Physiol Ther.* 1996;19(9):597–606.

37. Cassidy JD, Thiel HW, et al. Side posture manipulation for lumbar intervertebral disk herniation [see comments]. *J Manipulative Physiol Ther.* 1993;16(2):96–103.

38. Vernon H, Humphreys K, et al. Chronic mechanical neck pain in adults treated by manual therapy: a systematic review of change scores in randomized clinical trials. *J Manipulative Physiol Ther.* 2007;30(3):215–227.

39. Vernon HT, Humphreys BK, Hagino CA. A systematic review of conservative treatments for acute neck pain not due to whiplash. *J Manipulative Physiol Ther.* 2005;28(6): 443–448.

40. Martin Saborido CF, Garcia Lizana, et al. Effectiveness of spinal manipulation in treating whiplash injuries. *Aten Primaria.* 2007;39(5):241–246.

41. Coulter I. *The appropriateness of spinal manipulation and mobilization of the cervical spine: Literature review, indications and ratings by a multidisciplinary expert panel,* Santa Monica, CA: RAND, Monograph No. DRU-982-1-CCR; 1995.

42. Boline PD, Kassak K, et al. Spinal manipulation vs. amitriptyline for the treatment of chronic tension-type headaches: a randomized clinical trial. *J Manipulative Physiol Ther.* 1995;18(3):148–154.

43. Hurwitz EL, Aker PD, et al. Manipulation and mobilization of the cervical spine. A systematic review of the literature [see comments]. *Spine.* 1996;21(15):1746–1760.

44. Kjellman GV, Skargren EI, et al. A critical analysis of randomised clinical trials on neck pain and treatment efficacy. A review of the literature. *Scand J Rehabil Med.* 1999;31(3):139–152.

45. Bitterli J, Graf R, et al. [Objective criteria for the evaluation of chiropractic treatment of spondylotic headache (author's transl)]. *Nervenarzt.* 1977;48(5):159–162.

46. Hoyt WH, Shaffer F, et al. Osteopathic manipulation in the treatment of muscle-contraction headache. *J Am Osteopath Assoc.* 1979;78(5):322–325.

47. Bove G, Nilsson N. Spinal manipulation in the treatment of episodic tension-type headache: a randomized controlled trial [see comments]. *JAMA.* 1998;280(18):1576–1579.

48. Nilsson Christensen HW, et al. The effect of spinal manipulation in the treatment of cervicogenic headache. *J Manipulative Physiol Ther.* 1997;20(5):326–330.

49. Nilsson N. A randomized controlled trial of the effect of spinal manipulation in the treatment of cervicogenic headache. *J Manipulative Physiol Ther.* 1995;18(7):435–440.

50. Nelson CF, Bronfort G, et al. The efficacy of spinal manipulation, amitriptyline and the combination of both therapies for the prophylaxis of migraine headache. *J Manipulative Physiol Ther.* 1998;21(8):511–519.

51. Tuchin PJ, Pollard H, et al. A randomized controlled trial of chiropractic spinal manipulative therapy for migraine. *J Manipulative Physiol Ther.* 2000;23(2):91–95.
52. Turk Z, Ratkolb O. Mobilization of the cervical spine in chronic headaches. *Manual Med.* 1987;3:15–17.
53. Jensen IK, Nielsen FF, et al. An open study comparing manual therapy with the use of cold packs in the treatment of post-traumatic headache. *Cephalalgia.* 1990;10:243–250.
54. McCrory DC. *Evidence report: Behavior and physical treatments for tension-type and cervicogenic headaches.* Des Moines, IA: Foundation for Chiropractic Education and Research; 2001.
55. Winters JC, Sobel JS, et al. Comparison of physiotherapy, manipulation, and corticosteroid injection for treating shoulder complaints in general practice: randomised, single blind study. *BMJ.* 1997;314(7090):1320–1325.
56. Davis PT, Hulbert JR. Carpal tunnel syndrome: conservative and nonconservative treatment. A chiropractic physician's perspective. *J Manipulative Physiol Ther.* 1998; 21(5):356–362.
57. Davis PT, Hulbert JR, et al. Comparative efficacy of conservative medical and chiropractic treatments for carpal tunnel syndrome: a randomized clinical trail [see comments]. *J Manipulative Physiol Ther.* 1998;21(5):317–326.
58. Bonebrake AR, Fernandez JE, Marley RJ, Dahalan JB, Kilmer KJ. A treatment for carpal tunnel syndrome: evaluation of objective and subjective measures. *J Manipulative Physiol Ther.* 1990;13(9):507–520.
59. Bonebrake AR, Fernandez JE, Dahalan JB, Marley RJ. A treatment for carpal tunnel syndrome: results of a follow-up study. *J Manipulative Physiol Ther.* 1993;16(3): 125–139.
60. Sucher BM. Myofascial manipulative release of carpal tunnel syndrome. documentation with magnetic resonance imaging. *J Am Osteopath Assoc.* 1993; 93(12): 1273–1278.
61. Sucher BM. Palpatory diagnosis and manipulative management of carpal tunnel syndrome. *J Am Osteopath Assoc.* 1994;94(8): 647–663.
62. Wiberg JM, Nordsteen J, et al. The short-term effect of spinal manipulation in the treatment of infantile colic: a randomized controlled clinical trial with a blinded observer. *J Manipulative Physiol Ther.* 1999;22(8):517–522.
63. Illingworth RS. Infantile colic revisited. *Arch Dis Child.* 1985;60:981–985.
64. Lucassen PL, Assendelft WJ, et al. Effectiveness of treatments for infantile colic: a systematic review. *BMJ.* 1998;316:1563–1569.
65. Olafsdottir E, Forshei S, et al. Randomised controlled trial of infantile colic treated with chiropractic spinal manipulation. *Arch Dis Child.* 2001;84:138–141.
66. Fallon J. The Role of the chiropractic adjustment in the care and treatment of 332 children with otitis media. *J Clin Chiropr Ped.* 1997;2(2):167–183.
67. Fallon J, Edelman MJ. Chiropractic care of 401 children with otitis media: a pilot study. *Altern Ther Health Med.* 1998;4(2):93.
68. Thomasen PR, Fisher BL, et al. Effectiveness of spinal manipulative therapy in treatment of primary dysmenorrhea: a pilot study. *J Manip Physiol Ther.* 1979;2:140–145.
69. Kokjohn K, Schmid DM, et al. The effect of spinal manipulation on pain and prostaglandin levels in women with primary dysmenorrhea [see comments]. *J Manipulative Physiol Ther.* 1992;15(5):279–285.
70. Hondras MA, Long CR, et al. Spinal manipulative therapy versus a low force mimic maneuver for women with primary dysmenorrhea: a randomized, observer-blinded, clinical trial. *Pain.* 1999;81(1–2):105–114.
71. Nelson CD, McMillin DL, et al. Manual healing diversity and other challenges to chiropractic integration. *J Manipulative Physiol Ther.* 2000;23(3):202–207.

Chiropractic 199

72. Browning JE. Pelvic pain and organic dysfunction in a patient with low back pain: response to distractive manipulation: a case presentation. *J Manipulative Physiol Ther.* 1987;10(3):116–121.
73. Lauretti WJ. The comparative safety of chiropractic. In: Redwood D, Cleveland CS, eds. *Fundamentals of Chiropractic.* St. Louis, MO: Mosby; 2003.
74. Haldeman S, Carey P, et al. Arterial dissections following cervical manipulation: the chiropractic experience. *CMAJ.* 2001;165(7):905–906.
75. Gabriel SE, Jaakkimainen L, Bombardier C. Risk for serious gastrointestinal complications related to use of nonsteroidal anti-inflammatory drugs: a meta-analysis. *Ann Int Med.* 1991;115:787–796.
76. Cassidy JD, Boyle E, Cote P, et al. Risk of vertebrobasilar stroke and chiropractic care: results of a population-based case-control and case-crossover study. *Spine.* 2008;33(4S): S176–S183.
77. Rothwell DM, Bondy SJ, Williams JI. Chiropractic manipulation and stroke: a population-based case-control study. *Stroke.* 2001;32(5):1054–1060.

CHAPTER 11

Reflexology

Donald Bisson

Reflexology is a focused pressure technique, usually directed at the feet or hands. It is based on the premise that there are zones and reflexes in different parts of the body that correspond to all organs of the body.[1] Stimulation of these reflex areas assists the body to correct, strengthen and reinforce itself by returning to a state of homeostasis. In Asian cultures, some reflexologists also use electrical or mechanical devices; however, these approaches may be discouraged or banned in North America.

The oldest documentation of the use of reflexology is found in Egypt, with an ancient Egyptian papyrus depicting medical practitioners treating the hands and feet of their patients in approximately 2500 B.C.[2] Dr. William H. Fitzgerald, MD, (1872–1942) is credited with being a founder of modern reflexology.[3] His studies brought about the development and practice of reflexology in the United States.

Dr. Fitzgerald's studies found that pressure applied in the nose, mouth, throat, tongue, hands, feet, joints, and so forth, deadened definite areas of sensation and relieved pain. These findings led to the development of *Zone Therapy*. In the early years, Dr. Fitzgerald worked mainly on the hands. Later, the feet became very popular as a site for treatment, and over the years, hand reflexology was not used very much. In his book on zone therapy in 1917, Dr. Fitzgerald spoke about working on the palmar surface of the hand for any pains in the back of the body, and working on the dorsal aspect of the hands and fingers for any problems on the anterior part of the body. The distal joints were squeezed, then the medial, and then the proximal joints by clasping the hands.[4] Dr. Fitzgerald claimed to relieve pain in individuals by applying pressure to their hands and feet.

Dr. Joe Shelby Riley, MD, was taught zone therapy by Dr. Fitzgerald. Dr. Riley carried the techniques out to finer points, making the first detailed diagrams and drawings of the reflex points located on the feet and hands.[5]

In this chapter, reflexology as an alternative medical therapy is described, and the experiences with this technique to treat pain and neurological diseases is reviewed.

THEORY

Reflexology is based on the premise that there are zones and reflexes in different parts of the body that correspond to all parts, glands, and organs of the entire body. Manipulating specific reflexes removes stress, activating a parasympathetic response to enable the blockages to be released by a physiological change in the body. With stress removed and circulation enhanced, the body is allowed to return to a state of homeostasis.[1]

Conventional Zone Theory

Conventional zone theory (CZT) is the foundation of hand and foot reflexology. An understanding of the CZT and its relationship to the body is essential to understanding reflexology and its applications.[1,6,7]

Zones are a system for organizing relations between various parts, glands, and organs of the body and of the reflexes. There are 10 equal longitudinal or vertical zones running the length of the body from the tips of the toes and the tips of the fingers to the top of the head. From the dividing centerline of the body, there are five zones on the right side of the body and five zones on the left side. These zones are numbered 1 to 5 from the medial side (inside) to the lateral side (outside). Each finger and toe falls into one of the five zones, for example, the left thumb is in the same zone as the left big toe, Zone 1.

The reflexes are considered to pass all the way through the body within the same zones. The same reflex, for example, can be found on the front and also on the back of the body, and on the top and on the bottom of the hand or foot. This is the three-dimensional aspect of the zones.

Reflexology zones are not to be confused with acupuncture and acupressure meridians.

Pressure applied to any part of a zone will affect the entire zone. Every part, gland, or organ of the body represented in a particular zone can be stimulated by working any reflex in that same zone. This concept is the foundation of zone theory and reflexology.

In addition to the longitudinal zones of CZT, reflexology also uses the transverse zones (horizontal zones) on the body and feet or hands. The purpose is to help fix the image of the body by mapping it onto the hands or feet in a proper perspective and location. Four transverse zone lines are commonly used: transverse pelvic line, transverse waistline, transverse diaphragm line, and transverse neck line. These transverse zone lines create five areas: pelvic area, lower abdominal area, upper abdominal area, thoracic area, and the head area.

Internal Organs and the Three-Dimensional Body

It is important to remember that internal organs lay on top, over, behind, between and against each other in every possible configuration. The reflexes on the hands and feet corresponding to the parts, organs and glands, overlap as well. For example, the kidney reflexes on the foot chart (Figure 11.1) or hand chart (Figure 11.2) overlap with many other reflexes just as the kidneys overlap other organs and parts of the body when viewed from the back or the front.

Exception to the Zone Theory

The basic concept of the CZT is that the right foot or hand represents the right side of the body, and the left foot or hand, the left side. However, within the central nervous system, the right half of the brain controls the left side of the body and vice versa. In any disorders that affect the brain or the central nervous system, a reflexologist will emphasize the reflexes or areas of the disorder on the opposite hand or foot.[1] For example, the brain reflexes will be worked on the left foot or hand for strokes that caused paralysis on the right side of the body.

Zone Related Referral Areas

It is a common assumption that the hands and feet are the only areas to which reflexology can be applied. However, *there are reflexes throughout the 10 zones of the body,* and they may present unlikely relations within these zones.[7] For example, there is a zonal relationship between the eyes and the kidneys because both lie in the same zone. Working the kidney reflexes can affect the eyes.

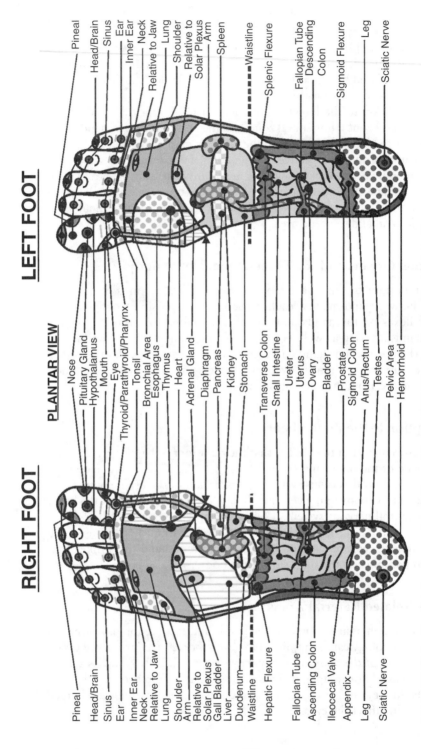

FIGURE 11.1 Foot reflexology chart. Copyright © 1999–Version 2.6 by Donald A. Bisson.

RIGHT FOOT

PLANTAR VIEW

LEFT FOOT

Right foot labels:
Pineal
Head/Brain
Sinus
Ear
Inner Ear
Neck
Relative to Jaw
Lung
Shoulder
Arm
Relative to Solar Plexus
Gall Bladder
Liver
Duodenum
Waistline
Hepatic Flexure
Fallopian Tube
Ascending Colon
Ileocecal Valve
Appendix
Leg
Sciatic Nerve

Center labels:
Nose
Pituitary Gland
Hypothalamus
Mouth
Eye
Thyroid/Parathyroid/Pharynx
Tonsil
Bronchial Area
Esophagus
Thymus
Heart
Adrenal Gland
Diaphragm
Pancreas
Kidney
Stomach
Transverse Colon
Small Intestine
Ureter
Uterus
Ovary
Bladder
Prostate
Sigmoid Colon
Anus/Rectum
Testes
Pelvic Area
Hemorrhoid

Left foot labels:
Pineal
Head/Brain
Sinus
Ear
Inner Ear
Neck
Relative to Jaw
Lung
Shoulder
Relative to Solar Plexus
Arm
Spleen
Waistline
Splenic Flexure
Fallopian Tube
Descending Colon
Sigmoid Flexure
Leg
Sciatic Nerve

204

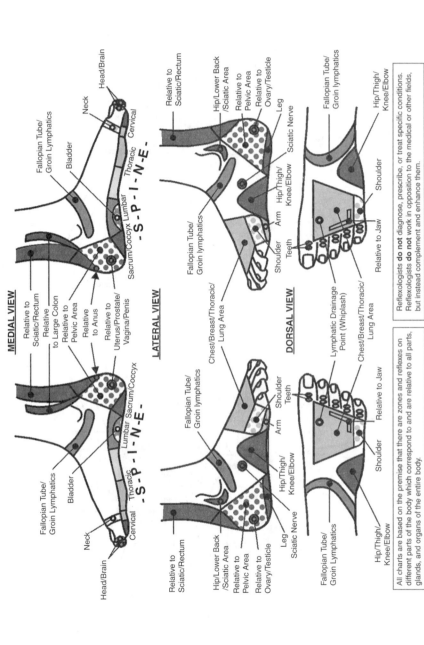

FIGURE 11.1 (Continued)

205

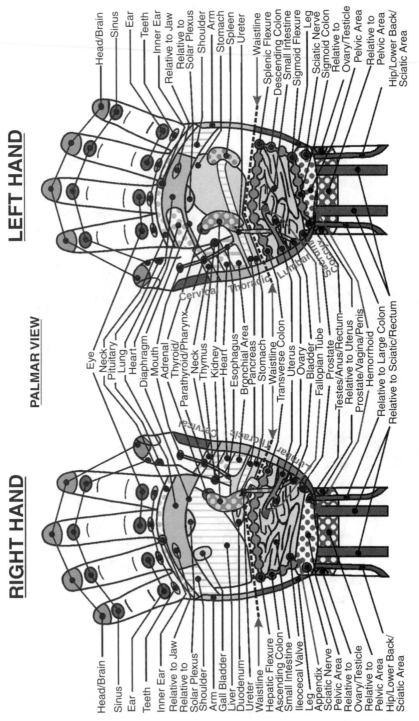

RIGHT HAND

PALMAR VIEW

LEFT HAND

Left hand labels (top, left to right):
Head/Brain — Sinus — Ear — Teeth — Inner Ear — Relative to Jaw — Relative to Solar Plexus — Shoulder — Arm — Stomach — Spleen — Ureter — Waistline — Splenic Flexure — Descending Colon — Small Intestine — Sigmoid Flexure — Leg — Sciatic Nerve — Sigmoid Colon — Relative to Ovary/Testicle — Pelvic Area — Relative to Pelvic Area — Hip/Lower Back/Sciatic Area

Center labels:
Eye — Neck — Pituitary — Lung — Heart — Diaphragm — Mouth — Adrenal — Thyroid/Parathyroid/Pharynx — Neck — Thymus — Kidney — Heart — Esophagus — Bronchial Area — Pancreas — Stomach — Waistline — Transverse Colon — Uterus — Ovary — Bladder — Fallopian Tube — Prostate — Testes/Anus/Rectum — Relative to Uterus — Prostate/Vagina/Penis — Hemorrhoid — Relative to Large Colon — Relative to Sciatic/Rectum

Right hand labels (bottom, left to right):
Head/Brain — Sinus — Ear — Teeth — Inner Ear — Relative to Jaw — Relative to Solar Plexus — Shoulder — Arm — Gall Bladder — Liver — Duodenum — Ureter — Waistline — Hepatic Flexure — Ascending Colon — Small Intestine — Ileocecal Valve — Leg — Appendix — Sciatic Nerve — Pelvic Area — Relative to Ovary/Testicle — Relative to Pelvic Area — Hip/Lower Back/Sciatic Area

Spine labels: Cervical — Thoracic — Lumbar — Sacrum — Coccyx

FIGURE 11.2 Hand reflexology chart. Copyright © 2000–Version 2.6 by Donald A. Bisson.

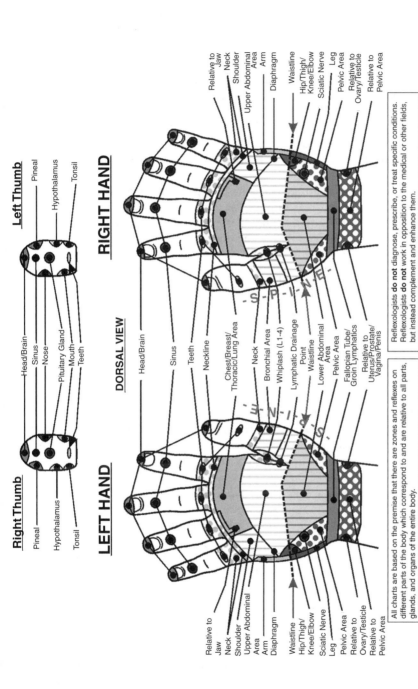

Right Thumb

Pineal
Hypothalamus
Tonsil

Head/Brain
Sinus
Nose
Pituitary Gland
Mouth
Teeth

Left Thumb

Pineal
Hypothalamus
Tonsil

LEFT HAND

DORSAL VIEW

RIGHT HAND

Relative to Jaw
Neck
Shoulder
Upper Abdominal Area
Arm
Diaphragm

Waistline
Hip/Thigh/ Knee/Elbow
Sciatic Nerve

Leg
Pelvic Area
Relative to Ovary/Testicle
Relative to Pelvic Area

Head/Brain
Sinus
Teeth
Neckline
Chest/Breast/ Thoracic/Lung Area
Neck
Bronchial Area
Whiplash (L1-4)
Lymphatic Drainage Point
Waistline
Lower Abdominal Area
Pelvic Area
Fallopian Tube/ Groin Lymphatics
Relative to Uterus/Prostate/ Vagina/Penis

Relative to Jaw
Neck
Shoulder
Upper Abdominal Area
Arm
Diaphragm

Waistline
Hip/Thigh/ Knee/Elbow
Sciatic Nerve
Leg
Pelvic Area
Relative to Ovary/Testicle
Relative to Pelvic Area

Reflexologists **do not** diagnose, prescribe, or treat specific conditions. Reflexologists **do not** work in opposition to the medical or other fields, but instead complement and enhance them.

All charts are based on the premise that there are zones and reflexes on different parts of the body which correspond to and are relative to all parts, glands, and organs of the entire body.

FIGURE 11.2 (Continued)

207

If there is an injury on the foot, the area should be avoided and not be worked. Alternate parts of the body in the same zones should be worked instead. For example, the arm is a reflection of the leg, the hand to the foot, the wrist to the ankle, and so forth. If any part of the arm is injured, the corresponding part of the leg can be worked and vice versa. Common problems such as varicose veins and phlebitis in the legs can be helped by working the same general areas on the arms.

This approach can be used to find other referral areas by identifying in which zone(s) an injury has occurred and tracing it to the referral area. Tenderness in the referral area will usually help the reflexologist find it.

Referral areas can give insights into problem areas by showing the relationships to the areas in the same zone(s) that may be at the root of the problem. For example, a shoulder problem may be due to a hip problem because the shoulder lies in the same zone as the hip.

Negative Feedback Loop

A reflexology session usually begins on the right foot or hand and finishes on the left foot or hand. In addition, the reflexes on both feet and hands are worked from the base of the foot/hand up to the top finishing with the toes or fingers.

To aid the body's self-regulation, a highly complex and integrated communication control system or network is required. This type of network is called a *feedback control loop*. Different networks in the body control diverse functions such as blood carbon dioxide levels, temperature, and heart and respiratory rates. Homeostatic control mechanisms are categorized as *negative* or *positive feedback loops*. Many of the important and numerous homeostatic control mechanisms involve negative feedback loops.

Negative feedback loops are *stabilizing mechanisms*, that is, maintaining homeostasis of blood carbon dioxide (CO_2) concentration. As blood carbon dioxide increases, the respiration increases to permit carbon dioxide to exit the body in increased amounts through expired air. Without this homeostatic mechanism, body carbon dioxide levels rapidly rises to toxic levels, and death results.

The blood circulation loop is from the left side of the body to the right side—fresh oxygenated blood enters the aorta from the left ventricle of the heart and travels to the body, and venous blood with carbon dioxide enters the vena cavae on the right side of the heart. By beginning a reflexology session on the right foot/hand, we are helping to "boost" the loop by pushing venous or deoxygenated blood into the heart/lungs so that fresh oxygenated blood will be available to the body cells. The same reason applies for the direction that we work on the foot/hand—*from the bottom of the foot upward*—to bolster the homeostatic loop.[1,6]

BENEFITS AND SCOPE

Reflexology demonstrates four main benefits: (a) relaxation with the removal of stress; (b) enhanced circulation; (c) assists the body to normalize the metabolism naturally; (d) complements all other healing modalities.

When the reflexes are stimulated, the body's natural electrical energy works along the nervous system to clear any blockages in the corresponding zones.

A reflexology session seems to break up deposits (felt as a sandy or gritty area under the skin), which may interfere with the flow of the body's electrical energy in the nervous system.

Reflexologists do not diagnose medical conditions unless qualified to do so. The only diagnosis made is a tender reflex. Nor are any blockages in any area of the body diagnosed other than in the reflexes. A reflexologist will refer to other qualified health care practitioners when services required are outside the reflexologist's scope of practice.

Similarly, reflexologists do not prescribe medications unless qualified to do so. The therapeutic intervention is limited to *working the reflexes.*

In randomized controlled trials, reflexology has been found to be effective in reducing pain in women with severe premenstrual symptoms[8] and in patients with migraine and tension headaches.[9] It has also demonstrated benefit in alleviating motor, sensory, and urinary symptoms in patients with multiple sclerosis.[10] Recent systematic reviews on the efficacy of reflexology with cancer patients found positive improvements in anxiety and pain.[11–13]

Siev-Ner et al.[10] conducted a randomized controlled trial to compare the effects of reflexology to nonspecific calf massage on 71 multiple sclerosis patients, using paraesthesiae, urinary symptoms, muscle strength, and muscle spasticity as the measurable outcomes. The reflexology group demonstrated significantly increased improvement in urinary and spasticity symptoms compared to those in the massage group, suggesting that reflexology was effective to some extent.[14]

Lafuente et al[15] did a randomized study with 32 headache sufferers to receive sham reflexology and Flunarizine (a migraine drug), or reflexology and a placebo. Over a 2- to 3-month period, reflexology/placebo was shown to be more effective than sham reflexology/Flunarizine, although the result is not statistically significant. It was concluded that reflexology was at least as effective as Flunarizine and may be an appropriate alternative treatment for patients with contraindications to pharmacological treatment.[14]

Reflexology is a useful complementary or alternative therapy to decrease anxiety and pain in patients with cancer.[16]

ADVERSE EFFECTS

The adverse effects of reflexology are minor and may include fatigue (increase in parasympathetic activity), headache, nausea, increased perspiration, and diarrhea.

CREDENTIALING AND TRAINING

No formal or standardized credentialing exists for reflexology in North America. Certification is provided by certain educational institutions specializing in this training. A patient should look for a therapist who is certified and/or registered as a qualified reflexologist by a reputable organization. Also select a reflexologist who presents a professional attitude.

There are many schools of reflexology that can provide adequate training, ranging from 100 to 1000 hours of instruction. Look for a school that is established and if possible, recognized by the local governing body.

In the United States and Canada, there are regulations for practicing reflexology with each state or province (not all) having its own set of educational or licensing requirements.

CONCLUSION

Reflexology is a form of manipulative therapy that has been used successfully to treat various neurological and non-neurological disorders along with pain management. There are many neurological conditions where reflexology can assist in healing, especially in pain management as confirmed by recent studies and publications.

Reflexology impacts the autonomic nervous system, more directly than many other therapies, balancing the parasympathetic nervous system and the sympathetic nervous system, the two subdivisions of the autonomic nervous system that exert opposite effects on the end organs to maintain or restore homeostasis.[17(pp38)]

Many of the benefits from reflexology come from the relief of tension and stress.[12,13] As with many alternative medical approaches, good

scientific studies to confirm its benefit are relatively sparse and more research is required. It does appear to relieve stress, which in turn could
reduce or minimize physical symptoms.[13] At best, reflexology should only
be used as an adjunct to proven therapies in the treatment of disease. The
profession of reflexology also needs to be regulated.

REFERENCES

1. Bisson DA. *101 Foot Reflexology Course.* New Liskeard, Canada: Ontario College of
   Reflexology; 1999.
2. Issel C. *Reflexology: Art, Science & History.* Sacramento, CA: New Frontier Publishing; 1990.
3. Marquardt H. *Reflexotherapy of the Feet.* Stuttgart, Germany: Georg Thieme Verlag;
   2000.
4. Fitzgerald WH, Bowers EF. *Zone Therapy, Relieving Pain At Home.* Columbus, OH:
   I. W. Long, Publisher; 1917.
5. Riley JS. *Zone Reflex.* Santa Cruz, CA: Daglish Health Food Service; 1924 (reprinted
   1942).
6. Bisson DA. *N201 Hand Reflexology Course.* New Liskeard, Canada: Ontario College
   of Reflexology; 2000.
7. Kunz K, Kunz B. *The Complete Guide to Foot Reflexology.* New York, NY: Prentice
   Hall Press; 1987.
8. Oleson T, Flocco W. Randomized controlled study of premenstrual symptoms treated
   with ear, hand and foot reflexology. *Obstet and Gynecol.* 1993;82(6):906–911.
9. Launso L, Brendstrup E, Arnberg S. An exploratory study of reflexological treatment
   for headache. *Alt Thera in Health and Med.* 1999;5(3):57–65.
10. Siev-Ner I, Gamus D, Lerner Geva L, Achiron A. Reflexology treatment relieves symp-
    toms of multiple sclerosis: a randomized controlled study. *Multiple Sclerosis.* 2003;9(4):
    356–361.
11. Solà I, Thompson E, Subirana M, López C, Pascual A. Non-invasive interventions for
    improving well-being and quality of life in patients with lung cancer. *Cochrane Data-
    base Syst Rev.* 2004;18(4):CD004282.
12. Andersen SG, Hodgson NA. Reflexology with nursing home residents: a case vignette.
    The Internet J of Geriatr and Gerontol. 2007;3(2). http://www.ispub.com/ostia/index.
    php?xmlFilePath=journals/ijgg/vol3n2/reflexology.xml. Accessed February 29, 2008.
13. Stephenson N, Dalton JA, (2003). Using reflexology for pain management: a review.
    J of Holistic Nurs. 2003;21:179.
14. Mackareth P, Tiran D, eds. *Clinical Reflexology: A Guide for Health Professionals.*
    Toronto, Canada: Churchill Livingstone; 2002.
15. Lafuente A, et al. Effekt der Reflex zonenbehandlung am Fuß bezuglich der prophylak-
    tischen Behandlung mit Flunarizin bei an Cephalea-Kopfschmerzen leidenden Patieten.
    Erfahrungsheilkunde. 1990;39:713–715.
16. Lacey MD. The effects of foot massage and reflexology on decreasing anxiety, pain,
    and nausea in patients with cancer. *Clin J of Oncol Nurs.* 2002;6(3):183.
17. Crane B. *Reflexology: The Definitive Practitioner's Manual.* Shaftesbury, Dorset,
    England: Element Books; 1997.

PART III

Asian Medical Therapies

CHAPTER 12

Acupuncture

Ravinder Mamtani and William H. Frishman

Acupuncture, an integral modality of Traditional Chinese Medicine (TCM), is performed by stimulating designated points along the energy anatomy of the body. This stimulation is done through the insertion of thin flexible needles, application of electricity, laser or heat, or a combination of these methods. According to Chinese medicine, good health is maintained by a constant flow of energy, called *Chi* or *Qi* in the body. This energy flows through certain pathways or channels called meridians. Appropriate balanced flow of Qi in meridians maintains homeostasis and body functions, and in turn promotes and preserves health. Any imbalance in the flow of energy disrupts body functions thereby creating a disease process. The application of acupuncture at chosen designated points can correct this imbalance. At first encounter with acupuncture, many Western physicians are understandably suspicious because explanations of how the procedure might work are bound up with mystifying concepts formulated 2,000 years ago. However, in light of recent advances in the neurophysiology of acupuncture and research on alternative medicine, suspicion is giving way to acceptance.

Research studies have validated acupuncture's beneficial clinical effects and safety for several conditions such as low back pain, dental pain, and nausea associated with anesthesia, chemotherapy, and pregnancy. The evidence concerning its benefits in the treatment of several other pain problems is encouraging and receiving serious consideration. Investigators have implicated therapeutic mechanisms involving the Melzack-Wall gate control theory of pain and the release of endogenous opioids. This chapter briefly describes traditional aspects of acupuncture and examines the scientific evidence concerning its usefulness in pain management and in the treatment of other neurological problems. It is beyond the scope of this chapter to examine the details and diverse aspects of the art and practice of acupuncture. The discussions on various topics are brief and focused to give the reader an overview of the subject material to stimulate clinical interest in managing chronic health problems associated with pain and other neurological symptoms.

TRADITIONAL ACUPUNCTURE

From the Latin *acus* (needle) and *punctura* (pricking), acupuncture was coined by Jesuit missionaries who returned from China reporting on the use of slender needles for medical treatment.[1] One of the most popular fields of complementary and alternative medicine (CAM), acupuncture accounts for approximately several million treatments given annually in the United States.[2] The demand for acupuncture is strong. Its use is growing and widespread worldwide.

TCM, of which acupuncture is a component, is based on the premise that good health is maintained by a constant flow of energy, called Chi or Qi in the body. This energy flows through certain pathways or channels called meridians. Appropriate balanced flow of Qi in meridians maintains homeostasis and body functions, and this in turns promotes and preserves health. TCM relies on cosmological theories. The first is tao, or the natural law described by fifth century B.C. philosopher Lao Tse. According to this theory, there are two opposing energy fields known as yin and yang. They are interdependent and work together to create homeostasis and balance. They are complementary such that one has no meaning without the other. The yin and yang are also descriptors of various body organs, nature, human experiences, and personal attributes. The heart, lungs, spleen, liver, kidney, and pericardium are grouped under yin, while the small intestine, large intestine, urinary bladder, stomach, and gall bladder are classified as yang organs. A second theory is based on the five elements—wood, fire, earth, metal, and water. Each one of the major organs of the body belongs to one of the five elements. Like the first theory, these five forces are also dynamically interactive; thus, the organs are also interdependent with each other.[3]

When these forces are in balance, Qi flows without obstruction through the meridians of the body. Qi is the energy that nourishes the organs and the body as a whole. This energy is divided into congenital (which is inherited and present since birth) and acquired (which is received from food). The meridians are pathways connecting a yin organ to its corresponding yang organ. Transversely running collateral pathways further interconnect these meridians. This system is comprised of 12 principal channels/meridians, 8 minor (extraordinary) meridians, 15 collateral connections, 12 divergent meridians, and 12 channel sinews, associated with body musculature. Principal meridians are associated and named after various organs of the body. These include urinary bladder (UB), kidney (Ki), heart (He), stomach (St), spleen (Sp), lung (Lu), large intestine (LI), liver (LV), gall bladder (GB), pericardium (PC), also called master of heart (MH), san jiao (SJ), also called triple heater or warmer (TH or TW). The san jiao is the only channel that is not associated with any organ. Along the principal meridians and two of the minor meridians (governing vessel = GV; conception vessel = CV) exist 361 acupuncture points.[4]

TCM and acupuncture diagnoses are based on determining the disturbance in the flow of energy (Qi) through this system, and the goal of treatment is to maintain this flow by keeping the forces in balance.[1] Conditions are classified as yin and yang; excess or deficient; interior or exterior; cold or heat. In traditional Chinese acupuncture, an evaluation includes taking a patient's history and detailed physical exam (appearance, speech quality, odor, local tenderness, tongue diagnosis, and pulse quality). This helps in identifying pathology and patterns of disharmony. The acupuncturist then determines appropriate acupuncture points.

ACUPUNCTURE: AN EVOLVING DISCIPLINE

Acupuncture is a ubiquitous term that refers to needling procedures explained by metaphysical concepts of TCM. In the broadest sense, it also includes acupressure, laser acupuncture, scalp acupuncture, auriculotherapy (ear acupuncture), electrical acupuncture, moxibustion, Korean hand acupuncture, and others.[2] Myofascially based acupuncture involves the assessment of meridians and the needling of carefully palpated tender points representing areas of unbalanced energy.[1]

French energetic acupuncture focuses on bioenergetics, viewing the body as a circulating electrolytic environment that requires needling to the correct blockage of flow. Korean hand acupuncture emphasizes the hands and feet, which are believed to be the origin of all the body's circulating energy. Auricular acupuncture correlates a somatotopic map on the ear with other anatomic regions and is often employed in conjunction with other acupuncture techniques.

As a result of advances in the neurophysiology of pain and acupuncture, the boundary between acupuncture and conventional medicine is constantly changing. For example, a simplified and more empirical Westernized form of acupuncture of local dry needling has been developed recently which is found very effective in the treatment of myofascial pain.[4] Needles used in such a treatment are at the site of the pain or at points in the vicinity of the pain, called trigger points (rather than at distant sites as commonly done in traditional Chinese acupuncture practice). In fact, many scientists and those engaged in acupuncture research think acupuncture (involving needling with or without stimulation) may refer to at-least four different distinct acupuncture therapies with different rationales and efficacies: (a) classical Chinese acupuncture; (b) scientific, evidence-based acupuncture; (c) trigger point acupuncture; and (d) acupuncture with electrical stimulation.[5] Chinese acupuncture is based on the TCM theory, while scientific, trigger point, and electrical acupuncture are based on the mechanism of neurotransmitter-mediated responses and other physiological models.

Acupuncture performed by physicians in a medical setting is considered medical acupuncture. The medical acupuncture approach utilizes conventional and TCM methods of evaluation and management to treat patients. Informing patients about benefits, limitations, and risks consistent with the allopathic standards of care is imperative. An integrative approach to medical acupuncture incorporates the science and art of acupuncture in a conventional medical setting so as to provide the best of both worlds to the patient.

NEUROPHYSIOLOGICAL MECHANISMS

Western medicine has been understandably suspicious of acupuncture because explanations of how the procedure might work are bound up with abstract and mystifying concepts formulated 2,000 years ago. However, in light of advances in understanding the neurophysiology of pain and of scientific explanations of how acupuncture relieves pain, acupuncture is becoming an accepted practice. Further, the idea that the body has an energetic field that influences health is consistent with contemporary concepts in biology and physics, while not yet included in the biomedical model.

Over the past three decades, increasing interest and scientific research have focused on the mechanism and utilization of acupuncture in pain control. Pain can be categorized as nociceptive and neurogenic. Nociceptive pain involves the activation of myelinated (A-delta) and unmyelinated (C-fiber axon) fibers present in the innervation to the skin and deep somatic and visceral structures. In normal, healthy tissue, both types of axons are insensitive to pain; however, in chronic pathologic processes, such as cancer, these axons become the source of extreme pain. Neurogenic pain is due to insults of the central or peripheral nervous system, resulting in altered pain sensation. Sympathetic pain is a type of neuropathic pain involving peripheral nerve injury, which results in severe burning, or causalgia of the region of the nerve. Based on several observations, nociceptive pain appears to be more responsive to acupuncture analgesia than does neurogenic pain.[6] The reasons for this distinction are not clear.

Somatosensory afferent nerves have been demonstrated to be essential for acupuncture pain relief. Procaine injection at acupuncture points, which abolishes afferent transmission from the stimulation site, results in a lack of analgesia from needling.[7,8] This phenomenon is often explained by the gate control theory, which states that nociceptive pain signals carried by small axons are blocked by acupuncture-induced impulses transmitted by large nerve fibers of the same spinal segment.[9] Afferent activity from various acupoints have been shown in experimental models to converge at the preoptic area of the anterior hypothalamus, posterior hypothalamus, the solitary nucleus, and the amygdala.[10]

Extensive review has shown that acupuncture is effective in treating pain.[9] Neurologic mechanisms of acupuncture analgesia are rapidly becoming apparent. Acupuncture activates small myelinated nerve fibers (A-delta or Group III) in skin and muscle, which transmit impulses to the spinal cord and activate centers in the spinal cord, midbrain, and pituitary hypothalamus. At the level of spinal cord level, the neurotransmitters involved in blocking incoming painful stimuli, by inhibiting the substantia gelatinosa (SG) cells, include enkephalins and dynorphins. At the level of the midbrain, two descending mechanisms are involved: the serotoninergic mechanism, which involves the raphe magnus; and the noradrenergic mechanism, which involves the paragigantocellular nucleus. The serotoninergic system releases serotonin that activates cells at the junction of lamina I and II in the spinal cord, releasing enkephalin, which in turn inhibits the SG cells. The noradrenergic mechanism, on the other hand, releases noradrenaline throughout the dorsal horn of the spinal cord, inhibiting the SG cells. Finally, at the level of hypopituitary axis, there is an involvement of generalized hormonal mechanism, which causes release of β-endorphin and adreno-corticotrophic hormone (ACTH).[11] The various mechanisms and/or neurotransmitters involved in acupuncture are listed in Table 12.1.

The role of endorphins in acupuncture analgesia is supported by the finding that naloxone, the opioid antagonist, blocks the effect and may cause hyperalgesia.[12,13] Similarly, lesions of the arcuate nucleus of the hypothalamus, the site of β-endorphin release, block analgesia.[14] In

TABLE 12.1 Neurotransmitter Mechanisms Proposed for Acupuncture

Neurotransmitter/mechanism	Effects
Needling causes A–delta fiber stimulation relaying information to spinal cord, midbrain and hypo-pituitary axis.	Segmental and hetero-segmental generalized effects. Segmental effects occur at the same spinal segment as the needle. The hetero-segmental effects occur through the brainstem and higher centers, and descending inhibition serotoninergic and adrenergic mechanisms.
Opioids- enkapahalin, dynorphins, β-endorphins.	Analgesia. Type of neurotransmitters released vary with the type of acupuncture used. For example, dynorphins release is predominant with high frequency acupuncture.
Gamma-amino butyric acid (GABA)	Pain relief. GABA is released with high-frequency electrical acupuncture.
Serotonin	Analgesia and mood enhancing effect.
Oxytocin	Analgesia and sedation.
Autonomic effects	Increases blood flow by vasodilatation, increases feeling of warmth, lowers blood pressure, and normalizes gastrointestinal motility.
Adrenocorticotrophic hormone	Anti-inflammatory; immunomodulatory effect.
Nerve growth factor	Trophic effect on sensory and autonomic nerves.
Cholecystokinin	Anti-epileptic and may contribute to acupuncture Tolerance.

Adapted from Filshie J. Acupuncture in palliative care. *Eur J Palliative Care.* 2000;7:41–44; and Ernst E. Clinical effectiveness of acupuncture—an overview of systematic review. In: Ernst E, White A, eds. *Acupuncture: A Scientific Appraisal.* Woburn, MA: Butterworth-Heinemann Publishers; 2000:107–127.

regard to monoamines, lesions of the nucleus raphe magnus, site of serotonin and norepinephrine secretion, also abolish the analgesic effect of acupuncture.[8]

Acupuncture also affects other systems and tissues. It affects the cardiovascular system in a variety of ways, and these effects are explained by both central and peripheral effects.[15]

It stimulates the β-endorphinergic system, which influences vaso-motor areas in the brain stem, thereby regulating the sympathetic tone. Acupuncture may also increase vagal (parasympathetic) activity. There is an indication that acupuncture may exert peripheral effects by increasing the release of neuropeptides, such as calcitonin gene-related peptide. Acupuncture has been reported to lower arterial blood pressure and cause vasodilation. Its role in the management of patients with hypertension and angina is under consideration.[16–23]

There are several reports that have documented beneficial effects of acupuncture in the treatment of symptoms such as nausea, asthma, allergies, paralysis, menstrual cramps, and dry mouth (xerostomia). Its mechanisms of action for various reported benefits remain unknown.[11]

MUSCULOSKELETAL AND NEUROLOGICAL CONDITIONS

It is quite common today for people to turn to acupuncture as a last resort to find relief from a chronic, nagging, debilitating pain. One of the difficulties in evaluating acupuncture clinically is that patients often come for acupuncture treatment only after the repeated failure of various mainstream medical treatments. Those suffering from long-standing chronic pain and debilitating conditions are likely users of acupuncture. Acupuncture has benefited many patients in the relief of both acute and chronic pain. Common applications include the following conditions: low back pain, neck pain, osteoarthritis, fibromyalgia, myofascial pain syndrome, headaches/migraine, and reflex sympathetic dystrophy.[6,24,25]

Ten years ago, the Consensus Development Conference Panel on Acupuncture, sponsored by the National Institutes of Health, acknowledged the proven efficacy of acupuncture for postoperative and chemotherapy-induced nausea and vomiting, the nausea of pregnancy, and postoperative dental pain.[24] In addition, acupuncture has been found to be an effective adjuvant treatment for many other conditions. These conditions include, but are not limited to, addiction, headache, stroke rehabilitation, menstrual cramps, carpal tunnel syndrome, and asthma. Electro-acupuncture has been shown to have positive results in treating depression and post-traumatic stress disorder. Beneficial results have been reported for osteoarthritis, as well as some intestinal problems (Table 12.2).

It has been shown that acupuncture is of documented benefit for low back pain, dental pain, fibromyalgia, nausea, headache, and osteoarthritis of knee.[26,27] In contrast, acupuncture has not yet been proven useful for weight reduction, rheumatoid arthritis, and smoking cessation, despite its success in helping to modify addictive behaviors.

TABLE 12.2 Evidence for Acupuncture in Various Conditions[16,24–27]

Conclusively positive	Useful as an adjunct	Inconclusive evidence	Conclusively negative
Chronic back pain	Neck pain	Angina	Weight loss
Post-operative Nausea/vomiting	Headache/ migraine	Hypertension	Smoking cessation
Fibromyalgia	Osteoarthritis	Tinnitus	
Osteoarthritis of knee	Addiction		
	Asthma		
	Stroke		
	Carpal tunnel syndrome		
	Tennis elbow		
	Menstrual cramps		

Cochrane Collaboration Study reviews report positive results for many conditions. In a recent review on low back pain, authors found that acupuncture was better for pain relief than no treatment or sham treatment. Additionally they reported that acupuncture in combination with conventional treatments produced superior results over conventional treatments alone. Dry needling was also found a useful complementary treatment.[28] In another recent review on neck pain, acupuncture was determined to be better for pain relief than sham treatments.[29] The strength of evidence was of moderate level. For other conditions such as lateral elbow pain and shoulder pain, the Cochrane Database of Systematic Review reports show that the evidence is insufficient to draw any conclusions. In examining the studies on epilepsy, the review found that the current evidence does not support acupuncture as a treatment for epilepsy.[30]

TREATMENT PROTOCOLS

Acupuncture is performed with extremely thin, flexible (filiform) needles made of steel alloy. There is nothing special about the needle, it is merely a tool to correct the energy imbalance in the body, and or release neurotransmitters. There is often a brief needle prick sensation as the needle passes through the skin. When placed correctly, the practitioner perceives the *de qi*, or "obtaining qi" effect. As the needle begins to work and effects start to occur the patient may feel numbness, heat, dull aching, or a tingling sensation in the vicinity of the needle insertion. Generally, the needles are left in place for about 15–30 minutes. They may be rotated by the practitioner or stimulated by electricity or heat. Side effects due to acupuncture appear to be minor and transient.

The acupuncture points used in the treatment of pain and neurological problems depend on a number of factors. Examples of such factors include:

1. the TCM and conventional diagnosis of the condition being treated,
2. nature of the problem (e.g., acute or chronic; musculoskeletal or neurogenic; inflammatory or degenerative).
3. site of pain and or other symptoms
4. presence of comorbidity
5. palpation and other examination findings (e.g., presence of tenderness points, if any)

In choosing points, consideration is also given to the properties of channels/meridians and points, and their relations to various tissues. For example, according to TCM, kidney and urinary bladder channels are associated with bone and joints. Therefore, points situated on them are used to treat joint diseases. Additionally there are specific points with special

TABLE 12.3 A Partial List of Common Acupuncture Points to Treat Pain and Neurological Conditions[31]

Property/function	Point(s)
Pain relieving property	LI 4, ST 44, ST 43
Help maintain homeostasis	LI 11, ST 36
Regional effects (including analgesia)	
• Anterior chest	PC 6
• Neck	LU 7
• Lower back	UB 40
Nourishes muscles and tendons	GB 34
Beneficial psychological and neurological effects	GV 20

Note: GV = governing vessel; PC = pericardium; UB = urinary bladder; ST = stomach; GB = gall bladder; Lu = lung; LI = large intestine.

attributes/ properties. Table 12.3 lists some commonly used points in the treatment of various pain producing conditions.[31]

SAFETY

Acupuncture is performed with a view to stimulate specific points in the body. The needle is merely a tool used to correct the energy imbalance in the body (and/or to release neurotransmitters in one biomedical model of mechanism of action). There is often a brief discomfort or a pricking sensation when the needle passes through the skin. As the effects begin to occur, the patient may feel numbness, heat, dull aching, or a tingling sensation at the site or in the vicinity of the needle insertion. Generally, the needles are left in place for only 15 to 30 minutes. They may be rotated by the practitioner or stimulated by electricity. Most side effects associated with acupuncture are minor and transient. They occur in up to 7%–11% of patients, including occasional dizziness, light-headedness, and slight bleeding after needles are withdrawn.[32,33] As with the use of the larger, hollow-point venipuncture needles for blood drawing, fainting can occur. Local infection and other serious side effects, such as lung or liver puncture, are exceedingly rare. Needles used in the United States are sterile and disposable.

Contraindications to acupuncture in patients might include a history of bleeding disorder, the use of anticoagulant medication, and the presence of a pacemaker implant when using electrical acupuncture. Some practitioners regard pregnancy (first trimester) and epilepsy to be contraindications. Caution should be exercised when putting needles in the thorax and abdomen.

RESEARCH CHALLENGES

Despite encouraging results, there are challenges in conducting better quality studies of acupuncture. One reason may be the difficult nature of conducting Western medicine's so-called gold standard—randomized, double-blind trial (designed to test drugs against placebo)—on a treatment modality that is not based on the same empiric system that can not be blinded using a placebo pill. Specific methodological research problems with regard to acupuncture include: (a) it is virtually impossible to construct an inert placebo that parallels the insertion of a needle 2–4 cm into the skin; (b) ascribing relief to acupuncture is not always certain because of the mediation of some nonspecific effects by endogenous opiates; (c) because the location of the insertion and manipulation of the needle are essential to successful acupuncture, the acupuncturist relies on individualizing treatment of each patient, so two subjects with the same diagnosis may be prescribed different puncture sites, confounding standardization of the evaluation results.

CONCLUSION

Although acupuncture is still relatively infrequently in this country today, it is likely to see substantial growth in the future. Despite skepticism concerning the validity of underlying Chi-based theories of acupuncture, many scientists and researchers have a great deal of respect for the observations and overwhelming experience of traditional Chinese doctors who have shown that acupuncture works time and again for a variety of problems. What these ancient and contemporary Chinese doctors observed and continue to see can no longer be questioned.

In light of recent advances in the neurophysiology of acupuncture and an objective attitude toward alternative medicine, suspicion is giving way to acceptance. Evidence documenting its benefit is becoming apparent.

Acupuncture shows promise as one of several options available to patients. Its role has been well documented as an effective modality for pain relief due to a variety of musculoskeletal problems such as low back pain, fibromyalgia, osteoarthritis (of the knee), idiopathic headache, dental pain, and nausea associated with chemotherapy and anesthesia. Additionally, its use as an adjunct in conditions such as neck pain, myofascial pain, addictions, cancer pain, elbow pain, Bell's palsy, shoulder pain, and general osteoarthritis is under active consideration. There is now sufficient evidence that this art of medicine, if appropriately used, can successfully complement conventional care in providing symptomatic assistance and in improving the quality of life for patients having pain and suffering associated with certain chronic pain and neurological conditions.

REFERENCES

1. Ceniceros S, Brown GR. Acupuncture: a review of its history, theories, and indications. *South Med J.* 1998;(91):1121–1125.
2. Ulett GA, Han J, Han S. Traditional and evidence-based acupuncture: history, mechanism, and present status. *South Med J.* 1998(91):1115–1120.
3. Hsu DT. Acupuncture: a review. *Reg Anesth.* 1996(21):361–370.
4. Baldry PE. Principles of trigger point acupuncture. In: Baldry PE, ed. *Acupuncture, Trigger Points and Musculoskeletal Pain.* 3rd ed. Philadelphia, PA, and London, UK: Elsevier Churchill Livingston Publishers; 2005:131–149.

5. Filshie J, White A. *Medical Acupuncture: A Western Scientific Approach.* London: Churchill Livingstone, 1998.
6. Mamtani R. Acupuncture for chronic pain management in the elderly. *Longterm Care Forum.* 1995;5:9–12.
7. Nathan PW. Acupuncture analgesia. *Trends Neurosci.* 1978;7:21–23.
8. Hans JS, Terenius L. Neurochemical basis of acupuncture analgesia. *Ann Rev Pharmacol Toxicol.* 1982;(22):193–220.
9. Melzac R, Wall P. Pain mechanisms: a new theory. *Science.* 1965;(150):971–973.
10. Wu DZ. Acupuncture and neurophysiology. *Clin Neurol Neurosurg.* 1990(92):13–30.
11. Pomeranz B. Scientific basis of acupuncture. In: Stux G, Pomeranz B, eds. *Basics of Acupuncture.* Berlin, Germany: Springer Verlag; 1997:1–72.
12. Pomeranz B, Chiu D. Naloxone blocks acupuncture analgesia and causes hyperalgesia: endorphin is implicated. *Life Sci.* 1976;(19):1757–1762.
13. Mayer DJ, Price DD, Raffi A. Antagonism of acupuncture analgesia in man by the narcotic antagonist naloxone. *Brain Res.* 1977(121):368–372.
14. Wang Q, Mao L, Han JS. The arcuate nucleus of hypothalamus mediates low but not high frequency electroacupuncture in rats. *Brain Res.* 1990(51):60–66.
15. Longhurst JC. Acupuncture's beneficial effects on the cardiovascular system. *Prev Cardiol.* 1998;4:21–33.
16. Meyer DJ. Acupuncture: An evidence-based review of the clinical literature. *Ann Rev Med.* 2000;(51):49–63.
17. Luundeberg T. Peripheral effects of sensory stimulation (acupuncture) in inflammation and ischemia. *Scand J Rehab Med S.* 1993;(29):61–86.
18. Ernst M, Lee MHM. Sympathetic effects of manual and electrical acupuncture of the Tsuanli knee point: comparison with Hoku hand point sympathetic effect. *Exper Neurol.* 1986;(94):1–10.
19. Yao T, Anderson S, Thoren P. Long lasting cardiovascular depression induced by acupuncture like stimulation on the sciatic nerve in unanesthetized spontaneously hypertensive rats. *Brain Res.* 1982;(244):295–303.
20. Goponjuk PJ, Leonova MV. Clinical effectiveness of auricular acupuncture treatment of patients with hypertensive states. *Acupuncture Res.* 1993;11:29–31.
21. Ballegaard S, Jensen G, Pedersen F, et al. Acupuncture in severe, stable angina pectoris: a randomized trial. *Acta Med Scand.* 1986;(220):307–313.
22. Ballegaard S, Pedersen F, Pietersen A, et al. Effects of acupuncture in moderate stable angina pectoris: a controlled study. *J Intern Med.* 1990(227):25–30.
23. Ballegaard S, Meyer CN, Trojaborg W. Acupuncture in angina pectoris: does acupuncture have a specific effect? *J Intern Med.* 1991;(229):357–362.
24. National Institutes of Health. National Institutes of Health Consensus Development Conference Statement. *Acupuncture.* 1997;15(5):1–34.
25. Ernst E. Clinical effectiveness of acupuncture: an overview of systematic review. In: Ernst E, White A, eds. *Acupuncture: A Scientific Appraisal.* Woburn, MA: Butterworth-Heinemann Publishers; 2000:107–127.
26. Haake M, Müller H-H, Schade-Brittinger C, et al. German acupuncture trials (GERAC) for chronic low back pain. *Arch Intern Med.* 2007(167):1892–1898.
27. Ernst E, Pittler MH, Wilder B. Acupuncture. In: Ernst E, Pittler MH, Wilder B, eds. *The Desktop Guide to Complementary and Alternative Medicine: An Evidence Based Approach.* Philadelphia, PA: Mosby Elsevier; 2006:292–297.
28. Furlan AD, van Tulder MW, Cherkin DC, et al. Acupuncture and dry needling for low back pain. *Cochrane Database of Systematic Reviews 2005.* 2005;(1). doi:10.1002/14651858.cd001351.

29. Trinh KV, Graham N, Gross AR, Goldsmith CH, Wang E, Cameron ID, Kay T. Cervical Overview Group. Acupuncture for neck disorders. *Cochrane Database of Systematic Reviews 2006.* 2005;(3). doi:10.1002/14651858.cd004870.

30. Cheuk DKL, Wong V. Acupuncture for epilepsy. *Cochrane Database of Systematic Reviews 2006.* 2006(2). doi:10.1002/14651858.cd005062.

31. Stux G. Acupuncture treatment. In: Stux G, Pomeranz B, eds: *Basics of Acupuncture.* Berlin, Germany: Springer Verlag; 1997:214–271.

32. White A, Hayhoe S, Hart A, Ernst E. Adverse events following acupuncture: prospective survey of 32,000 consultations with doctors and physiotherapists. *BMJ.* 2001; (323):485–486.

33. Melchart D, Weidenhammer W, Streng A, et al. Prospective survey of adverse effects of acupuncture in 97,733 patients. *Arch Intern Med.* 2004;(164):104–105.

CHAPTER 13

Auricular Acupuncture

Terry Oleson

The field of complementary and alternative medicine (CAM) is often recommended for the treatment of chronic pain. The limited ability of opioid and other pain medications to provide sustained pain relief without complications due to tolerance and constipation, as well as legal and regulatory complications, are well known. One CAM modality that is an intriguing area of integrative medicine for pain management is the use of auricular acupuncture. The stimulation of acupoints on the external ear is a style of traditional acupuncture that integrates both Asian and Western approaches to health care. While the earliest clinical records of ear acupuncture points can be traced back to ancient Chinese texts written 2,000 years ago,[1] the style in which auricular acupuncture is currently practiced in modern China and throughout the rest of the world originated with the pioneering discoveries of a French physician in 1957.[2]

Unlike the seemingly random array of acupuncture points on the ear that had been used by ancient Chinese doctors, Dr. Paul Nogier of Lyon, France, proposed that the auricle can be perceived as an inverted fetus. (see Figure 13.1).[3]

Medical conditions associated with the head and face are treated by ear reflex points on the lower regions of the auricle; dysfunctions of the neck and upper back are found on middle regions of the auricle; and pain or pathology in the lower back, leg, and foot are represented on the highest regions of the external ear.[4]

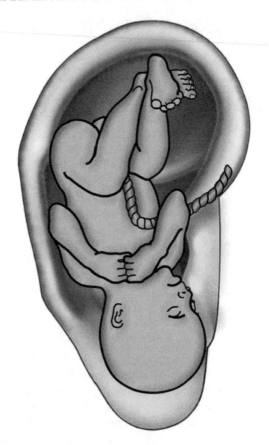

FIGURE 13.1   The concept of an inverted fetus pattern represented on the external ear was first described by Dr. Paul Nogier of Lyon, France.

Nogier's original report of an inverted, somatotopic pattern on the external ear (see Figure 13.2) was first presented at a scientific meeting in France, then distributed internationally by a German publication, next translated into Japanese, and finally printed in China. By 1958, the Nanjing Army Ear Acupuncture Research Team had conducted a clinical survey of 2,000 pain patients who had been successfully treated with auricular acupuncture alone.[1,3]

Scientific assessments of auricular acupuncture have been limited in number, but those studies which have been conducted are statistically supportive. A double blind, controlled evaluation of auricular diagnosis was conducted by the UCLA Pain Management Center in 1980.[5] We

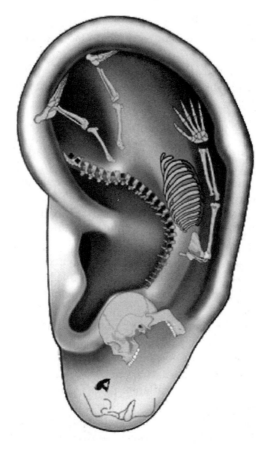

FIGURE 13.2 The curving ridges on the external ear correspond to a somatotopic pattern that shows specific areas of the auricle that represent specific areas of the body.

observed a statistically significant difference in the characteristics of electrically conductive ear points as compared to nonconductive ear points. High conductive ear points corresponded to areas of the body where musculoskeletal pain was present, whereas low conductive ear points represented regions of the body where there was no pain or pathology. The only other systematic study of auricular diagnosis was a double blind evaluation of coronary patients by Saku in Japan.[6] Patients with coronary disorders exhibited higher electrical conductance at auricular points that represent the heart, whereas nearby areas of the ear that correspond to other internal organs exhibited low electrical conductance. Many Western scientists remain skeptical of the concept that the organization of auricular acupoints exhibits a somatotopic arrangement. However, the currency of this concept is gaining ground among a wide-ranging group of practitioners and scientists. A human brain imaging study by Alimi[7] demonstrated greater fMRI responses in the somatic cortex area that represented the hand when activated by acupoint stimulation of the hand area of the auricle.

ENERGETIC AND NEUROPHYSIOLOGICAL THEORIES

Classical acupuncture theory attributes chronic pain and disease to the blockage of energy flow along acupuncture meridians, invisible lines of force extending over the surface of the body. Only the yang acupuncture meridians directly connect to the acupuncture points on the external ear.[1,3] As with body acupuncture, the purported ability of auricular acupoints to alleviate chronic pain and pathology is attributed to the increased flow of qi energetic forces throughout the body. While he was knowledgeable of the Chinese energetic perspective of the human body,[8] Nogier emphasized ontogenetic and neurophysiologic connections between auricular reflex points and the central nervous system to explain the somatotopic relations between auricular regions and body pathology.[2]

In his subsequent writings, Nogier proposed that there are three different territories on the external ear that are related to different types of neural innervation and three different types of embryological tissue.[9]

These three territories of the auricle can be viewed as three concentric rings (see Figure 13.3). The embryologically based endodermal organs are found at the central concha of the ear, the mesodermal tissue that becomes the somatic musculature is represented on the middle ridges of the auricle, and the ectodermal skin and nervous system tissue are represented on the outer ridges of the ear. The central concha of the ear is innervated by the actual vagus nerve and serves as the region for autonomic regulation of visceral pain and pathology associated with internal organs. The surrounding antihelix and antitragus ridges of the ear are innervated by the somatic trigeminal nerve and are used to treat myofascial pain that contributes to headaches, backaches, and body aches in the limbs. The outer rim of the auricle represents central nervous system pathways that affect neuropathic pain, such as peripheral neuropathies and trigeminal neuralgia. The ear lobe, at the bottom of the auricle, corresponds to the brain, whereas the outer helix tail of the auricle represents the spinal cord and spinal nerves (see Figure 13.4).

The remote relief of pain by stimulation of auricular acupuncture points can be conceptually explained by the theory of stimulation produced analgesia. Liebeskind and his colleagues developed this theory to

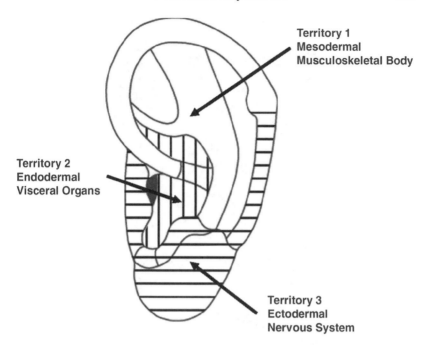

FIGURE 13.3 The external ear can be viewed as three concentric rings, each territory of the auricle corresponding to three embryological regions. The central valley of the external ear represents endodermal visceral disorders, the surrounding middle ridge of the auricle represents mesodermal myofascial tension, and the outer rim of the auricle represents ectodermal neuropathic pain.

explain the pain relieving effects produced by electrical stimulation of deep areas of the brain stem.[10] In addition to the classically known, ascending, pain sensation pathway, there is a descending pain control pathway that travels down the spinal cord to activate pain inhibitory cells in the dorsal horn of the spinal cord.[11] In their gate control theory of pain, Melzack and Wall had previously proposed that an inhibition of sensory input from nociceptive neurons was produced by sensory input from tactile neurons through spinal inhibitory interneurons. Melzack and Wall further allowed that supra-spinal gates in the brain could produce descending inhibition of the ascending pain messages.[12] Basbaum and Fields showed that lesions in the descending, dorsolateral tract in the spinal cord blocked behavioral analgesia from deep brain stimulation and have also been shown to block acupuncture analgesia.[13]

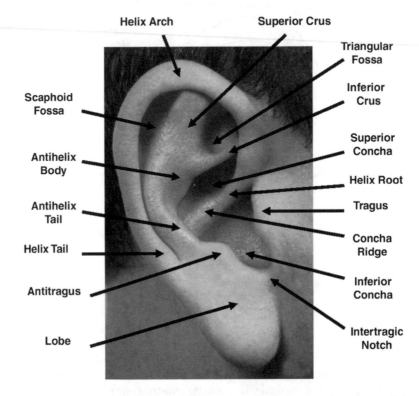

FIGURE 13.4   Nomenclature for the specific anatomical regions of the external ear that distinguish different auricular structures associated with different body areas.

A different, but complementary, perspective to the theory that acupuncture analgesia is based upon neurophysiological reflexes is suggested by the role of endorphin hormones. Both body acupuncture and auricular acupuncture have been found to raise serum endorphin levels, and both types of acupuncture analgesia are blocked by the opiate antagonist naloxone.[14–18] Animal research by Pert showed that 7 Hz auricular electrical stimulation through needles inserted into the concha of the rat produced an elevation of hot plate threshold, which was reversed by naloxone.[19] The behavioral analgesia to auricular electroacupuncture was accompanied by a 60% increase in radioreceptor activity in cerebrospinal fluid levels of endorphins, an effect not found in a control group of rats. Concomitant with these CSF changes, auricular electroacupuncture led to depletion in beta-endorphin radioreceptor activity in the ventromedial hypothalamus and the medial thalamus regions of these animals. Supportive findings in human back pain patients was obtained by Clement-Jones.[20] Low frequency electrical stimulation of the concha led to relief of pain within 20 minutes of the onset of electroacupuncture and an accompanying elevation of radioassays for CSF beta-endorphin activity in all 10 subjects. Abbate examined endorphin levels in 12 patients undergoing thoracic surgery.[21] Six patients were given 50% nitrous oxide combined with 50 Hz auricular electroacupuncture while six control patients underwent their surgery with 70% nitrous oxide but no acupuncture. The auricular acupuncture patients not only needed less nitrous oxide than the controls but they also showed a significant increase in beta-endorphin immunoreactivity.

Electro-stimulation was applied by Fedoseeva and colleagues to the auricular lobe of rabbits, an auricular area corresponding to the jaw and teeth in humans.[22] Auricular electroacupuncture produced a significant decrease in behavioral reflexes and in cortical evoked potentials following electrical stimulation of the teeth. The suppression of behavioral and neurophysiological effects was abolished by injection of naloxone. Naloxone reversibility of auriculotherapy analgesia in human volunteers was examined by Simmons and Oleson.[23] All 40 volunteers were first assessed for tooth pain threshold by a dental pulp tester. Subjects were assigned to one of four groups: true auricular electrical stimulation (AES) followed by an injection of naloxone; true AES followed by an injection of saline; placebo stimulation of the auricle followed by an injection of naloxone; or placebo stimulation of the auricle followed by an injection of saline. Dental pain thresholds were significantly increased by AES conducted at appropriate auricular points for dental pain. Pain thresholds were not altered by sham stimulation at inappropriate auricular points. Naloxone produced a slight reduction in dental pain threshold in the subjects given true AES, whereas the true AES subjects then given saline showed a further increase in pain threshold.

STIMULATION OF AURICULAR MASTER POINTS

Auriculotherapy treatments are achieved by the electrical stimulation of low electrical resistance acupoints on the ear, the insertion of half inch needles into ear points based upon established treatment protocols, or the application of pressure by small acubeads taped to the ear. The first set of ear acupoints considered for stimulation are referred to as master points and supportive points. (See Figure 13.5.)

These auricular points do not correspond to one specific body organ but affect many different medical conditions. The first two master points, Point Zero and Shen Men, are utilized in most auriculotherapy treatment

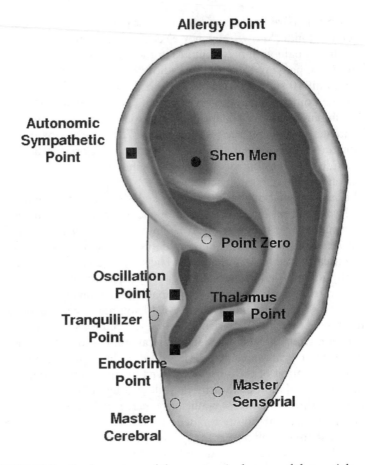

FIGURE 13.5   Surface view of the anatomical areas of the auricle that indicate the location of master points on the ear. An open circle represents raised ridges on the ear, a closed circle represents deeper areas of the ear, and a black square represents hidden, vertical areas of the ear.

plans for the alleviation of several health disorders. Point Zero was first described by Nogier and is found in a notch on the Helix Root as it rises from the Concha Ridge. Point Zero functions as a homeostatic balancing point that leads to normalizing of dysfunctional conditions. The Shen Men point is the most frequently utilized ear point found in most Chinese treatment protocols, serving to alleviate stress, pain, tension, anxiety, depression, and substance abuse disorders. The English translation of this Chinese ear acupuncture point is "Spirit Gate," suggesting that activation of this auricular point connects an individual to one's spiritual essence, enhancing the vital forces of life and one's general well-being. The physical location of this auricular point is toward the tip of the Triangular Fossa. Detection of auricular points by an electrodermal point finder typically reveals that Point Zero and Shen Men are electrically reactive in most medical patients.

Two master points used in many neurological pathologies and pain disorders are the Autonomic Sympathetic Point, referring to its use in regulating the autonomic nervous system, and the Thalamus or Subcortex Point, representing a brain region that serves as a higher brain center for the control of pain. The Autonomic Sympathetic Point is found on the underside of the Internal Helix where it meets the Antihelix Inferior Crus. The Thalamus Point is found on the base of the Concha Wall, behind the Antitragus. The Endocrine Point is a nearby region of the Intertragic Notch which represents the Pituitary Gland, the master control gland for all other endocrine glands. Stimulation of this auricular point affects circulating hormones, such as adrenocorticotropic hormone (ACTH), cortisol, and endorphins, whose levels are frequently altered during many conditions associated with pain and stress. At the center of the ear lobe, vertically below Point Zero, is the Master Sensorial Point, used to alleviate any disturbing somatic sensations. Central to this point on the ear lobe is the Master Cerebral Point, also referred to as the neurasthenia or worry point. Its stimulation is utilized to contain pathological obsessions, unwarranted worry thoughts, and generalized anxiety symptoms that are frequently found in chronic pain patients. Above the Master Cerebral point is an auricular point that represents the Cingulate Gyrus, an area of the Paleocortex Limbic System that affects emotional aspects of pain and suffering. Clinical reports from multiple practitioners have shown that all six of these Master and Supportive ear points are very effective in the treatment of acute and chronic pain disorders.

SOMATOTOPIC MUSCULOSKELETAL AURICULAR POINTS

In his original text, *The Treatise of Auriculotherapy*, Paul Nogier focuses on auricular representation of the musculoskeletal body because practitioners new to auriculotherapy can confirm for themselves that specific regions of electrical conductivity and tenderness on the external ear correspond to specific areas of the body where a patient feels myofascial discomfort.[2] This somatotopic relationship of specific points on the auricle to specific areas of the musculoskeletal body is depicted in Figure 13.6. The Cervical Vertebrae are represented on the Concha side of the Antihelix Tail, the

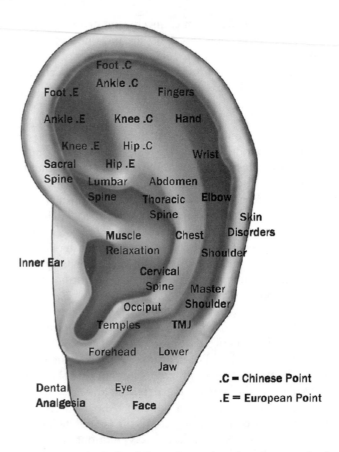

FIGURE 13.6   Musculoskeletal disorders related to the vertebral spine, head, and limbs are shown on specific areas of the Antihelix, Antitragus, Triangular Fossa, Scaphoid Fossa, and ear lobe. A designation of ".C" indicates the Chinese designation for the area of the ear which represents a specific area of the body, while a designation of ".E" indicates the European localization of the auricular region which corresponds to a given body area.

Thoracic Vertebrae are represented on the central side of the Antihelix Body, and the Lumbo-Sacral Vertebrae are represented on the Inferior Crus of the Antihelix. There are some differences between the somatotopic arrangement shown in many Chinese ear acupuncture charts, but with regard to the musculoskeletal system, the European and Chinese charts are relatively the same. The Posterior Groove behind each level of the Antihelix is also stimulated to effectively reduce pain from muscle spasms.

The Occiput is appropriately represented on the Antitragus region adjacent to the lowest portion of the Antihelix Tail that corresponds to the upper Cervical Spine. Toward the middle of the Antitragus is found the auricular microsystem point for the temples, whereas toward the base of the Antitragus, near the Intertragic Notch, is the forehead point. The most reactive of these Antitragus auricular points is utilized to treat both tension headaches and migraines. At the junction of the upper regions of the ear lobe and the lower sections of the Scaphoid Fossa is found the TMJ point that is used for the relief of tight and tense muscles of the lower jaw and upper jaw. In Chinese auricular charts, the hip, knee, ankle, and foot are represented in an upside down perspective on the Superior Crus of the Antihelix. The somatotopic presentation of these same leg points in the European system are also found in an inverted orientation, but they are located in the Triangular Fossa. As with vertebral points, stimulation of the Posterior side of the Triangular Fossa and the Superior Crus also serves to enhance the relief of myofascial pain in the legs or feet.

There is no discrepancy between European and Chinese ear charts which indicate auricular representation of the upper extremities. Treatment of shoulder problems is achieved by stimulation of a point in the Scaphoid Fossa peripheral to Point Zero. The shoulder point is logically located next to the junction of auricular representation of the cervical spine and the thoracic spine. Because the somatotopic system on the ear is an inverted orientation, the elbow point is found in the region of the Scaphoid Fossa above the shoulder point, and as one ascends higher in the Scaphoid Fossa, one arrives at the wrist point and above that are several points for the fingers. Both the front and the back side of the ear are stimulated to relieve tennis elbow, carpal tunnel syndrome, and arthritic pain in the fingers. In addition to auricular points for the arms and legs, Figure 13.6 indicates areas on the external ear which are utilized to treat sensory dysfunctions related to the eyes, nose, and inner ears.

AURICULAR TREATMENT OF VISCERAL DISORDERS

Visceral organs derived from endodermal embryological tissue are found in the central valley of the auricle, the Concha. Intriguingly, the autonomic vagus nerve, which regulates internal organs, only reaches the superficial skin in the region of the Concha floor. Near the opening to the to the actual auditory canal is the opening to the digestive system, the mouth. Extending peripherally from the auditory canal is the esophagus point, which leads to the stomach point found on the Concha Ridge.

Shiraishi and colleagues have demonstrated that stimulation of the auricular stomach point in animals reduces neuronal firing rates in the feeding center of the hypothalamus, whereas neuronal discharges in the satiety center of the hypothalamus are elevated by auricular stimulation.[24] On the Superior Concha is found auricular representation of the small intestines and the large intestines. Stimulation of these points are used to relieve physiological dysfunctions in each organ, such as nausea, diarrhea, or constipation, or they could alter the energetic function of the corresponding acupuncture meridian named for that organ. Several animal and human studies have shown that stimulation of ear reflex points for the stomach are able to alter physiological patterns in the nervous connections from the gastro-intestinal tract to the hypothalamus in the brain.[25-27]

The Five Element Theory of Traditional Oriental Medicine suggests that five Yin organs affect problems of energetic constitution other than the known physiological function of that organ. The kidney is energetically related to neurological and hearing disorders as well as physiological urinary dysfunctions, the liver can energetically affect tendon and ligament sprains as well as hepatitis, the spleen can energetically alleviate muscle spasms as well as affect lymphatic disorders, the lung is energetically used to treat skin disorders and drug detoxification as well as respiratory problems, and the heart is energetically utilized for mental calming as well as cardiovascular irregularities. The auricular point for the heart is found at the very center of the Inferior Concha, in the deepest region of the concha floor, but Nogier has shown an additional Heart point on the Antihelix area where the chest is represented. Coronary pain would be treated in both locations. (See Figure 13.7.)

AURICULAR TREATMENT OF NEUROPATHIC PAIN

Nervous system tissue is derived from ectodermal tissues that are represented on lower regions of the external ear. The ear lobe and the Antitragus above it represent the face and head as well as the brain inside the head. Shown in Figure 13.8 are locations for the Frontal Cortex, Parietal Cortex, Occipital Cortex, and Temporal Cortex. At the Intertragic Notch there is represented the Anterior Cingulate Gyrus, an area of the limbic system that has found to be very active in human pain patients and which is suppressed by body acupuncture stimulation.[3] Stimulation of the Cingulate Gyrus ear point is effective in relieving chronic pain in human patients. The other important auricular points for pain relief are the Thalamus Point and the Brain Point, both found on the Concha Wall behind the Antitragus.

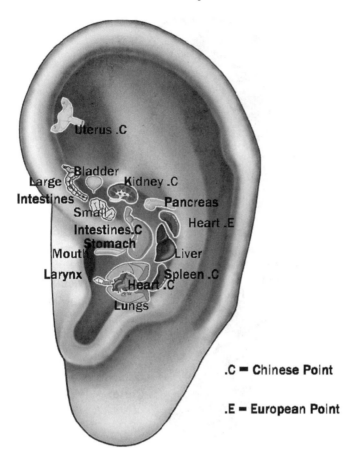

FIGURE 13.7   Visceral disorders related to problems with the gastro-intestinal tract, thoracic organs, and abdominal organs are shown on specific areas of the Inferior Concha, Concha Ridge, Superior Concha, the Triangular Fossa.

CONCLUSION

There is not yet the scientific research evidence that would lead to ready acceptance of the validity of the auricular acupuncture points which have been described. It may seem almost too good to be true that such a simple procedure as auriculotherapy could effectively alleviate pain and pathology in so many different parts of the body. Nonetheless, practitioners of this approach have repeatedly observed that specific areas of the auricle

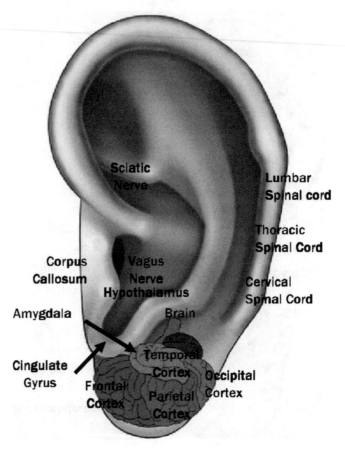

FIGURE 13.8   Localization of auricular points for the nervous system represented on the ear lobe, Antitragus, Inferior Concha, and Helix Tail.

are more sensitive to pressure and more electrically active in a predictable pattern that conforms to the inverted fetus perspective that Nogier first discovered in the 1950s. Activation of these auricular points with needle insertion, transcutaneous electrical stimulation, or application of pressure pellets, has been shown to alleviate physical symptoms in the corresponding part of the body. The growing use of auricular acupuncture for the relief of chronic pain and the treatment of substance abuse has occurred in China, Europe, and the United States because of the repeated clinical experience of the effectiveness of this technique. That neurological reflexes could connect distant regions of the body to somatotopic microsystems on the ear suggests a new kind of neuronal organization that required further elucidation by future studies.

REFERENCES

1. Huang H. *Ear Acupuncture.* Emmaus, PA: Rodale Press; 1974.
2. Nogier P. *Treatise of Auriculotherapy.* Moulins-les Metz, France: Maisonneuve; 1972.
3. Oleson T. *Auriculotherapy Manual: Chinese and Western Systems of Ear Acupuncture.* 3rd ed. London: Churchill Livingstone; 2003.
4. Oleson T. Differential application of auricular acupuncture for myofascial, autonomic, and neuropathic pain. *Medical Acupuncture.* 1998;9:23–28.
5. Oleson T, Kroening R, Bresler D. An experimental evaluation of auricular diagnosis: the somatotopic mapping of musculoskeletal pain at ear acupuncture points. *Pain.* 1980;8:217–229.
6. Saku K, Mukaino Y, Ying H, Arakwa K. Characteristics of reactive electrompermeable points on the auricles of coronary heart disease patients. *Clin Cardiol.* 1993;(16):415–419.
7. Alimi D, Geissmann A, Gardeur D. Auricular acupuncture stimulation measured on functional magnetic resonance imaging. *Med Acupunct.* 2002;13:18–21.
8. Helms J. *Acupuncture Energetics: A Clinical Approach for Physicians.* Berkeley, CA: Medical Acupuncture Publishers; 1995.
9. Nogier P. *From Auriculotherapy to Auriculomedicine.* Moulins-les Metz, France: Maisonneuve; 1983.
10. Liebeskind J, Mayer D, Akil H. Central mechanisms of pain inhibition: studies of analgesia from focal brain stimulation. In: Bonica JJ, ed. *Advances in Neurology.* Vol. 4. New York, NY: Raven Press; 1974.
11. Takeshige C, Sato T, Mera T, Hisamitu T, Fang J. Descending pain inhibitory system involved in acupuncture analgesia. *Brain Res. Bull.* 1992(29):617–634.
12. Melzack R, Wall P. Pain mechanisms: a new theory. *Science.* 1965;(150):197.
13. Basbaum A, Fields H. Endogenous pain control systems: brain stem spinal pathway and endorphin circuitry. *Annual Rev Neurosci.* 1979;7:513–532.
14. Kroening R, Oleson T. Rapid narcotic detoxification in chronic pain patients treated with auricular electroacupuncture and naloxone. *Intl J of Addict.* 1985;(20):1347–1360.
15. Ng L. Auricular acupuncture in animals: effects of opiate withdrawal and involvement of endorphins. *J Alt Compl Med.* 1996;2:61–64.
16. Ng L, Douthitt T, Thoa N, Albert C. Modification of morphine-withdrawal in rats following transauricular electrostimulation: an experimental paradigm for auricular electroacupuncture. *Biol Psychiatr.* 1975(10):575–580.
17. Sjolund B, Eriksson M. Electroacupuncture and endogenous morphines. *Lancet.* 1976;2:1985.
18. Sjolund B, Terenius L, Eriksson M. Increased cerebrospinal fluid levels of endorphins after electroacupuncture. *Act Physiol Scand.* 1977;(100):382–384.
19. Pert A, Dionne R, Ng L, Bragin E, Moody T, Pert C. Alterations in rat central nervous system endorphins following transauricular electroacupuncture. *Brain Res.* 1981(224):83–93.
20. Clement-Jones V, Mc Loughlin L, Lowery P, Besser G, Rees L, Wen H. Acupuncture in heroin addicts: changes in met-enkephalin and beta-endorphin in blood and cerebrospinal fluid. *Lancet.* 1979;2:380–383.

21. Abbate D, Santamaria A, Brambilla A, Panerai A, DiGuilio A. Beta-endorphin and electroacupuncture. *Lancet*. 1980;3:1309.
22. Fedoseeva O, Kalyuzhnyi L, Sudakov K. New peptide mechanisms of auriculo-acupuncture electro-analgesia: role of angiotensin II. *Acupunct & Elec-Ther Rex, Int J*. 1990;15:1–8.
23. Simmons M, Oleson T. Auricular electrical stimulation and dental pain threshold. *Anesth Prog*. 1993;(40):14–19.
24. Shiraishi T, Onoe M, Kojima T, Sameshima Y, Kageyama T. Effects of auricular stimulation on feeding-related hypothalamic neuronal activity in normal and obese rats. *Brain Res Bull*. 1995(36):141–148.
25. Asamoto S, Takeshige C. Activation of the satiety center by auricular acupuncture point stimulation. *Brain Res Bull*. 1992;(29):157–164.
26. Kawakaita K, Kawamura H, Keino H, Hongo T, Kitakohji H. Development of the low impedance points in the auricular skin of experimental peritonitis rats. *Am J Chin Med*. 1991;(19):199–205.
27. Lin X, Liang J, Rfen J, Mu F, Zhang M, Chen J. Electrical stimulation of acupuncture points enhances gastric myoelectrical activity in humans. *Am J Gastroenterol*. 1997;(92):1527–1530.

CHAPTER 14

Ayurveda and Yoga

Ravinder Mamtani and William H. Frishman

Is there anyone so wise as to learn from the experience of another?
—*Voltaire*

Ayurveda is an ancient philosophy of life and longevity, which also provides a fairly complete system of health. It is widely accepted and practiced in the Indian subcontinent. Those with chronic health conditions, such as chronic pain, degenerative and neurologic disorders, and digestive diseases are likely users of Ayurvedic treatments. Its origin goes back approximately 5,000 years to the Vedic Civilization of the Indus River Valley, and subsequently the Ganges River Valley, of India. Ayurveda comes from two Sanskrit words, *Ayus* and *Veda*, meaning "life" and "knowledge" respectively.[1] It literally means "knowledge of daily living." The literature, principles and practices of Ayurveda can be found in *Vedas*, the ancient religious Hindu books of knowledge. Unani, which in many ways is similar to Ayurveda and subsequently influenced by ancient Greek and Persian concepts of healing, is another system of health commonly practiced in India and other Asian countries. (See Box 14.7.)

Ayurveda is gaining acceptance worldwide. It is a holistic system, which focuses on the body, mind, and consciousness. As with traditional yoga practice, it values spirituality as an essential feature of optimum health and a noble way of life. Disease management in Ayurveda consists

245

of herbal preparations, diet, yoga, meditation, and other healthy practices such as good sleeping habits.

This chapter briefly describes Ayurveda and examines the scientific evidence concerning the usefulness of Ayurvedic herbal treatments and yoga for pain with a special focus on the principles of Ayurveda, herbs, and yoga.

THEORY AND PRINCIPLES

According to folklore, the Ayurvedic principles in the classical texts were developed and formulated in the foothills of the Himalayas where several noted sages *(vaidyas)* of the ancient Indus Valley civilization assembled to discuss and solve the problems faced of then prevalent diseases. It is believed that these sages were disgruntled with the prevailing system of health.[1] The sages went on to compile principles and practices of good health and disease management that emphasized optimum health and long life. These principles were documented in the *Vedas,* the divine Hindu books of knowledge. Thus came about the scriptures of Ayurveda. Unani, another system of medicine common in Pakistan and the Indian subcontinent, is similar to Ayurveda. It was founded by Hakim (Physician) Ibn Sina, although its threads can be traced back to Hippocrates.

It is the simplicity of Ayurveda that attracts people worldwide. Ayurveda is considered a natural system that aims at preserving wholeness. It has practical and spiritual components. It treats the individual as a whole entity and at the same time treats the root causes of the disease and not the symptoms alone. The Ayurvedic approach tailors treatment to the needs of the patient, which is particularly appealing to patients with chronic conditions such as pain. Chronic pain, as is well known, is not just correlated to physical factors, but also to social, environmental, physiological, pathological, and psychological factors. In some circumstances the Ayurvedic approach to treating chronic pain becomes an attractive option.

The basic philosophy of Ayurveda is that everything in the universe, including life, is composed of five elements, called *panchamahabhutas.* These five elements are space (ether), air, fire, water, and earth. These elements are not recognized as physical elements but rather they represent principles unique to the particular element.

In the beginning the world existed in an unmanifested state of pure consciousness.[1] From the vibration of the first sound O M (a word commonly recited and repeated during yoga sessions), the element of *ether* was born. With the movement of *ether,* the element of *air* was formed. The movement of *ether and air* created the element of *heat,* and heat in turn turned some *ether* into water, thus giving rise to the element *water.* The element of *water*

BOX 14.1

COMPARISON OF HEALING SYSTEMS

A Comparative Evaluation of Features of the Three Great Traditional Healing Systems With Western Medicine

	Unani	Ayurveda	Chinese	Western
Place & Date of Origin	Persia; circa 980 A.D.	India; circa 2000 B.C.	China; circa 2700 B.C.	Europe; United States; late nineteenth century.
Dynamic Elements	Ruh (soul; spirit).	Prana (energy).	Chi (life energy).	Natural Sciences
Correspondence with Elements of Nature	Four: Fire, Air, Water and Earth.	Five: Fire, Earth, Water, Air and Ether.	Five: Fire, Earth, Metal, Water and Wood.	Basic elements of chemistry.
Basic Cause of Disease	Imbalance of humoral temperament.	Ama the root cause of disease; dosha imbalance.	Systemic imbalances-Chi; yin/yang and five elements imbalance.	Physical, infective, vascular, degenerative, mental, neoplasia, and so on
Basis of Diagnosis	History, examination and humoral assessment: Blood, Phlegm, Yellow Bile; Black Bile.	History, examinations and Tridosha assessment: Vata, Kapha, Pitta.	History, examination and traditional Chinese medicine assessments.	Based on patient's history, physical examination, and laboratory and radiologic testing.
Diagnostic Models	Restore balance to humors, organ systems.	Concept of shiva-shakti; balance the tridosha or humor system.	Achieve balance of Chi, yin and yang, and five elements.	Specifically named pathology.
Main Dietary Influences	Non-alcoholic; regular fasting; non-pork.	Vegetarian.	Particular attention to diet.	Lifestyle habits influenced by modern and Western culture.

BOX 14.1 Comparison of Healing Systems *(Continued)*

	Unani	Ayurveda	Chinese	Western
Deity of System	Monotheistic; Abrahamic God of Islam, Christianity, Judaism.	Polytheistic; Hinduism.	Atheistic; Confucianism; Taoism; Buddhism.	Monotheistic; Abrahamic God of Islam, Christianity, Judaism.
Primary Treatment Modalities	Diet; herbs; fasting; cupping; purgation; baths; attars.	Panj Karma (detoxification); herbs; diet; emetic therapies.	Acupuncture, herbs; cupping; moxibustion; diet.	Pharmaceutical drugs; surgery and biomedical approaches.
Benefits	Evidence not conclusive; promising results have emerged for many herbs.	Evidence not conclusive; promising results have emerged for many herbs.	Evidence in favor of chronic pain conditions, nausea and dental pain.	Evidence for many conditions.
Side Effects	Overdose of herbal substances; incidence unknown.	Overdose of herbal substances; incidence unknown.	Side effects: transient and other symptoms from improper needle techniques; overdose of herbal substances: incidence unknown.	Iatrogenic; severe and frequent drug reactions.

Adapted from http://www.unani.com/comparison.htm. The American Institute of Unani Medicine. The above information is not comprehensive. It is intended to give the reader a flavor of comparative features of the four systems.

in turn after solidification gave rise to the fifth element, namely *earth*. And it is from this *earth* that all the substances arose: living and nonliving; organic and inorganic; vegetable, animal, and mineral kingdoms.[1,2]

It is important to remember that these elements are not to be taken in their literal sense. For instance, water does not mean the drinking water we see in a pitcher. It means and connotes cohesiveness. These five elements exist in all matter, and all have origins in the energy arising from cosmic consciousness. So, all five elements are present in the universe. It seems the knowledgeable sages who formulated the Ayurvedic scriptures studied nature very carefully and understood the basic forces of creation of all matter. The balancing of these five elements is essential in Ayurveda, and this is accomplished by use of herbs, exercise, meditation, yoga, and diet.

The five elements give rise to three basic type factors (or energies) that regulate the life cycle and control the entire human body. These factors, called *doshas,* are *vata, pitta,* and *kapha. Vata* arises from space and air; *pitta* from fire and water; and *kapha* from water and earth. A human body with balanced *doshas* is a healthy body. Although every individual has all three *doshas,* some *doshas* are more predominant than others in a given individual. *Doshas* contribute in various proportions to make up *prakruti* (the essential constitution) of an individual. *Prakruti* can be likened to genetics in nature. Just as the three *doshas* control regulatory aspects of the body, three *gunas (sattva, rajas, and tamas)* influence and control the mind. Ayurveda also recognizes seven *dhatus* (tissue elements): plasma, blood, muscle, fat, bone, nerve, and reproductive tissue; three *malas* (excretory products): feces, urine, and sweat; and *agni* (energy metabolism). Any disturbance in any of these factors can give rise to disease. Because *dosha* imbalance is at the core of every dysfunction, keeping *doshas* in balance will maintain good health.[2]

Like other alternative medicine systems, Ayurveda emphasizes the intrinsic relations between the body, mind, and consciousness. According to Ayurveda scholars, any imbalance in consciousness (or awareness) leads to undesirable personal lifestyle practices resulting in disharmony and disease process. That is why, in Ayurveda, mind-body interventions such as meditation and yoga are essential to disease treatment and prevention.[3]

Disease Management

Disease evaluation in Ayurveda is person specific. Treatments for pain and neurological conditions, as with any other problems, are individualized. A thorough Ayurvedic evaluation involves history taking, observation, palpation, and performing an examination of various organs and systems with emphasis on the heart, lungs, and intestines. Particular attention is paid to the examination of the pulse, tongue, eyes, and nails. Urine examination is also performed. The nature and the quality of the assessment are quite different from conventional biomedical assessment most physicians are used to. The findings have different interpretations and are based on the principles described above. For example, in Ayurveda, 12 different pulses are recognizable and they correlate with the functions of various internal organs.

There are four main categories of disease treatments in Ayurveda. They are *shodan* (cleansing), *shaman* (palliation), *rasayana* (rejuvenation), and *satvajaya* (mental health). These treatments include the use of herbal therapies, physical exercise and dietary regimens, meditation, and the use of certain practices. *Panchakarna purification therapy,* a well known Ayurvedic cleansing treatment, includes vomiting, purgation, use of medicinal enemas, blood letting, and administration of certain substances such as milk and herbal extracts via nasal passages.[1,2] Examples of commonly used practices and treatments appear in Table 14.1.

PLANT-BASED FOODS AND HERBS

The health benefits of plant-based foods and herbs have been known to the practitioners of Ayurveda and other systems of medicine for many centuries. Herbs and plant products have been an integral part of society. Various cultures around the world have valued them for their medicinal and culinary benefits. Many modern medications have been derived from plants. Digitoxin from *Digitalis purpurea* (foxglove) and salicin (aspirin) from *Salix alba* (willow bark) are examples of such medications. Aspirin is a commonly used pain medication worldwide. The scientific proof based on acceptable methods of research, establishing a direct relationship between food and health and disease, has become apparent only in recent years. For example, it was not until 1933 that a direct cause-effect relationship was observed between consumption of fruits and vegetable and cancer. Subsequent studies have confirmed lower rates of mortality and incidence of heart disease among those whose diets are rich in plant-based foods such as fruits and vegetables.[4] There are many reasons for these reported health benefits. Vegetarian foods are rich in vitamins, trace minerals, dietary fiber, and other non-nutritive, biologically active compounds called phytochemicals. Also, herbs commonly used in Asian and other cultures as food and for medicinal purposes possess antiplatelet, anti-inflammatory, and immune-stimulating properties that may be useful in reducing the risk of many cardiovascular and chronic neurodegenerative disease. The basic science of preventive mechanisms of plant-based diets rich in fruits and vegetables appear in Table 14.2.

The use of herbs and plant extracts remains an integral and significant part of the Ayurvedic approach to disease management. These extracts or their mixtures, based on Ayurvedic philosophy and principles, have been

TABLE 14.1 Common Treatment Strategies in Ayurveda[1,2,14]

Cleansing methods (*Shodan*)

The purpose of these methods is to remove excess toxins from the body. The main method is *Panchakarma*, which has the following five components. Examples are mentioned for each of the components.

Therapeutic vomiting (*vaman*). Vomiting is induced by the use of emetics such as licorice.

Purgation (*virechan*).

Medicated enema (*basti*). Sesame oil and milk are often used for this method.

Blood letting (*rakta moksha*). Sometimes leeches may be used. Blood-purifying herbs such as sandalwood and turmeric powders are also used.

Nasal administration or insufflation (*nasya*). Oils, certain herbs, and nasal massages may be used.

Palliation (*Shaman*)

This is done by use of herbs such as ginger, cinnamon, and black pepper and practices such as the following:

Fasting (*ksud nigraha*)

Observing thirst (*trut nigraha*)

Exercise: Yoga stretching (*vyayama*) *and* breathing exercises (*pranayama*)

Lying in the sun (*atap seva*)

Rejuvenation (*Rasayana*)

Rasayanas are Ayurvedic preparations used to revitalize the tissues, promote longevity and memory, and help in rejuvenation. MAK 4 and MAK 5 are examples of *rasayans*.

Spiritual healing (*Satvajaya*)

Mantras (sacred recitations) and meditation are examples of this type of treatment.

the subject of many studies in both animals and humans. Examples of herbs and various plant products of interest to researchers and practitioners in the management of neurological, pain, and painful inflammatory conditions are described below. Additionally, a listing of the herbs with reported beneficial effects in human studies appears in Table 14.3.

Allium sativum (Garlic)

Garlic has long been used in India as a medicinal food.[5] It was initially used as an anti-infective agent and subsequently became popular for its

TABLE 14.2 Potential Disease-Preventive Mechanisms of Plant-Based Foods as Identified in Human Studies[34]

- Antioxidant activity
- Decrease platelet aggregation
- Alteration of cholesterol metabolism
- Blood-pressure reduction
- Stimulation of the immune system
- Modulation of detoxification enzymes
- Modulation of steroid hormones concentration and metabolism
- Antibacterial and antiviral activity

antihypertensive and lipid-lowering effects. In the United States, the sales of garlic products have soared in recent years, generating over $60 million in the year 2000. Garlic has lipid-lowering, antithrombotic, antihypertensive, antioxidant, and immunomodulatory properties. Its role in specific neurologic conditions has not been explored (see Figure 14.1).

Several trials have shown the effectiveness of garlic in reducing total and low density lipoprotein (LDL)-cholesterol. Others, however, have failed to demonstrate and confirm these findings.[6-8] Garlic's reported antiplatelet, fibrinolytic, and antiatherosclerotic effects in some studies[7] need to be better defined and understood in terms of their benefits on various neurological and cerebrovascular conditions. In a recent analysis performed by the Agency for Healthcare Research and Quality (AHRQ), it was concluded that garlic may have short-term, positive lipid-lowering and encouraging antithrombotic effects.[9]

Boswellia serrata (Indian Frankincense)

Boswellia, also called H15, is a commonly used herb in Ayurvedic preparations. It comes from a gum tree that grows in South Asia and in Christian belief was one of the traditional gifts brought from the East by the Three Magi at Epiphany. Its effects are similar to those of corticosteroids but without the side effects. Boswellic acids are reported to have significant analgesic, anti-inflammatory, and complement-inhibitory properties.[10,11] The herb has been a subject of several controlled trials. In one trial involving 30 patients with osteoarthritis of the knee, those who received Boswellia tree extract reported a significant improvement in their knee pain, range of motion, and walking distance,

TABLE 14.3 Clinical Experiences Involving the Use of Plants/Extracts (in Ayurveda) Relevant to Inflammatory, Neurologic, Pain, and Vascular Disorders[7,10,12]

Genus, species Common Sanskrit name Common English name	Conditions and/or Results for which Human Studies are Reported (Proposed mechanism of action, if any)
Allium sativum Garlic Lahsoon	Hyperlipidemia. Results in improved levels of lipids (lipid lowering, antithrombotic, antihypertensive, imunomodulatory).
*Boswellia serrata** Indian Frankincense Shallaki	Arthritis. Some reports of beneficial effects. (anti-inflammatory).
*Capsicum annuum** Katuvitra Chili pepper, paprika	Cluster headaches, neuropathy, and arthritis. Improvement reported in some studies. External: rubifacient, blocks pain neurotransmitter-substance P, depletes substances P, desensitizes the sensory neurons. Internal: Reduces platelet aggregation and triglycerides, and improves blood flow.
*Curcuma longa** Haridra (Haldi) Turmeric	Functional gall bladder problems (Increase in secretin and bicarbonate output); Hyperlipidemia. Some studies report improvement in cholesterol levels. (Fatty acid metabolism alteration and decrease in serum lipid peroxide levels). Osteoarthritis. Some studies report positive results. (anti-inflammatory).
Commiphora (mukul) *guggulu* Guggulu Guggulu	Hyperlipidemia. Improved lipid levels noted. (antagonist of farnesoid X receptors).
*Withania somnifera** Ashwagandha Winter cherry	Arthritis. Some studies report improvement. (anti-inflammatory).
*Zingiber officinale** Ginger Sunthi	Antiemetic (carminative, local effect on stomach). Reduces nausea. Osteoarthritis. Some studies report benefit. (Anti-inflammatory; inhibits cyclo-oxygenase pathways, prostaglandin PGE2) and leukotriene (LTB4) synthesis.

*Some studies involved using preparations which contained several herbs. For example, *Boswellia*, has been used in conjunction with *Withania and Curcuma* to determine its effectiveness in the treatment of arthritic conditions.

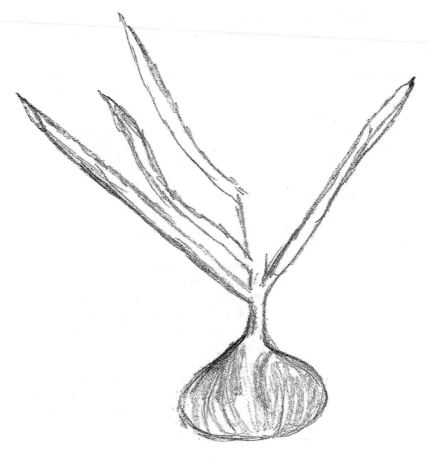

FIGURE 14.1   Garlic. (original line drawing by Alicia M. Micozzi.)

as compared to those in the control group.[12] In another study with a sample of 260 rheumatoid arthritis patients, a special gum extract of *Boswellia serrata*, resulted in a significant improvement of symptoms of pain and swelling.[10] These results are promising but need confirmation in larger trials.

Capsicum annuum (Chili Pepper)

Common names of this plant/herb include cayenne pepper, paprika, red pepper, bird pepper, and Peruvian pepper. The preparations of this plant are used in topical creams and ointments. It is commonly used for pain related to herpes zoster and diabetic neuropathy. Many use it for osteoarthritis pain. Some basic science studies have shown that it reduces pain by depleting Substance P. There are also reports of the herb desensitizing neurons.[7] More studies are warranted to confirm its beneficial effects.

Curcuma longa (Turmeric)

The active ingredient, curcumin, of turmeric, a commonly used spice in India, has anti-inflammatory and lipid-lowering effects. It is one of the three components of traditional curry spice. Curcumin's lipid-lowering effects observed in animal experiments are attributed to changes in fatty acid metabolism and facilitating the conversion of cholesterol to bile acids.[6] No human randomized trials could be found in prominent peer-reviewed literature. There are also reports of its benefit in patients with osteoarthritis. The benefit of turmeric is not conclusively proven; however, its use as a spice in overall healthy diet is prudent.

Withania somnifera (Ashwagandha)

Basic science studies suggest that this herb may have anti-inflammatory, antioxidant, immunomodulatory, and hemopoietic, as well as antiaging properties. It might also have a positive influence on the endocrine and central nervous systems. The mechanisms of these proposed actions require additional clarification. Several observational and randomized studies have reported its usefulness in the treatment of arthritic conditions.[10]

Zingiber officinale (Ginger)

Ginger is widely used in India, most commonly for control of nausea and osteoarthritis pain. Several randomized trials have shown its benefit in controlling nausea associated with pregnancy, motion sickness, and anesthesia, and some studies have demonstrated its usefulness in the treatment of osteoarthritis.[7,12] However, the evidence concerning its benefit for these conditions is not compelling (see Figure 14.2).

It should be mentioned that the methodology and quality of many studies aimed at determining the effectiveness of various herbs are less than satisfactory. Also, many studies involve the use of preparations that contain several herbs and other nutrients, which is quite common in day-to-day Ayurvedic practice. While such trials are useful, they do not, in and of themselves, identify and discern the beneficial effects of specific herbs. In one such trial involving a combination preparation of Withania somnifera, Boswellia serrata, Curcuma longa, and zinc, osteoarthritis

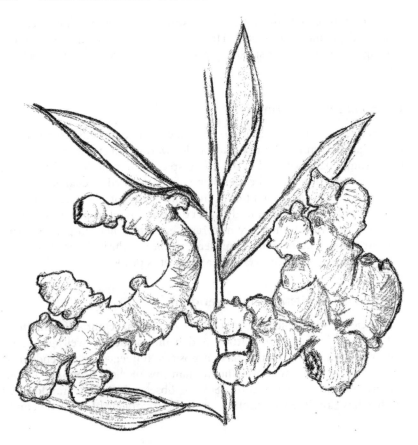

FIGURE 14.2   Ginger. (original line drawing by Alicia M. Micozzi.)

patients reported a significant reduction in their level of pain compared to those in the control group.[10]

LONGEVITY

Ayurveda consists of eight medical divisions, one of which is called *Rasayanatantra* that deals with aging. Ayurvedic practitioners commonly treat and advise people on various ways to combat the effects of aging. Their advice usually deals with ways and means to improve memory, restore youthfulness, overcoming weak states, and preserving sexual functions. The regimen for slowing aging and treating age-related problems

TABLE 14.4 Plants With a Potential for Antiaging Effects

Sanskrit name	Latin name
Vaccha	Acorus calamus
Kooshmand	Benincasa hispida
Jotishmati	Celastrus paniculadas
Shankhapushpi	Convolvulus microphyllus
Jataamansi	Nardostachys jatamansi
Tulsi	Ocimum gratissimum
Raasna	Plucha laceolata
Harikati	Terminalia chebula
Ashwgandha	Withania somnifera

Data from Dev Sukh. Ancient-modern concordance in Ayurvedic plants: some examples. *Environmental Health Perspectives.* 1999;107:783.

consists of counseling on diet, lifestyle choices, exercise, meditation and relaxation methods, yoga, and the use of specific herbs.

Various Ayurvedic treatments aimed at improving the quality of life of elderly patients are receiving a great deal of attention. This is due to several reasons. One, the number of elderly population with age-related problems such as dementia is increasing worldwide. Two, the available conventional biomedical approaches and drug treatments to treat such problems are either ineffective or inadequate. Three, some plants referred to as "medhya plants" have yielded positive results in memory and cognition problems commonly seen in the elderly.[13]

MEMORY AND COGNITIVE IMPROVEMENT

Table 14.4 lists plants and their products which have been reported to have antiaging effects. Examples of these effects include improvements in memory and cognition impairment. Based on the available scientific information, these herbs or their extracts have not been found to be of proven value. Additional studies are required to validate their reported benefits.

Examples of plants which have received attention for antiaging properties include *Shankapushpi, Ashwagandha,* and *Jataamans.*[13] Some basic science work has demonstrated that they may possess acetyl choline esterase inhibition or gamma-aminobutyric receptor binding properties, which might explain their beneficial effects.

Maharishi Amrit Kalash (MAK)

This Ayurvedic preparation comes in two forms, namely MAK 4 and MAK 5. These formulations are mixtures of many fruits and herbs. There are several studies that suggest that MAK preparations may have immune-enhancing, free radical scavenging, tumor regressing properties. Other studies indicate these preparations have the potential of reducing platelet aggregation and possibly slow the aging process.[14] All these findings, if true, have implications in the treatment of many neurologic conditions. More basic science and epidemiologic research is needed to confirm these findings.

PHYTOCHEMICALS

Plant-based foods have a wide range of aromas, colors, and tastes. These qualities make them distinctive and attractive for food consumption. These qualities are thought to be due to the presence of compounds called phytochemicals. Allylic sulfides responsible for the pungent odor of garlic, and anthocyanins, the red pigment in fruits such as strawberries, are examples of phytochemicals.

Many foods and herbs recommended by practitioners of Ayurveda contain phytochemicals that are possibly involved in optimizing health and preventing and/or treating cardiovascular diseases.[15] Phytochemicals are biologically active compounds that are present in small quantities in plants. While they are not nutrients, they seem to play a significant role in the prevention of several chronic diseases.

The health benefits of phytochemicals have not been proven conclusively; however, many herbs commonly used in Asian Indian cuisine and by Ayurvedic practitioners show promise for disease prevention.[15]

At the present time, the potential health benefits of phytochemicals are not attributed to any single compound, but rather to wholesome foods containing thousands of phytochemicals and other nutrients.[16] Also, no single disease entity or deficiency syndrome has been linked to any one or any group of phytochemicals. For these reasons, recommendations concerning their use as supplements, in place of a well-balanced healthy diet, is not appropriate.

Based on the limited number of studies, the evidence concerning the effectiveness of Ayurvedic herbs in the treatment of neurologic and pain disorders is not compelling. However, lack of compelling evidence of these herbs is not the same as their ineffectiveness. While more research is needed, there are inherent difficulties and problems in conducting research in alternative medicine systems such as Ayurveda. A brief description of such problems and difficulties appears further on in the chapter.

YOGA

Yoga is integrally related to Ayurveda, and its use in India is widespread. It is quite common to find people in India practicing yogic exercises in group-like situations in open areas or parks. The benefits reported by those who engage in yogic activity have been described in many ways (e.g., improved muscle strength, a state of relaxation, reduction in anxiety and sympathetic activity, general feeling of wellness, and attaining a higher state of enlightenment).[9,12,14,17-19]

It is gaining popularity in many other nations as well. According to one survey in the United Kingdom, the level of satisfaction associated with yoga is very high.[12] Its interest in the United States is growing, with training and certification programs in yoga emerging.

The origin of yoga dates back to ancient times, as early as 5,000 years ago. The word "yoga" comes from a Sanskrit word *yug*, meaning "to join" or "to yoke," as derived from Sanskrit in Old English. It connotes "the joining of the lower human nature to the higher."[17] It is claimed that the practice of yoga allows a person to alter his/her mental and bodily responses, normally thought to be beyond one's control. It facilitates an elevation of self-awareness and attainment of a state of enlightenment.[19] Simply put, yoga is a mind-body technique involving breath control, physical, and meditation that promotes physical, mental, social, and spiritual well-being.

Ancient Sanskrit Vedic texts have described several types of yogic practices. These include *bhakti* yoga (emphasizes spirituality and devotion), *jnana* yoga (emphasizes wisdom), *karma* yoga (emphasizes offering services without selfish motive), *raja* yoga (emphasizes mastering the mind by focused concentration), *dhyana* yoga (emphasizes meditation), *mantra* yoga (emphasizes repetition of sacred recitations), and *hatha* (emphasizes psychophysical energies of the body).[17,18]

Hatha yoga is the most popular form in the United States. It has three essential components: (a) physical exercises and postures (called *asanas*), (b) breathing techniques (called *pranayamas*), and (c) concentration and thinking techniques such as meditation.

Yoga Session

A hatha yoga session varies in content and duration. Yoga practice has undergone significant changes, some of which have been guided by the availability of new scientific information, and others by the emergence of new schools of thoughts. A typical 45–60 minute yoga session begins with breathing exercises requiring long and deep breaths through the nose.[3] Mental concentration of each breath as the air enters and exits the nostril is important. This allows people to relax their body and calm their mind. This phase could last anywhere between 15–20 minutes and can be done sitting or lying down. The next phase (usually of 20–25 minutes) involves gentle exercises and postural movements to facilitate relaxation of joints and muscles, followed by somewhat more difficult postures and exercises. Many difficult and cumbersome postures are contraindicated in certain musculoskeletal conditions and can be substituted by others. Physical damage to muscles, ligaments, and joints can occur. Those with balance and severe pain problems should be cautious. Practitioners are advised to exercise gently and slowly, and not stretch beyond their comfort level. Exercises and movements should be performed with ease. The last phase (10–15 minutes) involves meditation or a related technique such as visualization or guided imagery, and usually concludes with chanting, such as repeating *Om shanti* ("let there be peace").

Transcendental Meditation

Transcendental meditation (TM) is a variant of Ayurveda without the cumbersome physical and mental exercises often associated with yoga. Invented by an Indian practitioner, Maharishi Mahesh Yogi, this mind-body method of self-regulating attention has become quite popular in the United States. There are several reports of its benefits in reducing blood pressure and anxiety, and improving quality of life.[3]

Transcendental meditation is simple. Learners are asked to sit in a comfortable position and given a mantra (usually a sound or a word). They are instructed to repeat the mantra over and over again. Any intruding thoughts are acknowledged and the learner is asked to return his/her focus on mantra. Transcendental meditation is usually practiced for about 15–20 minutes.

Evidence Base

Yoga is a commonly used mind-body technique. Many mind-body interventions have demonstrated that their complementary use can be effective in the management of arthritis, low back pain, and headaches. The evidence concerning their benefit in improving mood and quality of life in those with chronic illnesses is considerable.[20] Conditions for which yoga is used include anxiety, back pain, arthritis, headache, insomnia, and other neurological conditions. Hatha yoga, the most common form of yoga practiced in the United States, has three components to it: stretching and exercises, breath control, and meditation. The routine practice of yoga produces a state of relaxation and improves muscle strength. It also induces a relaxation response associated with a lower level of anxiety and reduced sympathetic drive. Research findings have documented the usefulness of yoga for many pain and neurologic disorders. A brief summary of the evidence base follows.

Controlled Trials

Several controlled trials have shown that yoga reduces anxiety, stress, and symptoms of depression.[12,21,22] These finding are very important and relevant in the management of pain and neurologic conditions because constant and repeated cycles of stress (referred to as *allostatic load*) can compromise many normal physiological processes and contribute to the progression and development of many chronic diseases.[23] Stress and anxiety worsen chronic pain conditions. There are those who argue that allostasis may be an important etiologic entity responsible for many chronic conditions, such as atherosclerosis, metabolic syndrome, and Alzheimer's disease.

Other trials have demonstrated the usefulness of yoga in reducing the symptoms of osteoarthritis, carpal tunnel syndrome, and back pain.[12,18] There is also some evidence concerning the benefit of yoga in the treatment of those with obsessive compulsive and attention deficit disorders. The evidence for epilepsy is inconclusive.[12]

Many risk factors for cardiovascular diseases are also risk factors for neurologic conditions, such as cerebrovascular accident (CVA, or stroke). Many studies have shown that regular yoga practice can significantly improve cardiovascular risk factors, such as lipid profiles, body weight, and blood pressure, thereby helping reduce the risk of CVA.[18,24,25] There are several other controlled and uncontrolled studies that have demonstrated the long-term usefulness of yoga in the treatment of hypertension, another risk factor for stroke and other neurologic conditions.[14,18,26]

In a randomized trial of 33 hypertensive patients, subjects were assigned to one of three groups: those receiving yoga, those prescribed antihypertensive medication, or those receiving no treatment. Both yoga and antihypertensive medications were noted to reduce blood pressure over an 11-week period.[27] One randomized, controlled study suggests yoga is capable of producing a long-term beneficial effect in the treatment of hypertension.[3] Other studies involving the postural techniques of yoga (asanas) have demonstrated significant reductions in blood pressure.[3] Many scientists believe asanas restore baroreflex sensitivity, thereby reducing blood pressure.[27-29]

Neurophysiology

Meditation, as practiced in various mind-body techniques including yoga, elicits a relaxation response. A relaxation response is characterized by lower consumption of oxygen, lower heart and respiration, and changes in brain activity.[12,18,23]

Yoga alters various pulmonary, cerebral, mental and metabolic physiological functions, producing beneficial effects on the central nervous and cardiovascular systems. These beneficial effects include an increase in verbal creativity, a reduced visual reaction time and intraocular pressure, better breath holding ability, improved tidal volume and vital capacity, an improvement in physical fitness,[19,30] reduction in anxiety,[31] and improved sugar levels among diabetics. An association between increased cerebral blood flow and TM has also been observed.[14,32]

A very unique and a distinct phase of relaxation, referred to as "the fourth state of consciousness" (the other three being waking, dreaming and sleeping) has been described during TM.[19,32] This state is characterized by not only the usual changes seen in deep relaxation, such as reduced cortisol and plasma lactate levels, decreased muscle and red cell metabolism, and reduced breath rate, but also by an increased alpha brain wave activity and a distinctive pattern of enhanced cerebral blood flow.

The regular practice of yoga has also been shown to have positive effects on mood and emotional well-being.[17] Improved muscle strength and relaxation response have also been described.[3,17]

Although yoga cannot be recommended as a primary treatment for patients with pain and neurologic disorders, its use as an adjunct in these patients can be safely recommended. An adjustment of postures may be required for certain patients, such as pregnant women, who should avoid certain postural yogic techniques. Also, those with a history of psychosis should refrain from yoga. Excessive meditation may lead to mental disturbances.

Yoga is flexible and its techniques can be custom tailored to individual needs. It can be self-taught, although it is best learned with supervision in class situations. Yoga is a safe and inexpensive method for promoting general health and emotional well-being.

RESEARCH

Common to all areas of complementary, alternative, and integrative medicine, lack of funding, paucity of history of prior research, and absence of academic infra-structure make research in Ayurveda and yoga difficult.[33] There are also methodological challenges in applying research techniques developed for testing drugs on Ayurvedic medicine and yoga.

Incompatibility With Randomized Controlled Trial Methodology

Ayurveda and its practices are deeply rooted in the day-to-day, routine activities of Indian households. Diet, personal habits, hobbies, and spirituality are examples of such activities. In disease states, adjustments of these activities, the use of herbal preparations, and other practices are required to treat the whole person in terms of the mind, body, and spirit in order to create a balance to optimize health and well-being.

Ayurvedic treatment usually has several components and is not only disease-specific but also person-specific. Two persons with similar disease patterns could receive two entirely different treatments. Such a treatment approach cannot lend itself to a randomized controlled trial (RCT). This is so because in a RCT, all patients in the treatment group must receive the same treatment, while those in the control group receive an indistinguishable placebo. To fit into this research design, many research workers have chosen to test only specific herbal ingredients or plant products on a particular condition.[34] The reality of good Ayurvedic practice is that Ayurvedic physicians tend to use a wide range of Ayurvedic approaches, including the use of herbs, diet, meditative, and yoga practices, and a variety of other interventions. Similar variations are seen in yoga.

Problem of Designing Placebos

Given the wholesomeness and the complexity of the Ayurvedic approach, it is unthinkable to devise an acceptable placebo intervention. Also, designing placebos for specific Ayurvedic practices such as massage, fasting, vomiting, and yoga would be very cumbersome and difficult.

Rather, the instructive comparison is between traditional Indian and contemporary western European lifestyles and philosophies. How would you, for example, have a subject receive a sham massage or yoga? Complicated procedures can be devised to fool subjects into believing temporarily that they are receiving a true treatment. While such an approach may work for a treatment or two, but not when treatments are spread over one or more weeks in a true, complete Ayurvedic treatment protocol. This problem also illustrates a basic and serious limitation with how complementary/alternative medicine is experienced in the United States today. CAM is available on an outpatient basis using specific isolated treatment modalities. A real measure of the benefits of CAM and its full potential for disease treatments would come from residential CAM care where patients receive a total package of treatments over the course of several days. At present, we are seeing only the tip of the iceberg of the power and potential of CAM for management of medical conditions, effecting cures of chronic problems and achieving the highest levels of patient satisfaction and improvement in quality of life.

Research on meditation and yoga faces many challenges, as well. One, there is a lack of definition on what constitutes meditation. Two, there are many types of yogic and meditation practices with a wide range of variations. Three, due to a lack of definitions and heterogeneity in yoga practices, conducting meta-analysis and systematic reviews presents a challenge.

The methodological problems discussed previously can have the following effects on Ayurveda research data:

The treatment techniques used in RCTs are not representative of those used in the day-to-day practice of Ayurveda and yoga;

In typical RTCs in which herbal or yoga treatments are compared with placebo, and in which only short-term outcomes are assessed, the following questions may remain unanswered:

What are the long-term effects of Ayurvedic or yoga treatments compared to conventional treatments?

Are the RCT results, when put into practice, helping our patients, and if so, to what extent?

CONCLUSION

Based on the review of available studies, the evidence is not convincing that Ayurvedic herbal treatment is effective in the management of pain and neurologic disorders. The use of fresh chili pepper, garlic, ginger, and turmeric (curcurmin) as spices in the overall healthy diet is appropriate. Many studies reported in the literature suffer from various methodological problems. However, the lack of evidence regarding herbs should not necessarily be viewed as a lack of effectiveness. Several Ayurvedic herbs, such as pepper, ginger, turmeric, and Withania somnifera *(ashwagandha)* might be appropriate for additional and/or larger randomized trials in the future. Additional basic science work on antiaging herbs is also warranted.

Yoga has been shown to be useful to patients with musculoskeletal pain (e.g., low back pain), arthritis, anxiety disorders, and other neurologic conditions. Yoga reduces anxiety and stress, promotes well-being, and improves quality of life. Its safety profile is excellent. Its complementary use under medical supervision is appropriate and may be worth considering. Ayurveda is the oldest medical system in the world, dating back 5,000 years to the Vedic civilization of India. Ayurveda and yoga offer many challenges and opportunities, and are worthy of research and our attention.

REFERENCES

1. Gerson S. *Ayurveda: The Ancient Indian Healing Art.* 1st ed. Boston, MA: Elements Books Limited; 1993.
2. Lad V. An introduction to Ayurveda. *Altern Ther.* 1995;1:57–63.
3. *Alternative Medicine: Expanding Medical Horizons: A Report to the NIH on Alternative Medical Systems and Practices in the United States.* Bethesda, MD: National Institute of Health; 1992.
4. Drewnowski A, Gomez-Carneros C. Bitter taste, phytonutrients and the consumer: a review. *Am J Clin Nutri.* 2000;(72):1424–1435.
5. Frishman WH, Sinatra ST, Moizuddin M. The use of herbs for treating cardiovascular disease. *Sem Integrat Med.* 2004;2:23–35.
6. Low Dog T, Riley D. Management of hyperlipidemia. *Altern Ther.* 2003;9:28–40.
7. Blumental M. *The ABC Clinical Guide to Herbs.* New York, NY: The American Botanical Council, Thieme Publishers; 2003.
8. Stevinson C, Pittler MH, Earnst E. Garlic for treating hypercholesterolemia: a meta-analysis of randomized trials. *Ann Intern Med.* 2000;(133):420–429.
9. Mulrow C., Lawrence V. Ackerman R. *Evidence Report/ Technology Assessment Number 20: Garlic: Effects on Cardiovascular Risks and Diseases, Protective Effects Against Cancer and Clinical Adverse Effects.* Rockville, MD: Agency for Healthcare Research and Quality (AHRQ); 2000; Pub No 01-EO23.
10. Khan S, Balick MJ. Therapeutic plants of Ayurveda: a review of selected clinical and other studies for 166 species. *J Altern Complement Ther.* 2001;7:405.
11. Perlman A, Spierer M. Osteoarthritis. In: Rakel D, ed. *Integrative Medicine.* New York, NY, and St Louis, MO: Saunders; 2003:414–421.
12. Ernst E. *The Desktop Guide to Complementary and Alternative Medicine. An Evidence Based Approach.* 2nd ed. Philadelphia: Elsevier; 2006.
13. Bharani A, Ganguly A, Bhargava KD. Salutary effect of Terminalia arjuna in patients with severe congestive heart failure. *Int J Cardiol.* 1995;(49):191-199.
14. Sharma H, Clark C. *Contemporary Ayurveda. Medicine and Research in Maharishi Ayurveda.* 1st ed. Philadelphia, PA: Churchill Livingston; 1998.
15. Craig WJ. Health promoting properties of common herbs. *Am J Clin Nutr.* 1999; 70(suppl):491S–499S.
16. Micozzi MS. *Complementary and integrative therapies in cancer care and prevention.* New York: Springer Publishing; 2007:167–213.
17. Ananda S. *The Complete Book of Yoga: Harmony, of Body and Mind.* 1st ed. Delhi, India: Orient Paperbacks; 1981.
18. Raub JA. Psychophysiologic effects of hatha yoga on musculoskeletal and cardiopulmonary function: a literature review. *J Altern Complement Med.* 2003;8:797–812.

19. *Meditation Practices for Health: State of the Research.* Evidence Report/Technology Assessment, Number 155. AHRG Public Number 07-E010.
20. Mind Body Medicine: An Overview. National Center for Complementary and Alternative Medicine. http://nccam.nih.gov. Updated May 2007.
21. Shannoff-Khalsa D. An introduction to Kundalini yoga meditation techniques that are specific for the treatment of psychiatric disorders. *J. Altern Complement Med.* 2004;10:91–101.
22. West J, Otte C, Geber K, Johnson J, Mohr DC. Effects of Hatha yoga and African dance on perceived stress, affect and salivary cortisol. *Ann Behav Med.* 2004;28:114–118.
23. Benson H, Fricchione G, Sehlub E. Clinical training in mind body medicine. Presented at Harvard Medical School Mind Body Medicine Institute; June 19–23, 2006; Boston, MA.
24. Schmidt T, Wijga A, Von Zur Muhlen A. Changes in cardiovascular factors and hormones during comprehensive residential three months kriya yoga training and vegetarian nutrition. *Acta Physiol Pharmacol.* 1998(42):205–213.
25. Manchanda SC, Narang R, Reddy KS, et al. Retardation of coronary atherosclerosis with yoga lifestyle intervention. *J Assoc Physicians India.* 2000(48):687–694.
26. Patel C. Twelve month follow-up of yoga and bio-feedback in the management of hypertension. *Lancet.* 1975;1:62–64.
27. Marugesan R, Govindarajulu N, Bera TK. Effect of selected yogic practices on the management of hypertension. *Indian J Physiol Pharmacol.* 2000(44):207–210.
28. Selvamurthy W, Sridharan K, Ray US, et al. A new physiological approach to control essential hypertension. *Indian J Physiol Pharmacol.* 1998;(42):205–213.
29. Bernardi L, Porta C, Spicuzza L, et al. Slow breathing increases arterial baroreflex sensitivity in patients with chronic heart failure. *Circ.* 2002(105):143.
30. Benson H. The physiology of meditation. *Sci Am.* 1972;(226):84.
31. Fenwick PB, Donaldson L, Gillis L. Metabolic and EEG changes during transcendental meditation: an explanation. *Biol Psych.* 1977;5:101–118.
32. Jevning R, Wilson AF. Behavioral increase of blood flow. *The Physiologist.* 1978 (21):60.
33. Bodekar G. Evaluating Ayurveda. *J Altern Complement Med.* 2001;7:389–392.
34. Lampe JW. Health effects of vegetables and fruit: assessing mechanisms of action in human experimental studies. *Am J of Clin Nutri.* 1999;70(suppl):475S–490S.

Herbal Medicine, Plant-Based Therapies and Homeopathy

PART IV

Herbal Medicine,
Plant-Based Therapies,
and Homeopathy

CHAPTER 15

Herbal Remedies and Micronutrients

Marc S. Micozzi

Herbal and dietary supplement use is extremely common. According to an industry survey, sales of single herbal preparations in natural products stores grew by nearly 5% in 1 year to a total of over $400 million in 1998. Sales of these preparations in grocery, drug, and mass merchandise stores increased an average of 50% to reach a total of nearly $300 million.[1] A telephone survey of 2055 English-speaking adults found that over 40% had used at least one alternative therapy.[2] In the same survey, of adults who regularly take prescription medication, nearly 20% reported the concurrent use of at least one herbal product or high-dose vitamin. Nearly 40% of those surveyed who saw an unconventional practitioner discussed their experience with their regular physician. Interaction problems may arise when herbs are combined with other drugs.[3] The pharmacologic effect of herbs is not surprising since many of the drugs in clinical practice are derived from plants. Lidocaine and novocaine are derived from the coca plant (*Erythroxylum coca*), opioids from the poppy (*Papaver somniferum*), and aspirin from meadowsweet (*Spirea ulmaria*) whence the "spir" part of its name derives. Digoxin comes from foxglove (*Digitalis lanata*), and warfarin is a derivative of dicoumarin found in sweet clover (*Melilotus officinalis*).

The majority of herbal remedy use in the United States today involves botanical products purported to have therapeutic actions on the brain and central nervous system. Vitamins, amino acids, and other dietary supplements are also popular.[4] Some data indicate that dietary supplements hold promise for the treatment of pain and several neurologic problems. Following are summaries of selected trials in this area.

MIGRAINE HEADACHE

Magnesium

Magnesium, which is essential for all reactions using adenosine triphosphate (ATP), is the fourth most prevalent cation (or positive ion: Na+, K+, Ca++, Mg++) in the body. After calcium (Ca++), it is the second most common divalent cation (carrying two positive charges, Mg++). Magnesium deficiency is quite common. According to estimates of magnesium intake based on the Third U.S. National Health and Nutrition Examination Survey (1988 to 1994), magnesium intake was lower than the recommended daily allowance (RDA) in both males and females between 12 and 60 years of age in all racial and ethnic groups, except non-Hispanic white males.[5] The incidence of deficiency is even higher among hospitalized patients; 65% of those in intensive care, up to 12% in general wards, and 30% of hospitalized alcoholics have hypomagnesemia.[6]

Several trials have indicated that magnesium supplementation may be a helpful treatment for migraine as well as tension-type headaches.[7,8,9,10]

Although the exact mechanism of magnesium's effects is unclear, it may interrupt the process at the vasoconstriction stage by interacting with serotonin and N-methyl-D-aspartate receptors, nitrous oxide synthesis and release, other migraine-related receptors, and neurotransmitters.[11]

Some studies suggest that patients with low ionized serum magnesium levels are more likely to respond to initial magnesium treatment than those with normal serum magnesium levels. In one study of 40 patients with acute migraine attacks,[12] 35 had at least 50% pain relief within 15 minutes after IV infusion of 1g magnesium sulfate. In 18 of 21 patients whose pain relief lasted at least 24 hours, serum magnesium levels initially were below normal (0.54 to 0.65 mmol/l).

Excess magnesium causes diarrhea, an effect that was seen in every trial in which these data were collected. Inorganic forms of magnesium (magnesium oxide, magnesium chloride) may be more likely to cause diarrhea than organic forms (magnesium ci-trate, magnesium aspartate), but diarrhea can result from administration of any preparation.

Prevention

In another multicenter, randomized, double-blind study, 81 adult migraine patients, with a mean migraine frequency rate of 3.6 per month, received either oral magnesium (24 mmol trimagnesium dicitrate, equivalent to 600 mg/day) or placebo for 12 weeks.[13] In the last 4 weeks, frequency of migraine attacks was reduced by 41.6% in the magnesium group compared with 15.8% in the placebo group. The number of days with migraine was also significantly decreased in the magnesium group. No significant changes were noted in the duration or intensity of migraine attacks nor in drug consumption during an attack. Diarrhea was reported in 18.6% and gastric irritation in 4.7% of patients receiving magnesium.

A third placebo-controlled, double-blind trial of 69 subjects with migraine showed no benefit of magnesium supplementation over placebo.[14] Patients were treated for 12 weeks with either magnesium (10 mmol twice daily, equivalent to 500 mg/day) or placebo. Endpoints were reduction of intensity or duration of migraines by at least 50%. This trial, originally designed to enroll 150 patients, was stopped after the interim analysis of 69 patients showed no benefit for the patients receiving magnesium. An equivalent number of patients in each group (28.6% of those receiving magnesium and 29.4% of those receiving placebo) experienced a reduction in the intensity or duration of migraines. Mild adverse effects were experienced by 45.7% of those receiving magnesium and 23.5% of those on placebo. Diarrhea or soft stool was the most common complaint in the magnesium group. It is extremely unusual to stop a trial at interim analysis in such a case; usually trials are brought to an end only when there is such a large difference in either benefit or risk between the groups that it is deemed unethical to continue in the face of what is known at that point.

Prevention of Menstrual Migraine, PMS, and Menstrual Cramps

Researchers have noted lower levels of magnesium in the red blood cells of women with premenstrual syndrome.[15-17] Clinical trials have demonstrated the efficacy of magnesium for relief of menstrual pain. Magnesium also reduced the need for pain medication. There was no difference in adverse side effects of magnesium compared to placebo.[18]

In a randomized trial of 24 women with menstrual migraine,[19] the women received 360 mg/day of magnesium pyrrolidine carboxylic acid or placebo from the 15th day of their cycles until menses. During this phase of the trial, both groups reported a reduction in pain total index (a measure of both frequency and intensity of attacks). Women receiving magnesium had significantly less pain than the placebo group, and the number of days with headache decreased only in the magnesium group. After 2 months, the trial became an open-label trial in which magnesium was given to all patients for an additional 2 months. Significant decreases in pain total index were seen in both groups between the second and fourth months. Although subjects in this trial apparently were not routinely asked about side effects, two (one from each group) of four dropouts were attributed to side effects.

Riboflavin

Riboflavin is a B vitamin that is a necessary enzyme cofactor in the production of ATP. Although gross riboflavin deficiency is rare in Western countries, marginal deficiency is relatively common, especially among older adults and adolescents.

A randomized, placebo-controlled, 3-month trial of 55 patients with migraine found that 400 mg of riboflavin taken daily was superior to placebo in reducing attack frequency and headache days.[20] The proportions of patients who improved by at least 50% were 59% in the riboflavin group and 15% in the placebo group. Two of three patients who reported mild adverse effects of polyuria and diarrhea were in the treatment group. The dose of riboflavin used in this trial was quite high—about 300 times higher than the RDA. However, riboflavin is extraordinarily benign.

Feverfew (Tanacetum Parthenium)

Several trials indicate that feverfew may be effective in migraine prophylaxis. A small double-blind study tested feverfew withdrawal in regular users. Seventeen patients who regularly used feverfew to prevent migraine were randomized and given either freeze-dried feverfew powder or placebo.[21] Those who received placebo had a significant increase in the frequency and severity of headache, nausea, and vomiting, whereas those in the feverfew group showed no change in the incidence of migraines. In a larger crossover study, 72 migraine patients were given either one capsule of dried feverfew or placebo daily for 4 months, and then received the other therapy for 4 more months.[22] Patients receiving feverfew had fewer migraines, less severe attacks, and less emesis, although the duration of migraines that did occur remained the same. A review of five randomized, controlled trials of feverfew in migraine prevention found that although the majority of studies favored feverfew over placebo, the clinical effectiveness had not yet been proven beyond a reasonable doubt.[23]

CARPAL TUNNEL SYNDROME AND VITAMIN B$_6$

A review of the literature on vitamin B$_6$ and carpal tunnel syndrome[24] concluded that there is no convincing evidence that vitamin B$_6$ is adequate as the sole treatment of carpal tunnel syndrome but that it may be useful as adjunctive treatment to conservative therapy.

NEUROPATHY AND CHILI PEPPERS (CAPSICUM SPECIES)

Topical capsaicin may be useful in the treatment of diabetic neuropathy. One placebo-controlled study of 252 patients with diabetic neuropathy[25] found that 69.5% of patients treated with 0.075% capsaicin cream reported less pain compared with 53.4% of those on placebo. A controlled trial of 32 elderly patients with postherpetic neuralgia[26] found that almost 80% of the capsaicin-treated patients experienced some relief from their pain after 6 weeks.

A 4-week, placebo-controlled study found that, of 45 patients treated with 0.025% topical capsaicin or placebo for fibromyalgia,[27] those receiving capsaicin reported less tenderness at their trigger points. There was no significant difference in visual analog pain scores. A significant increase in grip strength in the capsaicin group was also noted.

A recent review found that topical capsaicin is effective for treatment of psoriasis, pruritus, and cluster headache and can help relieve itching and pain in patients with postmastectomy pain syndrome, symptoms of oral mucositis and cutaneous allergy, loin pain in those with hematuria syndrome, neck pain, amputation stump pain, and cutaneous pain associated with skin tumor. It may also be helpful for patients with neural dysfunction, including detrusor hyperreflexia and reflex sympathetic dystrophy.[28] The authors note that the placebo-controlled studies did not use a "burning" placebo and that this may have compromised blinding.

ANXIETY AND KAVA (PIPER METHYSTICUM)

A psychoactive member of the pepper family, the root of the Kava plant is used widely in Polynesia, Micronesia, and Melanesia as a ceremonial, tranquilizing beverage. It is used medicinally for anxiety and insomnia in Europe and the United States and is approved and registered in Germany for the treatment of "states of nervous anxiety, tension, and agitation" in doses of 60 to 120 mg of kavalactones for up to 3 months duration.[29,30] Kava appears to be a safe herbal remedy for short-term relief of stress and anxiety. Several placebo-controlled trials have shown significant anxiolytic activity.

In a randomized, double-blind, placebo-controlled trial, 58 patients with various anxiety and neurotic disorders as diagnosed per the International Classification of Diseases received 70 mg of kavalactones or placebo three times daily for 4 weeks. Compared with those receiving placebo, the kava group demonstrated a significant reduction in anxiety as assessed by the Hamilton anxiety scale.[31] In a second randomized, double-blind, placebo-controlled multicenter study, 101 outpatients with anxiety disorders (agoraphobia, specific phobia, generalized anxiety disorder, or adjustment disorder with anxiety) as diagnosed per the third, revised *Diagnostic and Statistical Manual of Mental Disorders (DSM-IIIR)* were treated with a kava extract for 24 weeks.[32] The results showed significant reductions in anxiety as assessed by the Hamilton anxiety scale in the kava group. Several other controlled, double-blind trials on kava extracts or the isolated compound DL-kawain have been published in the German literature.[29] In one placebo-controlled trial, 58 patients with anxiety received 210 mg kava or placebo daily for 1 month.[33] Compared with those receiving placebo, those receiving kava had significantly greater reductions in Hamilton Anxiety Scale (HAMA) scores, with improvements beginning within 1 week.

INSOMNIA AND VALERIAN (VALERIANA OFFICINALIS)

Valerian is a popular European medicine used for its mild sedative and tranquilizing properties. The drug's central nervous system activity is largely ascribed to the valepotriates and sesquiterpene constituents of the volatile oils. The German Commission E recommends 2 to 3 g of the dried root one or more times a day for "restlessness and nervous disturbance of sleep."[30] Valerian is a popular sleep remedy, despite the fact that few clinical trials on sleep or other parameters can be found in the literature.[34]

One study of 128 subjects compared the effects of an herbal preparation containing *Valeriana officinalis* as one of a mixture of herbs, a valerian-only extract (400 mg), and placebo in subjects with varying sleep difficulties.[35] Both valerian preparations produced a significant decrease in subjectively evaluated sleep latency scores and improved sleep quality. In another study, 27 patients with sleep difficulties received two pills that they took on consecutive nights.[36] Both pills contained hops and lemon balm, but one pill contained only 4 mg of valerian and the other contained a full 400-mg dose. Seventy-eight percent of the subjects preferred full-dose valerian, 15% preferred the low-dose valerian, and 7% had no preference.

DIABETIC NEUROPATHY

Vitamin E

In a randomized double-blind trial, 21 subjects with type II diabetes were assigned to receive either 900 mg vitamin E or placebo for 6 months.[37] Nerve conduction, measured by electrophysiologic tests, was the main outcome measure. Nerve conduction velocity in the median motor nerve fibers and tibial motor nerve distal latency improved significantly in the treatment group. The other 10 electrophysiologic parameters did not change.

Thiamine

In Tanzania, diabetic peripheral neuropathy is associated with thiamine deficiency. In a controlled study comparing thiamine (25 mg/day) and pyridoxine (50 mg/day) therapy with placebo (containing 1 mg each thiamine and pyridoxine), significant improvement in pain, numbness, parasthesia, and impairment of sensation in the legs was noted in the treatment group. The severity of signs of peripheral neuropathy decreased in 48.9% of the treatment group compared with 11.4% in the placebo group.[38]

ALPHA-LIPOIC ACID

In the study on alpha-lipoic acid use in patients with diabetic neuropathy, 328 patients with type II diabetes and symptomatic peripheral neuropathy were randomly selected to receive placebo or three different doses of intravenous alpha-lipoic acid (1200, 600, or 100 mg) over 3 weeks.[39] Total symptom scores were significantly reduced in groups receiving 600 or 1200 mg alpha-lipoic acid.

RESTLESS LEGS SYNDROME AND IRON

Iron deficiency, whether or not it results in anemia, appears to be an important factor in the development of restless legs syndrome (RLS) in older adults. In one study, 26 of 27 patients with severe RLS had ferritin levels less than or equal to 50 mcg/ml.[40] Lower ferritin levels correlated with greater severity of RLS symptoms and decreased sleep efficiency. In another study, serum ferritin levels were lower in 18 RLS patients (33 mcg/l) compared with 18 controls (59 mcg/l).[41] Lower serum ferritin levels correlated significantly with greater RLS severity, and improvement was noted after iron repletion.[41]

It must be kept in mind that excess body iron stores, or iron overload, is associated with increased risk of cancer and other chronic diseases, most likely related to the free radical generating properties of unbound, free iron in the body.

DISORDERS OF TASTE AND SMELL AND ZINC

Acute, severe zinc deficiency can cause hypogeusia (decreased sensitivity of taste). Two uncontrolled studies of patients with renal disease and hypogeusia found that taking 50 mg of elemental zinc a day significantly improved the patients' sense of taste. A single-blind study of 103 patients with idiopathic hypogeusia found that 100 mg zinc taken daily resulted in improvements.[42] However, an earlier double-blind crossover trial evaluated zinc (100 mg/day) in the treatment of hypogeusia in 106 patients with taste and smell dysfunction (of various etiologies) and found no effect.[43] It has been pointed out that these patients were on a variety of medications that may have affected the results.[42]

Zinc may be effective only in those individuals with low serum zinc levels. The 98 patients in one placebo-controlled trial were divided into four groups, depending on the etiology of their hypogeusia (zinc deficient, idiopathic, drug induced, and other). All received zinc gluconate (22.6 mg tid) for 4 months. Zinc benefited the zinc deficient and idiopathic groups but not the groups of patients whose conditions were drug induced or fell into other categories.[44]

In another study, patients with sensorineural olfactory disorder were treated with usual therapy, zinc sulfate, or both. Of patients with posttraumatic olfactory disorder, those in the zinc sulfate groups had significantly higher improvement rates than did those in the group that received the usual therapy.[45] For patients with disorders of postviral or unknown etiology, there were no significant differences in improvement among the three groups. In this study, pretreatment serum zinc concentrations were not significantly related to improvement rates.

Treatment for head and neck cancer often causes taste alterations. In a randomized, placebo-controlled study, 18 patients receiving external radiation to the head and neck were randomly chosen to receive zinc sulfate (45 mg tid) or placebo at the onset of taste alterations. The treatment was continued for 1 month after the radiation therapy had ended.[46] Patients treated with placebo experienced a greater loss in taste acuity during radiation treatment compared with those treated with zinc. In addition, those treated with zinc had a faster recovery of taste acuity than those receiving placebo.

DEMENTIA

Ginkgo (Ginkgo Biloba)

The ginkgo tree is one of the oldest living species. The use of ginkgo has greatly increased since 1994 when Germany approved a standardized form of leaf extract (EGb 761) for the treatment of dementia. The standardized extract contains 22% to 27% flavonoid glycosides (including quercitin and kaempferol and their glycosides) and 5% to 7% terpene lactones (consisting of 2.8% to 3.4% ginkgolides A, B, and C and 2.6% to 3.3% bilobalide).[29]

A randomized, double-blind, placebo-controlled trial of 309 patients with Alzheimer's disease or multi-infarct dementia found that patients who received EGb 761 (120 mg/day) scored higher on the Alzheimer's Disease Assessment Scale-Cognition subscale (ADAS-Cog).[47] After 1 year of treatment, 29% of patients receiving ginkgo showed at least a 4-point improvement on the test compared with 14% of those receiving placebo. Although improvement was not apparent according to the Clinician's Global Impression of Change, beneficial treatment effects were apparent to caregivers as measured by the Geriatric Evaluation by Relative's Rating Instrument.

A randomized, double-blind, placebo-controlled 6-month trial of 216 patients with Alzheimer's disease or multi-infarct dementia found that patients who were given 240 mg/day of a standardized ginkgo extract had significant improvements in memory, attention, psychopathology, and behavior compared with patients who were given placebo.[48]

In another randomized, double-blind, controlled trial of 40 Alzheimer's patients, those given 240 mg/day of standardized ginkgo extract for 3 months showed significant improvements in memory, attention, and psychopathology compared with those given placebo after 1 month.[49]

Ginkgo may also have beneficial effects on memory impairment that is not related to Alzheimer's disease. In one double-blind study, 31 outpatients who were older than 50 years and had mild to moderate memory impairment were given 120 mg of ginkgo a day. As evidenced by tests of digit copying and speed of response in a classification task, researchers noted a beneficial effect of the therapy; however, no improvement was noted on other tests of cognitive function at 12 and 14 weeks.[50]

A recent meta-analysis by Oken et al.[51] attempted a summary of all published studies in which ginkgo was given for dementia. Only randomized, double-blind, and placebo-controlled trials were included in the analysis. Analysis involved trials with patients who clearly met the criteria for a diagnosis of Alzheimer's disease, either (1) by *DSM-III*, (2) by National Institute of Neurological Disorders and Stroke-Alzheimer's Disease and Related Disorders Association criteria, or (3) by published studies in which the article contained sufficient clinical detail for the reviewer to assign diagnosis. The trials excluded patients with depression or other neurologic disease and excluded use of other central nervous system–active medications. They included studies that used standardized ginkgo extract at any dose, had at least one outcome measure that was an objective assessment of cognitive function, and contained sufficient statistical information for meta-analysis. Although more than 50 articles were identified, the majority did not meet inclusion criteria because of a lack of clear diagnoses of dementia and Alzheimer's. Of the four studies that met all inclusion criteria, there were 212 subjects in each of the placebo and ginkgo treatment groups. Overall, there was a significant effect (P < 0.0001) that translated into a 3% difference in ADAS-Cog scores. The authors concluded that 3 to 6 months of treatment with 120 to 240 mg ginkgo has a small but significant effect on objective measures of cognition in patients with Alzheimer's disease.

Choline and Lecithin

Neurochemical studies of Alzheimer's disease suggest a cholinergic deficit. Therefore there is a theoretical basis for treatments that enhance cholinergic activity. However, choline and lecithin supplementation has generally been ineffective.[52] Providing precursors of acetylcholine in this way is probably insufficient to boost cholinergic activity to a meaningful level; inhibiting the catabolism of acetylcholine with cholinesterase inhibitors is the current therapeutic alternative.

Phosphatidylserine

Although numerous studies, such as that by Cenacchi et al.[53] support a therapeutic effect of bovine-derived phosphatidylserine given to patients with dementia, these products are no longer available because of concerns about mad cow disease. Currently available preparations are derived from soy, but no studies involving these new products have been published in the scientific literature.

COGNITION AND VITAMIN STATUS

Subclinical malnutrition may play a small role in the reduced cognitive function in some older individuals. Folic acid deficiency, one of the most common nutritional deficiencies worldwide, has often been associated with cognitive disorders.[54] In elderly patients the incidence of deficiency is particularly marked and may be as high as 90%.[55]

Folate and vitamin B_{12} are required for the methylation of homo-cysteine to methionine and for the synthesis of S-adenosylmethionine. S-adenosylmethionine plays a role in numerous methylation reactions involving proteins, phospholipids, deoxyribo-nucleic acid, and neurotransmitter metabolism. Folate and vitamin B_{12} deficiency may cause similar neurologic and psychiatric disturbances, including depression, dementia, and a demyelinating myelopathy.[54,56] Supplementation may be beneficial in deficient individuals, but more definitive studies are ongoing.[57]

In an observational study, Goodwin et al.[58] evaluated the association between nutritional status and cognitive function in 260 noninstitution-alized men and women older than 60 years who had no known physical illnesses and were taking no medications. Nutritional status was evaluated based on 3-day food records and the participants' blood levels of specific nutrients. Cognitive status was evaluated by the Halstead-Reitan categories test (a nonverbal test of abstract thinking ability) and by the Wechsler memory test. Subjects with low blood levels of vitamins C or B_{12} had lower scores on both tests. Subjects with low levels of riboflavin or folic acid had lower scores on the categories test. These differences remained significant after controlling for age, gender, level of income, and amount of education.

TINNITUS

Ten ear, nose, and throat specialists conducted a multicenter, double-blind, placebo-controlled study involving 103 outpatients with tinnitus over a 3-month treatment period.[59] Patients, all of whom had had tinnitus for 1 year or less, were either given ginkgo or placebo. The groups were comparable in regard to duration and intensity of symptoms and degree of impairment. Comparison of the groups revealed that a significantly greater percentage of the ginkgo-treated group experienced either resolution of symptoms or distinct improvement, regardless of the duration of symptoms, whether the tinnitus was bilateral or unilateral, and whether symptoms were constant or intermittent.

Holgers et al.[60] designed a study in two parts. The first part was an open-label trial ($n = 80$) of ginkgo (Seredrin, approximately 30 mg/day) in subjects with persistent, severe tinnitus; the second part was a double-blind, placebo-controlled study ($n = 20$). Of 21 patients who reported that the ginkgo supplementation had a positive effect on their tinnitus in the open study, 20 were included in a double-blind, placebo-controlled crossover study ($n = 20$). Seven patients preferred ginkgo, 7 preferred placebo, and 6 had no preference. This study failed to confirm that consumption of ginkgo affects tinnitus; however, the dose was much smaller than that used in other studies.

Coles[61] published a brief correspondence describing an open trial of 23 tinnitus patients given 120 mg EGb 761 for 12 weeks. Eighteen of these patients had experienced tinnitus for more than 3 years; the median duration was 8 ½ years. Two patients did not complete the trial. Of the 21 who remained, 11 reported no change, 2 reported that severity of symptoms was lessened, and 2 reported that severity was slightly lessened. A total of 5 patients reported that their tinnitus was worse. There were no changes in audiometric measurements. The author concluded that ginkgo was ineffective in this trial.

Von Wedel and colleagues[62] reported a placebo-controlled trial in 155 patients with chronic tinnitus of at least 6 months duration and one or more failed treatments. The design included four groups treated with one of the following: an investigational technique involving soft-laser irradiation of the cochlea, a ginkgo extract given intravenously, both treatments combined, or a double-placebo control. Nineteen patients in the combined therapy group dropped out; 6 of them did so because the tinnitus worsened. The dropouts were not included in the analyses. Treatment consisted of 12 sessions 2 to 3 days apart. Patients in the combined-therapy group received 5 ml ginkgo intravenously (concentration or formulation was not provided) before the laser treatment. There were no differences among the groups, including the group receiving placebo. The conclusion of the authors was that neither treatment was effective.

There are mixed data on the efficacy of ginkgo in patients with tinnitus. There is a possibility that ginkgo may have significant potential only in patients with recent-onset tinnitus, such as those in the Meyer study.[59]

ACUTE HEARING LOSS

In a therapeutic trial of acute cochlear deafness, Dubreuil[63] reported a randomized, double-blind, controlled study of EGb 761 (320 mg/day) and a standard alpha-blocker (nicergoline) given for 30 days. The rationale for the study was that ischemia may underlie acute cochlear deafness, regardless of the triggering event. Nine patients in each group, which were comparable in pathology at the beginning of the study, completed the treatment. From the tenth day until the end of the trial, improvement appeared to be greater in the ginkgo group, although both groups improved. The audiometric gain in the ginkgo group ranged between 6 and 15 decibels greater than in the nicergoline group; however, no formal statistical analysis was performed.

Hoffmann and colleagues[64] reported the results of a randomized comparison study on 80 patients with idiopathic sudden hearing loss (of no more than 10 days' duration). EGb 761 (175 mg intravenous infusion plus 160 mg oral/day) was compared with the vasodilating, anti-serotonergic drug, naftidrofuryl (400 mg intravenous infusion plus 400 mg oral/day). The primary outcome was audiometric data, measured as relative hearing gain. After 1 week of observation, 40% of the patients in each group showed a complete remission of hearing loss. This percentage is consistent with expected rates of spontaneous recovery. After 2 and 3 weeks of observation, there was no difference between groups in relative hearing gain, yet there was a borderline benefit of ginkgo ($p = 0.06$) over naftidrofuryl. Although no side effects were attributed to ginkgo, some patients in the naftidrofuryl group developed orthostatic blood pressure changes, headache, or sleep disturbances.

VERTIGO

Haguenauer and others[65] enrolled 70 patients with vertigo of recent onset and undetermined origin in a multicenter study. In a randomized, double-blind trial conducted over a 3-month period, subjects received either 160 mg/day EGb 761 or a placebo. The effectiveness of ginkgo on the intensity, frequency, and duration of the disorder was statistically and clinically significant by the end of the first month. After 3 months, 47% of the ginkgo-treated patients were asymptomatic, compared with 18% of those who received placebo.

OMEGA-3 FATTY ACIDS

Omega-3 polyunsaturated fatty acids are long-chain, polyunsaturated fatty acids (PUFAs) found in plant and marine sources. These essential fatty acids, particularly docosahexaenoic acid (DHA), are necessary for proper membrane function and may be etiologic factors in depression, bipolar disorder, schizophrenia, and other psychiatric and neurologic disorders.[66-70] The Western diet contains considerably high amounts of omega-6 fatty acids and lesser amounts of omega-3 fatty acids. Fish oil is high in PUFAs, DHA, and eicosapentaenoic acid. Neuronal membranes contain high concentrations of DHA, as well as arachidonic acid (AA). Both of these acids are crucial components of the phospholipid bilayer; each comprises approximately 25% of the phospholipid content.[71] Neurotransmitter receptors lie embedded in the matrix of this membrane, and their three-dimensional conformation is dependent on the fatty acids that give structure to the membrane.[72]

Biochemical studies have shown that high doses of omega-3 fatty acids lead to the incorporation of these compounds into the neuronal membrane phospholipids, which are crucial for cell signaling.[73,74] Phosphatidylinositol-associated second messenger activity is also suppressed.[75] Dietary supplementation with large amounts of omega-3 fatty acids is related to a general dampening of signal transduction pathways associated with phosphatidylinositol, AA, and other systems.[74,76]

Some have suggested an association between depression and multiple sclerosis.[77] This relationship is based on a meta-analysis of published studies and is consistent with essential fatty acid depletion, especially DHA and to a lesser extent AA, in both white matter[78-80] and plasma.[81] DHA is apparently completely absent in the adipose tissue of patients with multiple sclerosis.[82]

The relationship between abnormal concentrations of omega-3 and omega-6 fatty acids and the occurrence of other neurologic disorders, such as Huntington's disease and tardive dyskinesia, also has been noted.[83,84]

CONCLUSION

Intriguing evidence is available regarding the possible benefits of certain alternative therapies as sole or adjunctive therapy in patients with some neurologic disorders. Magnesium (for migraine), ginkgo (for various vascular disorders), and essential fatty acids (for psychiatric and neurologic disorders) seem particularly promising. Naturally, more research must be done in these areas. Although these treatments may be considered alternative or complementary, testing them would be quite straightforward. These treatments would all lend themselves to standard clinical trial design, and perhaps testing them should be considered a higher priority.

REFERENCES

1. Johnson BA. Herbal formulas show market growth. *Herbal Gram.* 1999;46:57.
2. Eisenberg DM et al. Trends in alternative medicine use in the United States, 1990–1997: results of a follow-up national survey. *JAMA.* 1998;280:1569–1575.
3. Fugh-Berman A. Herb-drug interactions. *Lancet.* 2000;355:134–138.
4. Fugh-Berman A, Cott J. Dietary supplements and natural products as psychotherapeutic agents. *Psychosom Med.* 1999;61:712–728.
5. Shils ME. Magnesium. In: Shils ME, et al. *Modern Nutrition in Health and Disease.* 9th ed. Baltimore, MD: Williams & Wilkins; 1999.

6. Weisinger JR, Bellorin-Font E. Magnesium and phosphorus. *Lancet.* 1998;352:391–396.

7. Bigal ME, Bordini CA, Tepper SJ, et al. Intravenous magnesium sulfate in the acute treatment of migraine with and without aura. *Cephalalgia.* 2002;22:345–440.

8. Blumental M. *The American Botanical Council Guide to Herbs.* Austin, TX: ABC; 2003:138–142.

9. Ernst E, Pittler MH. The efficacy and safety of feverfew (Tanacetum partheniium L.) *Public Health Nutr.* 2004;3(4a):509–514.

10. Pfaffenrath V, Diner HC, Fisher M, et al. The efficacy and safety of feverfew in migraine prophylaxis. *Cephalalgia.* 2002;22:523–532.

11. Mauskop A, Altura BM. Role of magnesium in the pathogenesis and treatment of migraines. *Clin Neurosci.* 1998;5:24–27.

12. Mauskop A et al. Intravenous magnesium sulfate relieves migraine attacks in patients with low serum ionized magnesium levels: a pilot study. *Clin Sci.* 1995;89:633–636.

13. Peikert A, Wilimzig C, Kohne-Volland R. Prophylaxis of migraine with oral magnesium: results from a prospective, multi-center, placebo-controlled and double-blind randomized study. *Cephalalgia.* 1996;16:257–263.

14. Pfaffenrath V et al. Magnesium in the prophylaxis of migraine—a double-blind, placebo-controlled study. *Cephalalgia.* 1996;16:436–440.

15. Sherwood RA, Rocks BF, Steward A, et al. Magnesium and premenstrual syndrome. *Ann Clin Biochem.* 1986;23:667–670.

16. Rosenstein DL, Elin RJ, Hosseini JM, et al. Magnesium measures across the menstrual cycle in premenopausal syndrome. *Biol Psychiatry.* 1994;35:557–561.

17. Bigal ME, Rappaport AM, Sheftell FD, et al. New migraine prevention options. *Rev Hosp Clin.* 2002;57:293–298.

18. Wilson ML, Murphy PA. Herbal and dietary therapies for primary and secondary dysmenorrhoea. *The Cochrane Library.* 2002;(2).

19. Facchinetti F, et al. Magnesium prophylaxis of menstrual migraine: effects of intracellular magnesium. *Headache.* 1991;31:298–301.

20. Schoenen J, Jacquy J, Lenaerts M. Effectiveness of high-dose riboflavin in migraine prophylaxis. *Neurol.* 1998;50:466–470.

21. Johnson ES, et al. Efficacy of feverfew as prophylactic treatment of migraine. *BMJ.* 1985;291:569–573.

22. Murphy JJ, Heptinsall S, Mitchell JRA. Randomized double-blind placebo-controlled trial of feverfew in migraine prevention. *Lancet.* 1988;2:189–192.

23. Vogler BK, Pittler MH, Ernst E. Feverfew as a preventive treatment for migraine: a systematic review. *Cephalalgia.* 1998;18:704–708.

24. Jacobson MD, Plancher KD, Kleinman WB. Vitamin B$_6$ (Pyridoxine) therapy for carpal tunnel syndrome. *Hand Clin.* 1996;12:253–257.

25. Capsaicin Study Group. Treatment of painful diabetic neuropathy with topical capsaicin. *Arch Intern Med.* 1991;151:2225–2229.

26. Watson CPN, Evans RJ, Watt VR. Post-herpetic neuralgia and topical capsaicin. *Pain.* 1988;33:333–340.

27. McCarty DJ, et al. Treatment of pain due to fibromyalgia with topical capsaicin: a pilot study. *Semin Arthritis Rheum.* 1994;23(suppl 3):41–47.

28. Hautkappe M, et al. Review of the effectiveness of capsaicin for painful cutaneous disorders and neural dysfunction. *Clin J Pain.* 1998;14:97–106.

29. Schultz V, Hansel R, Tyler VE. *Rational Phytotherapy: A Physician's Guide to Herbal Medicine.* 3rd ed. Berlin, Germany: Springer-Verlag; 1998.

30. Blumenthal M, Goldberg A, Brinckmann J. *Herbal Medicine: Expanded Commission E Monographs.* Newton, MA: Integrative Medicine Communications; 2000.

31. Lehmann E, Kinzler E, Friedemann J. Efficacy of a special Kava extract (Piper me-thysticum) in patients with states of anxiety, tension, and excitedness of non-mental origin—a double-blind placebo-controlled study of four weeks treatment. *Phytomed.* 1996;3:113–119.

32. Volz HP, Kieser M. Kava-kava extract WS 1490 versus placebo in anxiety disor-ders—a randomized placebo-controlled 25-week outpatient trial. *Pharmacopsychiatry.* 1997;30:1–5.

33. Kinzler E, Kromer J, Lehmann E. Wirksamkeit eines Kava-Spezial-Extraktes bei Pa-tienten mit Angst-, Spannungs-und Erregungszustanden nicht-psychotischer Genese, *Arzneimittelforschung.* 1991;41:584–588.

34. Wagner J, Wagner ML, Hening WA. Beyond benzodiazepines: alternative pharmaco-logic agents for the treatment of insomnia. *Ann Pharmacother.* 1998;32:680–691.

35. Leathwood PD et al. Aqueous extract of valerian root improves sleep quality in man. *Pharmacol Biochem Behav.* 1982;17:65–71.

36. Lindahl O, Lindwall L. Double blind study of a valerian preparation. *Pharmacol Bio-chem Behav.* 1989;32:1065–1066.

37. Tutuncu NB, Bayraktar M, Varli K. Reversal of defective nerve conduction with vita-min E supplementation in type 2 diabetes: a preliminary study. *Diabetes Care.* 1998;21: 1915–1918.

38. Abbas ZG, Swai AB. Evaluation of the efficacy of thiamine and pyridoxine in the treat-ment of symptomatic diabetic peripheral neuropathy. *East Afr Med J.* 1997;74:803–808.

39. Ziegler D, Gries FA. Alpha-lipoic acid in the treatment of diabetic peripheral and car-diac autonomic neuropathy. *Diabetes.* 1997;46(suppl 2):S62–66.

40. Sun ER, et al. Iron and the restless legs syndrome. *Sleep.* 1998;21:371–377.

41. O'Keefe ST, Gavin K, Lavan JN. Iron status and restless legs syndrome in the elderly. *Age Ageing.* 1994;23:200–203.

42. Heyneman CA. Zinc deficiency and taste disorders. *Ann Pharmacother.* 1996;30:186–187.

43. Henkin RI, et al. A double-blind study of the effects of zinc sulfate on taste and smell function. *Am J Med Sci.* 1976;272:285–299.

44. Yoshida S, Endo S, Tomita H. A double-blind study of the therapeutic effect of zinc gluconate on taste disorder. *Auris Nasus Larynx.* 1991;18:153–161.

45. Aiba T, et al. Effect of zinc sulfate on sensorineural olfactory disorder. *Acta Otolaryn-gol Suppl (Stockh).* 1998;538:202–204.

46. Ripamonti C, et al. A randomized, controlled clinical trial to evaluate the effects of zinc sulfate on cancer patients with taste alterations caused by head and neck irradiation. *Cancer.* 1998;82:1938–1945.

47. Le Bars P, et al. A placebo-controlled, double-blind, randomized trial of an extract of Ginkgo biloba for dementia. *JAMA.* 1997;278:1327–1332.

48. Kanowski S, et al. Proof of efficacy of the Ginkgo biloba special extract EGb 761 in outpatients suffering from mild to moderate primary degenerative dementia of the Alz-heimer type or multi-infarct dementia. *Pharmacopsychiatry.* 1996;29:47–56.

49. Hofferberth B. The efficacy of Egb 761 in patients with senile dementia of the Alz-heimer type, a double-blind, placebo-controlled study on different levels of investiga-tion. *Hum Psychopharmacol.* 1994;9:215–222.

50. Rai GS, Shovlin C, Wesnes KA. A double-blind, placebo-controlled study of Ginkgo biloba extract ("Tanakan') in elderly outpatients with mild to moderate memory im-pairment. *Curr Med Res Opin.* 1991;12:350–355.

51. Oken BS, Storzbach DM, Kaye JA. The efficacy of Ginkgo biloba on cognitive function in Alzheimer disease. *Arch Neurol.* 1998;55:1409–1415.

52. Rathmann KL, Conner CS. Alzheimer's disease: clinical features, pathogenesis, and treatment. *Drug Intell and Clin Pharm.* 1984;18:684–691.

53. Cenacchi T, et al. Cognitive decline in the elderly: a double-blind, placebo-controlled multicenter study on efficacy of phosphatidylserine administration. *Aging (Milano.)* 1993;5:123–133.

54. Reynolds EH. Interrelationships between the neurology of folate and vitamin B_{12} deficiency. In: [[editor, ed.]] *Folic Acid in Neurology, Psychiatry, and Internal Medicine.* New York, NY: Raven; 1979.

55. Thornton WE, Thornton BP. Geriatric mental function and serum folate: a review and survey. *South Med J.* 1977;70:919–922.

56. Hutto BR. Folate and cobalamin in psychiatric illness. *Compr Psychiatry.* 1997;38: 305–314.

57. Nilsson-Ehle H. Age-related changes in cobalamin (vitamin B_{12}) handling: implications for therapy. *Drugs Aging.* 1998;12:277–292.

58. Goodwin JS, Goodwin JM, Garry PJ. Association between nutritional status and cognitive functioning in a healthy elderly population. *JAMA.* 1983;249:2917–2922.

59. Meyer B. Multicenter randomized double-blind drug vs. placebo study of the treatment of tinnitus with Ginkgo biloba extract. *Presse Med.* 1986;15:1562–1564.

60. Holgers KM, Axelsson A, Pringle I. Ginkgo biloba extract for the treatment of tinnitus, *Audiol.* 1994;33:85–92.

61. Coles R. Trial of an extract of Ginkgo biloba (EGB) for tinnitus and hearing loss. *Clin Otolaryngol.* 1988;13:501–502.

62. Von Wedel, et al. Soft-laser/Ginkgo therapy in chronic tinnitus: a placebo-controlled study. *Adv Otorhinolaryngol.* 1995;49:105–108.

63. Dubreuil C. Therapeutic trial in acute cochlear deafness: a comparative study of Ginkgo biloba extract and nicergoline. *Presse Med.* 1986;15:1559–1561.

64. Hoffmann F et al. Ginkgo extract EGb 761 (Tebonin)/ HAES versus naftidrofuryl (Dusodril)/HAES: a randomized study of therapy of sudden deafness. *Laryngorhinootologie.* 1994;73:149–152.

65. Haguenauer JP. Treatment of equilibrium disorders with Ginkgo biloba extract: a multicenter double-blind drug vs. placebo study. *Presse Med.* 1986;15:1569–1572.

66. Hibbeln JR, Palmer JW, Davis JM. Are disturbances in lipid-protein interactions by phospholipase-A2 a predisposing factor in affective illness? *Biol Psychiatry.* 1989;25: 945–961.

67. Hibbeln JR, Salem N Jr. Dietary polyunsaturated fatty acids and depression: when cholesterol does not satisfy. *Am J Clin Nutr.* 1995;62:1–9.

68. Hillbrand M, Spitz RT, VandenBos GR. Investigating the role of lipids in mood, aggression, and schizophrenia. *Psychiatr Serv.* 1997;48: 875–876.

69. Hibbeln JR et al. Do plasma polyunsaturates predict hostility and depression? *World Rev Nutr Diet.* 1997;82:175–186.

70. Stoll AL et al. Omega-3 fatty acids in bipolar disorder: a preliminary double-blind, placebo-controlled trial. *Arch Gen Psychiatry.* 1999;56:407–412.

71. Mahadik SP, Evans DR. Essential fatty acids in the treatment of schizophrenia. *Drugs of Today.* 1997;33:5–17.

72. Mitchell DC, et al. Why is docosahexaenoic acid essential for nervous system function? *Biochem Soc Trans.* 1998;26:365–370.

73. Medini L, et al. Diets rich in n-9, n-6 and n-3 fatty acids differentially affect the generation of inositol phosphates and of thromboxane by stimulated platelets, in the rabbit. *Biochem Pharmacol.* 1990;39:129–133.

74. Sperling RI, et al. Dietary omega-3 polyunsaturated fatty acids inhibit phosphoinositide formation and chemotaxis in neutrophils. *J Clin Invest.* 1993;91:651–660.

75. Kinsella JE. Lipids, membrane receptors, and enzymes: effects of dietary fatty acids, *J of Parenteral and Enteral Nutr.* 1990;14:200s–217s.
76. Tappia PS, et al. The influence of membrane fluidity, TNF receptor binding, cAMP production and GTPase activity on macrophage cytokine production in rats fed a variety of fat diets. *Mol Cell Biochem.* 1997;166:135–143.
77. Schubert DS, Foliart RH. Increased depression in multiple sclerosis patients. A meta-analysis. *Psychosomatics.* 1993;34(2):124–130.
78. Gerstl B, et al. Alterations in myelin fatty acids and plasmalogans in multiple sclerosis. *Ann NY Acad Sci.* 1965;122:405–407.
79. Kishimoto Y, et al. Gangliosides and glycerophospholipids in multiple sclerosis white matter. *Arch Neurol.* 1967;16:41–54.
80. Wilson R, Tocher DR. Lipid and fatty acid composition is altered in plaque tissue from multiple sclerosis brain compared with normal brain white matter. *Lipids.* 1991; 26:9–15.
81. Cunnane SC, Ho SY, Dore-Duffy P, Ells KR, Horrobin DF. Essential fatty acid and lipid profiles in plasma and erythrocytes in patients with multiple sclerosis. *Am J Clin Nutr.* 1989;50(4):801–806.
82. Nightingale S, Woo E, Smith AD, et al. Red blood cell and adipose tissue fatty acids in mild inactive multiple sclerosis. *Acta Neurol Scand.* 1990;82(1):43–50.
83. Nilsson A, et al. Essential fatty acids and abnormal involuntary movements in the general male population: a study of men born in 1933. *Prostaglandins Leukot Essent Fatty Acids.* 1996;55:83–87.
84. Vaddadi KS. Essential fatty acids and movement disorders. In: Peet M, Glen I, Horrobin DF, eds. *Phospholipid Spectrum Disorder in Psychiatry.* Carnforth, United Kingdom: Marius; 1999.

CHAPTER 16

Aromatherapy

Alan R. Hirsch

> The fundamental premises (of alternative medicine) are an advocacy of nature, vitalism, science, and spirituality.
>
> —*Ted Kaptchuk*[1]

Why is the concept of aromatherapy under consideration today? One reason is its antiquity. Throughout history, odorants have been used to treat various diseases. More than 5,000 years ago Egyptians treated disease using odors,[2] and 3,500 years ago Babylonians used odors to exorcise demons of disease.[3] Ancient Aztecs also used odors to treat disease. Aromatherapy has known no cultural or geographic boundaries. Virtually all cultures have fumigated the sick.[4]

One of the difficulties in understanding aromatherapy is that it means different things to different people. The one part of its definition that is agreed upon is that aromatherapy uses aromatic compounds to promote health and healing.[5] Beyond this, opinions differ. Aromatologists speak of using aromas not to treat disease but to promote wellness. Aromatologists sometimes believe in ingestion of the substance being used as well as its inhalation.[5] Many aromatherapists believe in using massage coincident with inhalation.[6] In this chapter, aromatherapy is defined as the use of odorants as inhalants to treat underlying medical or psychological conditions. This definition excludes any effects of ingestion or percutaneous absorption, although they may be significant depending upon the method of application.[7] As defined, aromatherapy use is also independent of any effects of coincident, noninhalational therapy, such as massage, interpersonal interaction, or bathing.

This definition is consistent with the literature indicating that so-called real aromatherapy involves the uptake of fragrant compounds *only* through inhalation, not by other methods.[4]

Many in the aromatherapy community believe that natural or essential oils are effective and that artificial synthesized compounds are not. However, in the treatment of neurologic and psychological disorders, literature does not differentiate between them.[8] No distinction is made herein between the use of synthesized as opposed to naturally occurring oils.

ANATOMY OF OLFACTION

Neuroscience provides insight into the mechanisms by which odors may impact behavior and neurologic functioning. There is an anatomic basis for the belief that odors can affect the brain and behavior.[9,10] Once an odor passes through the olfactory epithelium, it must stimulate the olfactory nerve, which consists of unmyelinated olfactory fila. The olfactory nerve has the slowest conduction rate of any nerve in the body. The olfactory fila pass through the cribiform plate of the ethmoid bone and enter the olfactory bulb. During trauma, much damage occurs in this bulb.[11] Different odors localize in different areas of the olfactory bulb.

Inside the olfactory bulb is a conglomeration of neuropil called the *glomeruli*. Approximately 2,000 glomeruli reside in the olfactory bulb. Four different cell types make up the glomeruli: processes of receptor cell axons, mitral cells, tufted cells, and second-order neurons that give off collaterals to the granule cells and to cells in the periglomerular and external plexiform layers. The mitral and tufted cells form the lateral olfactory tract and establish a reverberating circuit with the granule cells. The mitral cells stimulate firing of the granule cells, which in turn inhibit firing of the mitral cells.

A reciprocal inhibition exists between the mitral and tufted cells. This results in a sharpening of olfactory acuity. The olfactory bulb receives several efferent projections, including the primary olfactory fibers, the contralateral olfactory bulb and the anterior nucleus, the prepiriform cortex (inhibitory), the diagonal band of Broca (with neurotransmitters acetylcholine and GABA), the locus coeruleus, the dorsal raphe, and the tuberomamillary nucleus of the hypothalamus.

The olfactory bulb's efferent fibers project into the olfactory tract, which divides at the olfactory trigona into the medial and lateral olfactory stria. These project to the anterior olfactory nucleus; the olfactory tubercle; the amygdaloid nucleus (which in turn projects to the ventral medial nucleus of the hypothalamus, a feeding center); the cortex of the piriform lobe; the septal nuclei; and the hypothalamus, in particular the anterolateral regions of the hypothalamus, which are involved in reproduction. The neurotransmitters by which the olfactory bulb conducts its information include glutamate and aspartate.

NEUROTRANSMITTERS

The anterior olfactory nucleus receives afferent fibers from the olfactory tract and projects efferent fibers, which decussate in the anterior commissure and synapse in the contralateral olfactory bulb. Some of the efferent projections from the anterior olfactory nucleus remain ipsilateral and synapse on internal granular cells of the ipsilateral olfactory bulb.

The olfactory tubercle receives afferent fibers from the olfactory bulb and the anterior olfactory nucleus. Efferent fibers from the olfactory tubercle project to the nucleus accumbens as well as the striatum. Neurotransmitters of the olfactory tubercle include acetylcholine and dopamine.

The area on the cortex where olfaction is localized, that is, the primary olfactory cortex, includes the prepiriform area, the periamygdaloid area, and the entorhinal area. Afferent projections to the primary olfactory cortex include the mitral cells, which enter the lateral olfactory tract and synapse in the prepiriform cortex (lateral olfactory gyrus), and the corticomedial part of the amygdala. Efferent projections from the primary olfactory cortex extend to the entorhinal cortex (area 28), the basal and lateral amygdaloid nuclei, the lateral preoptic area of the hypothalamus, the nucleus of the diagonal band of Broca, the medial forebrain bundle, the dorsal medial nucleus and submedial nucleus of the thalamus, and the nucleus accumbens.

It should be noted that the entorhinal cortex is both a primary and a secondary olfactory cortical area. Efferent fibers from the cortex project via the uncinate fasciculus to the hippocampus, the anterior insular cortex (next to the gustatory cortical area), and the frontal cortex. This may explain why temporal lobe epilepsy that involves the uncinate often produces parageusias of burning rubber, uncinate fits.[12]

Some of the efferent projections of the mitral and tufted cells decussate in the anterior commissure and form the medial olfactory tract. They then synapse in the contralateral parolfactory area and contralateral subcallosal gyrus. The exact function of the medial olfactory stria and tract is not clear. The accessory olfactory bulb receives afferent fibers from the bed nucleus of the accessory olfactory tract and the medial and posterior corticoamygdaloid nuclei. Efferent fibers from the accessory olfactory bulb project through the accessory olfactory tract to the same afferent areas, for example, the bed nucleus of the accessory olfactory tract and the medial and posterior corticoamygdaloid nuclei. It should be noted that the medial and posterior corticoamygdaloid nuclei project secondary fibers to the anterior and medial hypothalamus, the areas associated with reproduction. Therefore the accessory olfactory bulb in humans may be the mediator for human pheromones.[13]

Some unique aspects of the anatomy of the olfactory system are worth mentioning. Smell is the only sensation to reach the cortex before reaching the thalamus, although a thalamic relay is present.[14] The only sensory system that is primarily ipsilateral in its projection, olfaction does not depend upon the cortex, as has been demonstrated in decorticated cats.

Neurotransmitters of the olfactory cortex are multiple, including glutamate, aspartate cholcystekinin, LHRH, and somatastatin. Furthermore, perception of odors causes modulation of olfactory neurotransmitters within the olfactory bulb and the limbic system. Virtually all known neurotransmitters are present in the olfactory bulb. Thus odorant modulation of neurotransmitter levels in the olfactory bulb, tract, and limbic system intended for transmission of sensory information may have unintended secondary effects on a variety of different behaviors and disease states that are regulated by the same neurotransmitters. For instance, odorant modulation of dopamine in the olfactory bulb/limbic system may affect manifestations of Parkinson's disease. Mesolimbic override to many of the components of Parkinson's disease have been well documented, for example, motoric activation associated with emotional distress and fear of injury in a fire.

EMOTIONAL AND BEHAVIORAL EFFECTS

Odors can affect behavior by acting as alternative sensory stimuli. The phenomenon of visual system mediation of the movements of Parkinsonian gait through the visual stimuli of lines placed on the floor[15] is an example of alternative stimuli. Other sensory input, including pain, has been shown to inhibit the Jacksonian march in epilepsy.[16] Similarly, odors may act as competing sensory stimuli during an uncinate seizure.[17] It seems possible that other sensory input, including odors, could modify Parkinson's disease as well as other neurologic conditions by acting as competing sensory stimuli. Alternatively, aromas may function to preferentially activate a non-olfactory sensory system, which would then induce analgesia through reduction of attention to other nonpainful sensations.[18]

That odors could act to affect non-olfactory sensory perception has been demonstrated at the primary level in the effect of olfactory stimuli on hearing, touch, gustation, and vision[19,20] and with complex integrated sensory perception with estimation of room size,[21] age,[22] and weight.[23]

Using another mechanism of action, odors can affect behavior and mood by producing secondary effects on the emotions of the individual. This is different from a direct neurophysiologic effect of the limbic system. Rather, the odor can change the mood of the individual, which then has secondary neurologic effects. For instance, the mood or level of alertness can affect a variety of neurologic conditions, including the perception of pain. A soldier who is severely wounded in battle may continue to fight and not feel pain until the battle is over. Studies also suggest that persons in a positive state of mind are less bothered by pain.[24]

Substantial evidence exists that odors can affect mood. As early as 1908, Freud[25] stressed the importance of olfaction on emotion in his description of a patient with an obsessional neurosis. Freud began his career as a neuropathologist, searching for organic causes and pathologic lesions for mental illness. Because the brains of people with mental illness are normal anatomically and pathologically sound, Freud embarked on the pursuit of more ethereal causes.

SIGMUND FREUD ON SMELL

By his own account, when a child, he recognized every one by their smell, like a dog, and even when he was grown up he was more susceptible to sensations of smell than other people:

"and I have come to recognize that a tendency towards osphresiolagnia which has become extinct since childhood may play a part in the genesis of neuroses.

In a general way I should like to raise the question whether the inevitable shunting of the sense of smell as a result of man's turning away from the earth and the organic repression of smell pleasure produced by it does not largely share in his predisposition to nervous diseases. It would thus furnish an explanation for the fact that with the advance of civilization it is precisely the sexual life which must become the victim of repression. For we have long known what an intimate relation exists in the animal organization between the sexual impulse and the function of the olfactory organs."

Of all the sensations, olfaction is the one most intertwined with limbic system functioning.[26] The profuse anatomic and physiologic interconnections through the olfactory bulb, stria, and nuclei to the olfactory tubercle, and from there to the prepiriform cortex, the amygdala, and numerous other limbic system structures support this.[27]

Smells are described differently from other sensory modalities, adding credence to their connection to emotion. Other sensory modalities are first described cognitively; a picture, for instance, is identified as being of a ship, a woman, or a house and only secondarily is it described affectively: "I like it," or "I dislike it."[28] But odors are first and foremost described affectively: "I like it," or "I dislike it."

The olfactory/limbic/hippocampal connections help to explain olfactory-evoked nostalgia, the phenomenon whereby an odor induces a vivid recall of a scene from the distant past.[29] In 86% of 989 subjects queried, certain odors triggered vivid associations analogous to a flashbulb memory. Classically an event must induce strong emotions for deposition of such memories to occur.[30,31] By directly stimulating the limbic system, odors likewise can act as the inducing agent. This phenomenon was vividly described by Proust,[32] who wrote that the aroma of madeleine dipped in tea evoked his flood of memories and nostalgic feelings. Olfactory-evoked recall is usually a positive experience, but it can be negative, as in the olfactory flashbacks of posttraumatic stress disorder.[33,34] Hence, it seems possible that olfactory-evoked nostalgia may affect behavior because approximately 90% of these memories are associated with strong affective tones.[35]

The facts bring to the forefront the question of how odors impact on behavior or mood. The answer can be represented by either of two constructs: the lock and key theory or the general affective theory of odors.

THE LOCK AND KEY THEORY

The lock and key theory of odors (also called the *systemic effect theory*)[4] suggests that odor acts very much like a specific neurotransmitter, a drug, or an enzyme. In this paradigm, an odorant has a specific effect on behavior or emotion—one odor for one emotion or one odor for, at most, a few emotions. Thus an odor could be viewed like a medication in the pharmacopeia. For instance, in the world of neurology, propranolol is used for modulation of essential tremor, migraine headache, and anxiety; however, one would not use propranolol as a treatment for insomnia, dementia, or multiple sclerosis. The lock and key theory suggests that specific odors have specific effects. This theory has been proposed in virtually every book about aromatherapy in which specific odors are recommended for specific health effects.[5,36-41]

An argument supporting the lock and key theory is that odorants exert central nervous system (CNS) effects outside a subject's conscious awareness as has been demonstrated on EEG with varying concentrations of the odorant galaxide.[42] In test animals, the more lipophilic an odor is, the greater its sedative effect. In addition, steric differences in odors create different effects despite similarities in perceived odor and volatility.[4,43]

According to the lock and key theory, odors act as a drug[44] with a potentially pharmacologic mechanism of action. The odorants are integrated in the membrane of the cells, causing an increase in membrane volume due to disruption of the membrane lipids. This leads to electrical stabilization of the membrane, thus blocking the inflow of calcium ions and suppressing permeability for sodium ions. As a result, action potential production is inhibited, which induces narcosis or local anesthesia. At higher concentrations of odorant, the conductivity of potassium ions is reduced. It is also possible that the odorants act on protein kinase C, which could impact upon the spontaneous rhythm of nerve cells.[4]

This mechanism of action is further supported by established physiology for the action of an odor on the target organ—in this case the brain. Inhalation of an odorant would have to produce measurable levels in the blood, sufficient to pass through the blood brain barrier. Stimpfl[45] demonstrated that this does occur. One subject inhaled 1,8-cineol for 20 minutes, which produced a linear increase of 1,8-cineol in the blood, up to 275ng/ml, a level high enough to allow penetration of the blood brain barrier.[45]

THE GENERAL AFFECTIVE THEORY

An alternative theory, the general affective theory of odors, also called the *reflectorial effect theory*,[4] holds that an odor experienced as hedonically positive induces a positive, happy mood and when in a happy mood, an individual does almost everything better. For instance, when a person feels happy, it is easier to learn and to sleep, and headaches are less frequent. According to the general affective theory, a single odor could have a multitude of diverse effects, thus affecting virtually all behaviors.

The major premise that hedonically positive odors induce happier moods was demonstrated by Alaoui-Ismaili.[46] Forty-four subjects inhaled five odorants, namely, vanillin, menthol, eugenol, methyl methacrylate, and propionic acid. Six autonomic nervous system parameters were recorded: skin potential, skin resistance, skin temperature, skin blood flow, instantaneous respiratory frequency, and instantaneous heart rate. Evaluation of these parameters demonstrated a pattern consistent with known emotional states. Hedonically pleasant odors evoked mainly happiness and surprise, and unpleasant ones induced mainly disgust and anger.[46,47]

Milter also showed that exposure to odors could change emotions in the same direction as the hedonic valence of the odor.[48] Using the startle reflex amplitude as a physiologic indicator of emotional valence, he found that the odor of hydrogen sulfide (H_2S) increased the startle reflex amplitude and the odor of vanillin reduced it.

Aromatherapists recognize the affective impact of odors as the mechanism of action. Buchbauer notes:

> A pleasant odor has always been, and still is, an important factor for people to feel good, and feeling well is synonymous with good health. Therefore we can conclude that all substances which are able to create a certain amount of well-being and well-feeling possess therapeutic properties and, therefore, can be called therapeutic agents.[49]

Reliance on the general affective theory of odors implies that virtually any sensory stimulus could be used as a therapeutic tool. This largely trivializes the definition of therapy.

Assuming the general affective theory of odors is valid, the challenge to assessing the validity of aromatherapy arises due to the intensity effect. This suggests that the hedonics towards an aroma varies inversely with the concentration. This is most prominent with an aroma like H_2S, which at low levels is perceived as sweet and at high levels is like rotten eggs. Similar negative effects of intensity on hedonics has been demonstrated with a wide variety of odorants including galbanum, jasmine, lavender, natural green odor, and indole.[50-53] Thus, in assessing aromatherapy studies, the perceived intensity of the aroma must be addressed in that it may be as important, if not more important that the actual aroma itself!

Another problem with the general affective theory of odors is that the same odor, in different contexts, may induce opposite emotional tones.[54]

Similarly, perception of source, in the absence of change in context, can influence odor hedonics and somatic conditions.[56] This source effect was demonstrated with 30 men and 30 women in response to 4-acetyl carene when it was suggested this was of natural origin. Subjects who were told the aroma was synthetic had higher levels of irritation and annoyance, stress, and health symptoms during exposure. To complicate the matter further, hedonics to the same aroma shifted depending upon the underlying psychological and emotional states of the rater. For

In *The Invalid's Story,* Mark Twain compares the disgust at the odor of a rotting corpse to the delight at the smell of cheese (both associated with the break-down products of nitrogen-containing proteins and amino and nucleic acids). The odors were the same but perceived to be from different sources. This suggests that an odor that is contextually appropriate in one situation might be considered totally inappropriate in another. Smelled in a positive context, it would be appreciated as hedonically positive and would enhance a positive affective state; smelled in a negative context, it would be perceived as hedonically negative and would, thus, induce a negative affective state.[55] Therefore the same odor could produce opposite mood states and opposite effects.

instance, when hungry and after a fast, food odors are rated hedonically more positively. And, in pregnancy, fruit is judged to be more hedonically positive.[57] Whereas degree of depression directly correlates with hedonics toward the aroma of feces.[58]

Güra's basic challenge to the General Affective Theory of Aromas involves the concept of odor hedonic mood congruence. While this is a common experience, not all experiments supported this, and even suggest negative associations. Among 20 healthy young subjects of equal gender, a significant improvement in most $(p < 0.05)$ was seen upon exposure to the self-rated hedonically negative odor of 3-methyl-2 hexenoic acid.[59] Such mood odor hedonic uncoupling calls the entire General Affective Theory of Aromas into doubt.

A variant of the general affective theory is that odors may induce a mood more congruent with the demands of the external environment whereby odorants act as "catalysts," facilitating response to external stimuli.[3] For instance, if the external environment requires that the individual be alert, the odor induces awareness of this. Therefore the individual responds by becoming more alert. Alternatively, if the external environment is such that it is more appropriate to be relaxed, the odor induces that awareness and the individual responds by becoming more relaxed. Evidence for the validity of this variant comes from studies of muguet odor. Where the external demand is for a greater degree of relaxation, individuals do become more relaxed, and in an environment where they are required to be more alert and vigilant, they become more alert. Warm et al.[60] demonstrated this effect of odorant-induced recognition of affective demands. Forty subjects underwent vigilance tasks for 40 minutes during which they received periodic 30-second whiffs of air or one of two hedonically positive fragrances: muguet (independently judged as relaxing) or peppermint (independently judged as alerting). Those who received either the relaxing or alerting fragrance detected more signals during the vigilance task than the unscented air controls ($p = .05$).

A corollary to the general affective theory is that hedonically negative odors or malodors have a negative effect on mood. If this is true, the simple elimination or masking of malodors with neutral or hedonically positive odors would induce positive effects.

Literature supports the negative effects of hedonically negative odors.[61] In 1980, Miner[62] described some effects of exposure to the odor of livestock waste. They included annoyance, depression, nausea, vomiting, headache, shallow breathing, coughing, insomnia, and impaired appetite.

One of the malodorous pollutants that has been studied, trichloroethylene, a universally present air pollutant, can cause cephalgia.[63] Acute exposure to nitrogen tetroxide can cause cephalgia[64] and chronic neurotoxicity.[65] Acute exposure to chlorine gas can cause neurotoxicity.[66] In 1991, Neutra[67] reported that people living near hazardous waste sites suffer more physical symptoms during times when they can detect malodors than when they are unaware of them. Shusterman[68] demonstrated that even at levels considered nontoxic, chemical effluviums can cause physical symptoms.

HEALTH EFFECTS OF MALODORS

Health effects of malodors can be divided into six categories: respiratory, chemosensory, cardiovascular, immune, neurologic, and psychologic.

> *Respiratory.* Asthmatics are especially affected by malodors. Any strong odor may induce an attack in persons with unstable asthma and, even in nonasthmatics, malodors have been demonstrated to affect the cardiorespiratory system. Increased ambient oxidant levels correlate with slower cross-country running times in high school students.[69]
>
> *Chemosensory.* Chronic exposure to malodors from pulp mills can cause permanent olfactory loss.[70]
>
> *Cardiovascular.* Certain malodors can induce an adrenocortical and adrenomedullary response leading to elevated blood pressure and a subsequent increase in stroke and heart disease.[71,72] The unpleasant aroma of rotting Welsh onion for instance, compared to a blank odor condition increased stress associated autonomic nervous system discharge as manifested by elevated heart rate variability and systolic and diastolic blood pressure.[73]

Immune. Immune function may be compromised either directly, as a result of olfactory/neural projections to lymphoid tissue,[71] or indirectly, as a result of malodor-induced depression or other negative mood states.[74,75]

Neurologic. Chronic exposure to intermittent malodors from a U.S. Navy dump site in Port Orchard, Washington, induced cortical and subcortical dysfunction, which was manifested by encephalopathy: limbic encephalopathy, and cephalgia.[76] Both ambient NO_2 and SO_2 impair visual adaptation to darkness and sensitivity to brightness, and increase alpha wave desynchronization on EEG.[77]

Psychologic. Recognized for centuries and noted by Freud and others, psychologic effects of odors vary widely among individuals. Persons under major stress are particularly vulnerable to the psychologic effects of ambient malodors.[71] Persons with a distorted or impaired olfactory sense may be annoyed by odors that other persons usually consider pleasant.[71]

Certain bad odors irritate nasal passages and may act as chemical irritants in the respiratory tract. Resultant trigeminal stimulation releases adrenaline, leading to a tense and angry state. Thus bad odors can trigger aggression that may then be covertly expressed. For example, in one experiment college men were instructed to apply electric shocks of varying intensity to their colleagues, supposedly for the purpose of training them. When bad odors were present, the subjects chose to inflict greater degrees of pain upon their colleagues.[78] Another example involves air pollution. On days when malodorous air pollution is high, the number of motor vehicle accidents increase, indicating that people drive more aggressively in a polluted environment.[79]

Various studies show how mood and well-being suffer in the presence of malodors. Residents exposed to the effluvium from nearby commercial swine operations reported that they suffered increased tension, fatigue, confusion, depression, and anger and that their vigor decreased.[80] According to one study[81] ambient pollutants decreased personal attraction. In a German urban area, the moods of young adults fluctuated in synchrony with the daily fluctuations in quality of environmental air, a pattern especially marked among more emotionally unstable individuals.[82] Further, daily diary entries of women in Bavaria showed that variations in their psychologic well-being coincided with variations in ambient air quality. The correlation was particularly marked among women suffering from chronic diseases, such as diabetes.[83,84] In Israel negative health effects were significantly associated with levels of urban pollution.[85]

The number of family disturbances and the number of 911 emergency psychiatric calls were also linked to malodors in the environment, as determined by ozone levels.[86] In several cities the number of psychiatric admissions paralleled the quality of environmental air.[87]

In a study of the malodorous emanations from a mulching site southeast of Chicago, it was found that on days when the miasma wafted from the site to the school across the street, children at the school demonstrated increased behavioral problems.[88]

Malodorous ambient SO_2 levels correlate with psychiatric admissions, child psychiatric emergencies,[89] and behavioral difficulties with decreased cooperation.[90] Ambient NO_2 levels covary with psychiatric emergency room visits.[91] In nonsmokers the odor of cigarette smoke has been demonstrated to exacerbate aggressive behavior.[92]

The fatigue and annoyance caused by ambient malodors undoubtedly reduce individuals' capacities to function normally. Their abilities to tolerate frustration, to learn, and to cope with other stressors are impaired. In one laboratory study, subjects exposed to unpleasant odors experienced increased feelings of helplessness.[93]

CONTRADICTORY THEORIES

If the general affective theory of odors is true, a single odor can induce a positive mood in one person and a negative mood in another. This paradox negates the lock and key theory in which odors' effects are produced outside of conscious awareness. Robin et al demonstrated this using eugenol.[94] Eugenol, which is often associated with the smell of dental cement, was rated pleasant by nonfearful dental subjects and unpleasant by fearful subjects ($p = 0.036$). Changes in subjects' autonomic nervous system measurements were consistent with their emotional states.[94,95] Nineteen subjects were exposed to eugenol while recording six autonomic nervous system parameters, including two electrodermal, two thermovascular, and two cardiorespiratory. The results of 7 subjects with high dental fear were compared with those of 12 without such fear. Those with dental fear had a stronger electrodermal response ($p = 0.006$), suggesting that eugenol triggered different emotional responses depending upon the unpleasantness of the subject's past dental experiences. Thus the same odor can have different effects depending upon the past experience of the individual.[95] And the same odor, in the same concentration, exposed to different people may be judged to be hedonically opposite, depending on their past experience with the odor and learned association with the odor[96] inducing a hedonic congruent mood state.[97] The aromas may even become paired with somatic symptoms, which recur upon re-exposure to the odor. Examples could include feeling the need to cough in response to the smell of a cherry cough drop or allergic symptoms in response to an aroma that had been perceived coincident with past allergic episodes.[98]

On the other hand, if the lock and key theory is true, and an odors' behavioral effects are produced outside of awareness and independent of affective reaction, this negates the general affective theory of odors. Ludvigson and Rottman do just that, demonstrating that the scent of lavender enhances mood state while impairing arithmetic reasoning ($p = 0.01$).[99]

Given the previous information, several factors must be taken into account in reviewing the literature regarding efficacy of aromatherapy in the treatment of neurologic disease. Can odors elevate mood as the general affective theory maintains or do they act in lock and key fashion? Were the odors tested considered hedonically positive by each subject? This question is essential because what is hedonically positive for one person can be hedonically negative for another, and an odor that is hedonically positive at one concentration may be hedonically negative at another.[100] Was an associated change in mood independent of the desired effect? Was there a control group? Was the procedure single blinded or double blinded? Was the subject size sufficient to obviate falsely positive test results? Did the subjects of the experiment have a normal or near-normal sense of smell? Olfactory ability must actually be tested since recognition of olfactory loss is poor in those who suffer from this condition: 42%–70% cognitively normal elderly and 70% of elderly with senile dementia of the Alzheimer's type were unaware of their olfactory loss.[101,102]

Could suggestion have an effect? This is particularly relevant because various studies suggest that, as in traditional pharmacologic intervention,[103–105] odors have both placebo and nocebo effects as demonstrated by Knasko et al.[106] Knasko subjected 90 subjects to water vapor sprayed in a room; 30 subjects were told that the water vapor odor was pleasant, 30 that it was unpleasant, and 30 that it was neutral. Those who had been told that the odorant was pleasant reported being in a better mood than did the other two groups ($p = 0.05$). Subjects who been told the odor was unpleasant, reported having more health symptoms ($p = 0.0003$).

Were the experiments controlled not only for the effect of suggestion but also for the effect of expectation of outcome?[107] It seems possible that persons with a positive view of aromatherapy who believe that odors can have a positive effect will experience a positive effect because of their bias.

The effect of expectation has been demonstrated neurophysiologically by Lorig and Roberts,[108] who measured the contingent negative variation (CNV) of the EEG in 18 subjects presented with a mixed odor of lavender, jasmine, and galbanium. They found CNV amplitude for the mixed odors varied depending on what the subjects were told about it ($p = 0.05$).

Did the experimenter consider the effect of social desirability whereby subjects try to please the examiner by biasing their answers?[109]

In light of such questions, one must be circumspect regarding articles touting aromatherapeutic efficacy in the treatment of neurologic disease. Because the basic physiologic mechanism of aromatherapy intervention has not been fully established, skepticism seems all the more appropriate.

NEUROLOGIC DISORDERS

As a general rule, neurologic diseases can be positively influenced by improving the patient's mood or allaying anxiety. Virtually all neurologic diseases are made worse with depression and/or high anxiety. If moods can be ameliorated by aromatherapy, it would suggest that aromatherapy could have a positive role in treating neurologic disease. The medical literature discusses the effects of aromatherapy in specific neurologic complaints and diseases.

Headache

Since more than 30% of patients are unresponsive to pharmacologic interventions,[110] nontraditional therapies are frequently used in the management of headache, such as acupuncture, massage, and biofeedback. Nineteen percent of patients seen in a neurology clinic for headache have used aromatherapy.[111] Of 11 professional aromatherapy organizations in the United Kingdom who responded to a survey regarding CAM usage, headache/migraine were among the top five conditions treated.[112,113]

Historically, odors have been recognized to have analgesic effects. When Roman soldiers returned from battle, they placed bay leaves in their baths to reduce their pains.[114] In ancient Greece, the Corinthian physician, Philonides, recommended pressing cool, scented flowers against the temples to relieve headaches.[114]

In contemporary lay literature, a multitude of unsupported claims are made for headache and pain reduction using specific odorants. These claims do not indicate whether the mechanism of action is primarily analgesic, soporific, or anxiolytic. Suggested odorants include cloves for dental pain;[5] wintergreen for muscle pain;[5,115] menthol, ginger, lemon grass, rosewood, clary sage,[36] cajeput, tea tree, juniper, and pepper[116] for headaches;[5] lavender,[117] lavandula angustifoia, chamaemelum mobile, ocimium basilicum, origanum majorala, rosmarinus officinalis,[118] eucalyptus,[36] true Melissa,[39] basil, anise, German chamomile, peppermint, rose extract, and otto[119] for migraine; mentha x piperila for "headache caused by digestive disorder,"[118] peppermint and eucalyptus for tension headache.[120]

Experimental studies of odors for pain management are few. Hirsch and Kang[121] studied 50 chronic sufferers whose headaches met International Headache Society criteria. Upon olfactory testing, only 31 demonstrated normal olfactory ability. Green apple odor was given in an aromatherapy inhaler. Only 15 subjects found the odor hedonically pleasant. In this open-label, nonblinded study, subjects served as their own controls. The control condition consisted of resting in a dark, quiet room, and the experimental condition involved inhaling the green apple odor while resting in the same dark, quiet room. Results indicated that green apple odor produced *no* statistically significant improvement over simple resting in a dark, quiet room. However, in the subgroup of 15 subjects who liked the odor, there was a statistically significant reduction in the severity of the headache (p = 0.03). Therefore the efficacy of the green apple odor was hedonically dependent. Subjects who liked the smell experienced a statistically significant reduction in the severity of the headaches, but patients who disliked the smell experienced no significant improvement.

The mechanism of the odor's action in reducing headaches in these 15 patients is subject to speculation. The odor may have induced a variety of psychologic effects. The therapeutic result may have been mediated through Pavlovian conditioning. For example, the respondents may have consciously or unconsciously associated[122] the green apple odor with past anxiolytic or pain-alleviating experiences so that the association reproduced this same effect during the headache episodes. The odor might also have worked through olfactory-evoked recall, because olfactory-evoked recall is usually pleasant and associated with a positive mood state. The green apple scent, by inducing a positive mood state in the 15 patients, could thus have reduced perception of pain.[24] This corresponds with the general affective theory of odors described previously.

The lack of response in those who found the green apple scent unpleasant indicates that hedonics were more important than the particular odor used. This does not preclude the possibility of a neurophysiologic effect of the odor, inducing a change in serotonin, dopamine, acetylcholine, norepinephrine, GABA, gastrin, beta endorphin, or substance P, all of which are known to be modulators of headache, including migraine. Because these neurotransmitters exist within the olfactory bulb, they could, theoretically, be influenced by odors.[123–138]

Green apple odor may have worked somewhat like pharmacologic agents used in the treatment of headache, for example, amitriptyline or propranolol, by modifying the neurotransmitters in the pain pathway. In the patients who disliked the odor, a strong negative mood state may have been induced that overwhelmed the odor's neurophysiologic effect. Therefore their pain was not alleviated.

Gobel also studied the effects of odors on headaches.[115,139] In that study, 32 healthy subjects underwent a double-blind, placebo-controlled, randomized crossover study of the effects of peppermint oil, eucalyptus, and ethanol. The odors were used in different combinations on various measures of headache pain, including the relaxation of pericranial muscles and contingent negative variation. In this study, three applications of odorant were placed on the skin of the forehead and temples at 15-minute intervals using a small sponge. After 45 minutes, parameters were assessed. To avoid factors of circadian rhythm, all testing took place between 3 P.M. and 6 P.M. To prevent subjects from recognizing the presence versus the absence of odors and thereby breaking the double-blind nature of the study, traces of peppermint oil and eucalyptus oil were added to all applications.

Eucalyptus had no effect. Peppermint combined with eucalyptus and ethanol relaxed pericranial muscles ($p = 0.05$) as did a combination of peppermint and ethanol. The most reduction of pain sensitivity as measured by algesimetry was from a combination of peppermint oil and ethanol. Regulation of pericranial muscles was a postulated mechanism of action of the peppermint.

This study has several potential problems. Because the traces of peppermint and eucalyptus were sufficient to cause olfactory response, they may also have been sufficient to produce an effect, although they were described as inert. Hence the authors may not have tested the particular odors they thought they tested. Furthermore, no parameter was measured to determine whether the effect was based on hedonics, to eliminate any influence of the general affective theory of odors. No assessment was made of subjects' olfactory abilities, nor was the anticipation effect (belief versus nonbelief in aromatherapy) addressed.

The author postulated that the odors, through a peripheral mechanism in the gate control theory of pain, acted by segmental inhibition of the posterior horn.[115] However, this same pathway could have been activated totally independently of the odors. The experimental procedure of applying the odors by rubbing cold oils on the skin may, in and of itself, have influenced the pain pathway. The cold stimuli could have induced firing of A delta fibers, which would have increased blood flow in the skin and created a counterstimulus to reduce the headache pain. Alternatively, the inhalation of odors may have affected central serotonergic systems, leading to a change in mood state and thus a reduction in pain (general affective theory of odors).

In another study, Gobel et al. found aromatherapy with peppermint oil was effective in treating tension headaches meeting IHS classification.[140] Peppermint oil was applied locally in a randomized, placebo-controlled, double-blind, crossover fashion. Ten grams of peppermint oil and 90% ethanol was used. Placebo was 90% ethanol solution to which traces of peppermint oil were added for blinding purposes. During their headache attacks, peppermint oil was applied across the forehead and temples of 41 patients. The application was repeated after 15 and 30 minutes. Compared with the placebo, peppermint oil significantly reduced headache intensity after 15 minutes ($p = 0.01$). The analgesic effect equaled that of 1000 mg of acetaminophen. Very few studies that claim to have demonstrated efficacy of aromatherapy have been as carefully performed.[141]

Another possible mechanism by which peppermint may relieve headache is by noncompetitive inhibition of serotonin and substance P.[120]

Odors may inhibit headaches by acting as calcium channel blockers. *Romarinus officinalis*, for example, has been demonstrated to relax tracheal smooth muscle by way of its calcium antagonistic property.[142]

An often quoted study validating use of eucalyptus oil for sinus headache does *not* actually involve use of aromas, but rather, involved ingestion of cineole capsules.[143]

Chronic Pain

Opinion regarding relief of nonheadache pain is mixed. In an experimental model of pain, the cold pressor test, inhalation of a sweet odor induced subjects to tolerate pain for significantly longer duration.[144] However, retronasal application of peppermint and cinnamon odors showed no analgesic effect on the cold pressor test.[145] Gedney found no analgesic effect of lavender oil or rosemary in a paradigm of pain using contact heat, pressure, and ischemic pain tasks.[146] In this sex controlled, balanced, crossover study of 26 subjects, no statistically significant analgesic was produced by either aroma.[147] Similarly, Saeki did not find a statistically significant analgesic effect of inhalation of lemon, grapefruit, sweet orange, eucalyptus, rosemary, or lavender.[148] This was based on a Visual Analogue Scale of pain sensation of 25 women who were inflicted with standard electrical shocks to the forearm, designed as a paradigm for sharp, pin prick–like sensation. In a blinded study by Dale[149] of 635 postpartum women, use of lavender in the daily bath was compared with an aromatic placebo consisting of 2-methyl-3-isobutyl tyrosine diluted in distilled water. Of the women, 217 received lavender, 213 synthetic, and 205 control. This study demonstrated no statistically significant effect of using lavender in treating peroneal pain. In a study that was not randomized, not double blinded, and not age controlled, Woolfson and Huet gave aromatherapy and massage in 20-minute sessions twice a week to 12 patients. Another 12 patients received massage only. The aromatherapy patients were massaged with lavender oil in an almond oil base. The other patients were massaged with almond oil only. Observations were recorded at the beginning and end of each 20-minute session and 30 minutes after treatment. All sessions were conducted in midafternoon. Approximately 50% of the patients were in the coronary care unit and the others were in intensive-care units. Fifty percent of the patients were artificially ventilated. The authors state that 50% of the aromatherapy patients and 41% of massage-only patients reported a decrease in pain. This could be misleading, however. That six patients responded to aromatherapy and five patients responded to massage without aromatherapy is clearly not a statistically significant difference. If anything, these results indicate that aromatherapy was no better than massage alone. Given their selection of patients, however, one would not anticipate that aromatherapy would be effective, because the pathway for olfactory input was compromised by artificial ventilation.

In a study by Burns and Blamey[150] of 585 women, no statistically significant effects were described, but analgesia was noted in 4 women who inhaled lavender, 1 who inhaled eucalyptus, 3 who inhaled clary sage, 1 who inhaled jasmine, 2 who inhaled chamomile, and 1 who inhaled lemon.

Use of combinations of aromas including geranium, lavender, and roman chamomile for periarticular pain in Guillian Barré Syndrome has been advocated.[151] However, in the first case study presented, the aromas were applied coincident with 15 minutes of massage and passive range of motion exercise for each joint. In the subject of questionable olfactory ability, these concurrent therapies may have been more accurately identified as the analgesic agent.

In a rehabilitation hospital, among three patients who reported pain, a blend of lavender, bergamot, sweet orange, and marjoram were applied along with massage, Pain and anxiety were reduced in all subjects. Any improvement due to aromatherapy as opposed to massage remains speculative.[152]

In 100 patients with pain of the periarticular system,[153] treatment of from 10 to 20 days compared the efficacy of mint oil with that of hydroxyethylsalicylate gel. The mint oil was put into a gel and applied topically. Of the patients and physicians, 78% thought that mint therapy was highly effective, and 50% of patients and 34% of physicians thought that hydroxyethylsalicylate gel was highly effective. None of the confounding parameters previously mentioned, such as olfactory ability, expectation, and hedonics, were addressed in this study.

Multiple Sclerosis

Of 848 patients with clinically definite multiple sclerosis (MS) who responded to a mail survey in British Columbia, 52 (6.1%) admitted to using aromatherapy to help manage their conditions.[154] Yet no scientific studies support the use of aromatherapy in the treatment of MS and because 23% of MS patients experience olfactory deficit,[155] the efficacy of aromatherapy for this condition would be questionable.

Epilepsy

Aromatherapists suggest the use of a variety of odorants as anticonvulsants, including chamomile, clary sage, and lavender,[6] but few studies have been performed.

Yamada et al.[156] found that inhaling lavender oil vapor blocked pentatetrazol and nicotine-induced convulsions in mice. Gowers noted that the olfactory and trigeminal countermeasures—ammonia and amyl nitrite—inhibit seizure induction, especially in patients with olfactory auras.[16] Efron[17] described a patient with uncinate fits that were inhibited within 8 seconds of inhaling dimercaprol (Bal). Other odorants found to be effective seizure abortants included hydrogen sulfide, n-ethyl butyrate, skatole, the haptenes, and pure jasmine. All were strong and unpleasant, an indication that their effect may have been based on their trigeminal stimulating properties.

More recently, Betts et al.[157] described the inhalation of aromatherapy oil as a countermeasure against epileptic seizures. This was an open-label study of 30 patients but neither the percent success nor the exact odors used were described.

Movement Disorders

Several odorants have been advocated for the treatment of movement disorders, including bergamot, chamomile, clary sage, fennel, marjoram,[158] white birch, rosemary,[38] and mandarin[39] for muscle spasms; lavender for leg cramps;[38] and marjoram for tics.[6] These must be viewed skeptically because no scientific studies have been performed, and many movement disorders, including Parkinson's disease[159] and Huntington's disease,[160] are associated with olfactory impairment, which would render any odorant superfluous. Despite this, 10% of 80 Parkinson's disease patients surveyed admitted to using aromatherapy in the management of their disease.[161]

Alcoholism

Many odorants have been suggested for use in alcohol recovery to help alleviate both the physical and emotional problems associated with the desire to drink[162] (see Box 16.1). However, both acute intoxication[163] and chronic alcoholism[164] are associated with olfactory loss, and no formal studies have been performed. Therefore aromatherapy for alcoholism cannot be recommended at this time.

Nicotine Addiction

Early work by Westman et al has demonstrated that the aroma of cigarette smoke, when delivered through a cigarette-like device, could provide the sensory experience of smoking without the nicotine or carcinogens. With such a device, cigarette craving was reduced significantly.[165] However, such a contraption has not been of practical utility in the treatment of nicotine addiction. Other odors have also been studied to stimulate the trigeminal and olfactory sensory system of smokers with the aim of reducing nicotine cravings. Felbaum used peppermint, which is both a trigeminal and olfactory stimulant, to curb cigarette craving and withdrawal symptoms.[166]

Insomnia

A multitude of odorants have been touted for use as hypnotics in the treatment of insomnia, including valerian,[167] asafetida,[167] musk,[167] lavender,[36,38,167,168] basil, chamomile, clary sage, everlasting, mandarin, marjoram, neroli, sandalwood, ylang-ylang,[36] bergamot, celery, hops, hyacinth, jasmine,[169] camphor, cypress, frankincense, geranium, lemon, melissa, myrrh, nutmeg, patchouli, petitgrain, rose, sage,[41] orange,[116] and juniper berry.[119]

Animal studies support the use of odorants as hypnotics. Decreased motility, an indication of sedation, was produced in mice after inhalation of the essential oils of lime blossoms and Herba Passiflora.[168] In young albino rats, inhalation of valerian and asafetida induced sedation, compared with control conditions.[167] Odorants that were not found to be significantly sedating included musk, lavender, violets, oil of roses, incense, gum olibanum, gum galbanum, Hinode, and sandalwood. Due to the low levels used, the mechanism of action was postulated to be due not to systemic absorption but rather to the olfactory sensation with secondary effects from olfactory CNS projections.[167]

BOX 16.1

Oils Used in Aromatherapy Treatment of Alcohol Recovery

Rose otto	Rosemary	Cedarwood, Atlas	Patchouli
Ginger	Lemongrass	Myrrh	Petitgrain
Grapefruit	Mandarin	Pimento berry	Rose absolute
Chamomile, Roman	May chang	Spruce	Ylang-ylang
Neroli	Nutmeg	Thyme linalool	Cardamom
Juniper	Black pepper	Yarrow	Chamomile, German
Lavender	Geranium	Carrot	Eucalyptus citriodora
Frankincense	Benzoin	Coriander	Eucalyptus globules
Marjoram	Melissa	Hyssop	Myrtle
Peppermint	Ravensara	Kanuka	Niaouli
Lavandin	Thyme thujanol	Linden absolute	Pine
Lemon	Bergamot	Manuka	Rosewood
Angelica	Clary sage	Orange, sweet	Sandalwood
Almond	Cypress	Hyacinth absolute	Turmeric
Cinnamon leaf	Fennel	Immortelle	Verbena lemon
Jasmin Sambac (Abs)	Palmarosa	Spikenard	Tea tree
Vetiver	Violet leaf absolute	Valerian	Tea tree, lemon

Sedation was produced in Swiss mice by inhalation of lavender oil and its components linalool and linalyl acetate.[168] Based on studies with rats, Elisabetsky et al postulated that linalool's hypnotic properties are mediated through inhibition of glutamatergic transmission in the CNS.[170,171]

Buchbauer et al [43] exposed Swiss mice to more than 40 odorants. In general, the more lipophilic, the greater the biologic effect (Table 16.1). It was suggested that the sedative effect of these essential oils was due to their interactions with lipids of the neural cell membranes in the cortex.

Experiments with humans have also been performed to assess the soporific effects of odors, with mixed results. While heliotropin has been

TABLE 16.1 Effects of Fragrance Compounds and Essential Oils on the Motility of Mice After a 1-h Inhalation Period

Compound	Motility %	Caffeine %
Anethole	−10.81	−1.26
Anthranillic acid methyl ester	+17.70	+38.22
Balm leaves oil (Austria)	−5.21	+16.29
Benzaldehyde	−43.69	−34.28
Benzyl alcohol	−11.21	−23.68
Borneol	−3.05	−1.88
Bornyl acetate	−7.79	+2.27
Bornyl salicylate	−17.29	−2.99
Carvone	−2.46	−47.51
Citral	−1.43	+17.24
Citronellal	−49.82	−37.40
Citronellol	−3.56	−13.71
Coumarin	−15.00	−13.75
Dimethyl vinyl carbinol	+5.36	−2.11
Ethylmaltol	+9.73	+2.09
Eugenol	+2.10	−38.73
Farnesol	+5.76	+36.34
Farnesyl acetate	+4.62	−30.71
Furfural	+3.04	−4.51
Geraniol	+20.56	+1.20
Geranyl acetate	−29.18	−7.46
Isoborneol	+46.90	−11.23
Isobornyl acetate	+3.16	−22.35
Isoeugenol	+30.05	−74.34
Beta-Ionone	+14.20	−27.97

TABLE 16.1 (*continued*)

Compound	Motility %	Caffeine %
Lavender oil (Mont Blanc)	−78.40	−91.67
Lime blossoms oil (France)	−34.34	+30.41
Linaloof	−73.00	−56.67
Linalyl acetate	−69.10	−46.67
Maitol	+13.74	−50.04
Methyl salicylate	+16.64	−49.88
Nerol	+12.93	+29.31
Neroli oil	−65.27	+1.87
Orange flower oil (Spain)	−4.64	−14.62
Orange terpenes	+35.25	−33.19
Passion flower oil (USA)	+8.15	−27.93
2-Phenyl ethanol	+2.67	−30.61
2-Phenylethyl acetate	−45.04	+12.42
Alpha-Pinene	+13.77	+4.73
Rose oil (Bulgaria)	−9.50	+4.31
Sandalwood oil (East India)	−40.00	−20.70
Alpha-Terpineol	−45.00	−12.50
Thymol	+33.02	+19.05
Valerian root oil (China)	−2.70	−12.01

touted for its soporific qualities, formal evaluations demonstrate no statistically significant effects on sleep.[172] Hudson[173] evaluated nine older patients, many with dementia, in a hospital setting. Her assumption was that lavender inhalation would promote sleep and that, secondarily, it would reduce confusion and enhance alertness the next day. The effects of the application of one drop of lavender oil on the pillow each night for 1 week were compared with a 1-week baseline period with no odor. Nocturnal sleep improved 2% and daytime wakefulness increased 3% with lavender.

A conclusion that all elderly patients would benefit from nocturnal inhalation of essential oil of lavender must be viewed with some reservation for the following reasons:

- No statistical analysis was performed on the results.
- It would be expected that with time, patients would adjust to the hospital surroundings and their sleeping patterns would improve.

- No tests for hedonics or olfactory ability were performed. Being elderly,[174] on medication,[175] and demented[176] is apt to impair olfactory ability, bringing into question whether these subjects could even detect an odor.
- The nurse observers were not blinded to the intent of the study and, hence, may have been inadvertently biased in their observations. This bias has been demonstrated to occur in other aromatherapy studies.[109]

Because changes of only 2% to 3% were observed, a more accurate interpretation of this study might be that the lavender did *not* promote sedation.

However, other investigators also believe that odorants have a soporific effect on humans. Karamat et al[177] evaluated the effects of inhaling lavender oil on 24 subjects undergoing vigilance tasks. A significant increase in their reaction time was found, consistent with a sedative effect. But, no *p* value was noted for significance, nor were hedonics, blinding, or olfactory ability assessed.

Kikuchi et al[178] claim rose odor induced sedation as demonstrated by an inhibition of heart rate deceleration on a reaction time test. However, essential methodology including sample size, blinding, controls, and statistical significance were not provided. Thus, the sedation influence of rose odor remains elusive. EEG indicators of sedation include a reduced frontal beta wave activity. Sugara et al[179] measured such change associated with an arithmetic mental stress test in response to linalool, an ingredient of lavender oil. Large individual variation was noted and while a tendency for a reduction of beta waves was seen, no statistically significant effect was reported.

Miyake et al[180] used EEGs to assess sleep latency of subjects who inhaled spike lavender, sweet fennel, bitter orange, linden, valerian, and marjoram compared with those given no odors. The one odor found to significantly reduce sleep latency was bitter orange. Neither the number of subjects nor further details regarding blinding, subjects' expectations, hedonics, or olfactory ability were provided.

Aromatherapy must be tried judiciously in patients with insomnia because of the huge comorbidity of insomnia and respiratory disease. Insomnia is present in 53% of patients with chronic bronchitis and 55% of those with primary emphysema.[181] The inhalation of odorants by these patients could worsen their respiratory status and thus exacerbate, rather than relieve, their insomnia.

Aggression

Just as malodors increase aggressive feelings, evidence also exists that odors can reduce aggressive behavior. Although aromatherapists advocate using a variety of pleasant odors to reduce aggression and hostility, including chamomile, cypress lavender, marjoram, ylang-ylang,[36] sandalwood, cedarwood, rose extract, and jasmine,[119] studies suggest very different odors act to reduce aggression. In a double-blinded study of 18 undergraduate women, Benton[182] found that inhalation of 5-alpha-androst-16-en-3 alpha-ol (a potential human pheromone, androstenol) reduced aggression and increased submission ($p = 0.01$) compared with inhalation of the 70% ethanol control.

Hinoki essential oil was similarly demonstrated to reduce anger-hostility scores on the profile of mood state (POMS, which increases mental task performance).[10,183]

Anger and hostility, as measured by the POMS demonstrated a significant ($p < 0.05$) reduction in response to 5 minutes of inhalation of jasmine tea odor as compared to H_sO.[184] This was measured 54 minutes after exposure had ceased and only occurred in those who were hedonically positive toward the jasmine tea odor, or in those with negative hedonics towards the jasmine tea odor (n = unknown). No significance was seen with a higher level of jasmine tea odor, with green tea odor, or in those with negative hedonics towards jasmine tea odor. While other aspects of the POMS, including tension and anxiety and vigor also showed hedonically dependent changes, the results remain suspect since the subject size of the group with such changes may have been only one!

Hirsch[185] studied the effects of the odor of garlic bread on family interactions at dinner. Among the 50 families in this single-blinded, randomized, crossover study, there were 22.7% fewer negative remarks per family member per minute ($p = 0.05$) and 7.4% more positive comments per family member per minute ($p = 0.04$) when the aroma of garlic bread was present. The decrease in negative remarks was more pronounced among older rather than younger family members, among male rather than female members, among those who liked the aroma, and among those who had nostalgic feelings evoked by the aroma.

For family members who liked garlic bread, the aroma of garlic bread enhanced their mood so they became more positive and less critical of others and therefore made fewer negative comments. This supports Baron's demonstration that a positive mood can cause reduced critical appraisals both of products and of people.[186,187] The garlic bread aroma may have evoked nostalgic feelings that are usually associated with happy memories of childhood. Happy family members have more positive interactions.[188] The appetizing aroma and satisfying taste of garlic bread may induce generous feelings so family members reduce critical comments and increase pleasant and positive ones.[189] Just as a bad odor can cause aggressive feelings,[88] a pleasant aroma of garlic bread can enhance harmonious and agreeable feelings among family members, leading to more positive and fewer negative interactions.

In clinical practice, treatment with aversion aromas have been used to reduce both aggressive behavior[190] and deviant sexual behavior.[191] Tanner and Zeiler[192] describe the use of an odorant to treat for pathologic aggression in a 20-year-old autistic woman. In a nonblinded, open-label, single-case study, treatment with aromatic ammonia was found to reduce her self-injurious behavior from a baseline of 36.2 slaps per minute to 1.3 slaps per minute. Whenever self-injurious behavior was noted, the ammonia was thrust under the patient's nose and then withdrawn at cessation of the aggressive behavior. Statistical significance of the odor was not determined. When the routine application of aversive stimuli was discontinued, self-injurious behavior recurred. Moreover, frequent use of the odorant caused nasal irritation and scabbing at the tip of the nose.

Suppression of aggressive self-injurious behavior using aromatherapy was reported also by Baumeister and Baumeister.[193] Two severely retarded children, 4 and 7 years of age, demonstrated a reduction of their self-injurious behavior contingent with inhalation of aromatic ammonia, which persisted for at least 6 months after discontinuation of the inhalation.

In another experiment, four severely demented geriatric inpatients inhaled lavender with and without massage, to reduce agitated and self-aggressive behavior.[194] On individualized agitation scales, no benefits were demonstrated from the combined massage and aromatherapy as opposed to aromatherapy alone. One patient benefited from the aromatherapy, whereas for two, agitated behavior actually worsened as compared with the no-treatment control periods.

The staff providing care, blinded to the objectives measures, thought that aromatherapy reduced agitation and self-injurious behavior in all four patients. This experiment demonstrates the importance of scientific methods and techniques for objective measurements and the need to consider the examiners' preexisting bias and the effects of social desirability.[109] On the other hand, lavender oil was found to reduce agitated behavior amongst 9 of 15 patients on a long-stay psychogeriatric ward.[195] In this placebo controlled trial with blinded observer raters, a statistically significant reduction in agitation on the Pittsburgh Agitation Scale was observed ($p = 0.016$). The aroma was administered to the ambient environment of the ward through a steam aerosolizer for a total of five 2-hour periods whereby the severely demented participants were exposed to the lavender. Of those who improved, five had vascular dementia, three had senile dementia of the Alzheimer's type, and one had fronto-temporal lobe dementia. Because both being elderly and suffering from these diseases are associated with a higher incidence of olfactory impairment,[196–199] and because olfactory ability was not assessed in this study, an alternative explanation for the positive results must be explored. It is possible that the lavender aroma had no effect at all on the patients, but rather, the lavender indirectly changed behavior in the presumably normosmic ward medical personal, which engendered the patients to respond in a less aggressive manner to them. Because the staff was not blinded to the study, it is possible that their bias expectations toward the lavender may have influenced their behavior with resultant changes in patient behavior. Thus, conclusions of this study remain in question. On the other hand, lemon balm (Melissa officinalis) when applied to 36 severely demented and clinically agitated residents of long-term care facilities reduced agitation by 30% on the Cohen-Mansfield Agitation Inventory, compared to the no odor control. In the absence of assessment of olfactory ability in the subjects, it is unknown how much of an effect the aroma was on the study participants as opposed to the staff.[200]

Ten residents of a long-term care facility with dementia and extreme agitation underwent exposure over a 6-month period to a number of aromas including tangerine, orange, ylang ylang, patchouli, blue tansy, basil, cardamom, rosemary cineol, peppermint, rosewood, geranium, lemon, palmarosa, bergamot, Roman chamomile, and jasmine. Agitation was monitored using the Minimum Data Set assessment tool. While four patients' behavior improved, statistical significance was not provided. It remains unknown whether the positive effect of the aroma affected these demented (and likely anosmic) patients, or whether the effect was on the evaluators. This question is particularly relevant given that the fan diffusers were not only placed in the patient room but also in the nursing station.[201]

Anxiety

Patients with DSM-III-R generalized anxiety disorder are known to have impaired olfactory ability.[202] Still, aromatherapists recommend numerous odors, including chamomile, cypress, orange blossom, lavender, marjoram, rose, sandalwood, clary sage,[6] basil, bergamot, cedarwood, geranium, jasmine, juniper, neroli, petitgrain, ylang-ylang,[36] melissa,[38] benzoin, camphor, cardamom, fennel, frankincense, nutmeg, patchouli, peppermint, pine, rosemary, rosewood,[41] mandarin, lemon verbena,[40] neroli, juniper berry,[39] grapefruit, olibanum, and thyme.[119]

Studies of the effects of odorants on anxiety have relied primarily on individuals' self-appraisals of their feeling state. In one instance, apple/nutmeg odor associated with the task of performing certain mathematical calculations led to an attenuated increase in anxiety as determined by subjects' self-reports and blood pressure measurements.[203] Contrarily, as reported on a visual analog scale, sense of calmness was not necessarily enhanced amongst 20 subjects exposed to the aroma of (–)-limonene, (+)-limonene, (–)-carvone, and (+)-carvone. Rather, it was dependent on presentation order, intensity, and hedonics.[204]

The odor of green apple eased the anxiety of being in a space-deprivation booth for six normosmic subjects as demonstrated in a double-blind, controlled, randomized experiment.[21]

Along with massage, the aroma of lavender, sweet marjoram, and cypress was assessed in 11 subjects in an open label controlled study regarding its anxiolytic and antidepressant qualities.[205] The anxiogesic stimulus was serial subtraction and differential anxiety and depression score was measured with the Anxiety Inventory and the Self Rating Depression Scale. Compared to the no odor condition, no significant anxiolytic or antidepressant effect was found.

Physiologic evidence is even less conclusive regarding the potential of odorants on anxiolytics. Lavender odor was found to reduce the CNV among perfumers, and the lavender correlated with a more relaxed state.[206] This change on the CNV, however, may also indicate a distracting effect of the odorant.[207] Mild reduction in systolic blood pressure, an indicator of anxiolysis,[207] with inhaled odors was assessed in a double-blind, controlled, randomized fashion in normosmic and anosmic, awake and anesthetized adults.[208] No significant effect was noted with inhalation of hedonically positive odors, but inhalation of an irritant (ammonia) caused an increase in blood pressure. However, anxiolysis, as represented by a reduction in serum cortisol was demonstrated amongst 22 volunteers exposed to both lavender and rosemary.[209]

Studies have also addressed the anxiolytic effects of aromatherapy in the clinical setting with, at best, ambiguous results. In a case-controlled study of 36 men with public speaking anxiety, jasmine and apple spice were no more effective than the odorless control condition in reducing speech anxiety.[210] On the other hand, a double-blind randomized trial of 66 women in the state of high anxiety (preoperative) assessed anxiolysis using a verbal analogue anxiety scale. After 10 minutes of inhalation of a mixture of vertivert, bergamot, and geranium, anxiolysis was actually greater than with inhalation of the placebo (hair conditioner).[211]

Likewise, no clear efficacy has been demonstrated for aromatherapy for anxiety reduction in patients confined to the hospital. Aromas of marjoram, lavender, rose, eucalyptus, geranium, chamomile, and neroli were used in combination with massage and music therapy to treat 69 terminally ill patients.[212]

An 80% rate of success in this experiment, defined as "deriving benefit in some way," must be viewed critically for the following reasons:

- Statistical significance was not determined.
- Treatments ancillary to the aromatherapy including talking, massage, or music may have been the true agents.
- Concomitant medical treatment, for example, to decrease pain, may have been the agent of beneficial effects ascribed to aromatherapy.
- Different odors were used for each subject.
- No consideration was given to hedonics, anosmia, a control group, expectation bias, or examiner bias

In 122 intensive-care patients, aromatherapy with massage was no more effective than either massage alone or no treatment (the control subgroup) in either subjective perception of aromas ($p = 0.05$) or physiologic parameters of anxiety (systolic blood pressure, respiratory rate, and heart rate).[213,214]

Similarly, a randomized, double-blind trial of aromatherapy with two different species of lavender and massage was performed on 24 postoperative intensive-care cardiac patients. No statistically significant self-perceived anxiolytic effect for either species of lavender was found ($p = 0.09$).[215]

The same results were documented with inhaled neroli aroma combined with massage in 100 one-day postoperative intensive-care cardiac patients.[216] In this randomized, controlled study, again, no statistical significance was found in physiologic parameters of anxiety (heart rate, systolic blood pressure) or subjects' self-perceptions of anxiety as reported in a modified Spielberger State-Trait Anxiety Inventory (STAI) State Self-Evaluation Questionnaire.

Wilkinson[217] also used the STAI and the psychologic scale of the Rotterdam Symptom Checklist (RSCL) to assess anxiolytic effects of aromatherapy. Fifty-one cancer patients receiving palliative care were randomly assigned to receive three sessions of either full body massage with carrier oil only or full body massage with carrier oil and 1% Roman Chamomile essential oil. Upon completion of the sessions, there was no statistically significant effect ($p = 0.8$) of aromatherapy with massage as opposed to massage alone on the psychologic scale of the RSCL or the STAI. In a study of the practical application of aromatherapy for anxiolysis in children, essential oil of sweet orange was applied to a breathing filter during general anesthesia induction with sevoflurane. Compared to the control group, the 50 exposed to the orange aromas were more relaxed during induction,[218] facilitating smooth induction in 85% ($p < 0.05$). The mechanism may have been through anxiolysis or through hedonic transformation of the unpleasant sevoflurane to pleasant, sweet orange, thus enhancing acceptability of induction. Definitive evidence validating aromatherapy in anxiolysis remains to be seen.

Depression

A variety of odorants, including basil, bergamot, chamomile, frankincense, geranium, jasmine, lavender, neroli, patchouli, peppermint, rose, sandalwood, ylang-ylang,[218] clary sage, grapefruit, lemon, mandarin orange,[36] camphor, hyssop, melissa, petitgrain, pine, thyme,[38] coriander, helichrysum, rosewood, vetivert,[41] marjoram, thyme,[116] benzoin, and olibanum[119] have been advocated for the treatment of depression.[6] However, scientific studies have yielded disappointing results. Lucks tested the essential oil of the leaf of vitex agnus-castus in 14 menopausal women. It was reported that 80% felt improvement in mood swings, depression, and personality changes.[220] However, analysis of the data reveals it is possible that as few as 4 subjects (or 23%) reported such response on the mail-in survey forms. From this non-IRB approved study, it is even unclear if subjects just inhaled the aroma or actually ingested it. In a crossover design, 11 volunteers received aromatherapy with tree oil foot baths and massage with lavender, sweet almond oil, cypress oil, and sweet marjoram oil, counterbalanced with carrier oil. Mood state was assessed using the Self-rating Depression Scale and the State-trait Inventory Anxiety Inventory. No significant effects on either anxiety or mood were found.[221] Citrus odor (a combination of lemon oil, orange oil, bergamot oil, and cis-4-hexenol) was applied to the ambient air for 4 to 11 weeks in the rooms where 12 men were hospitalized for DSM-III-R major depression.[222] During this time, antidepressant medications were reduced or eliminated for 11 of the 12 men and kept constant for another 8 control patients whose rooms were not perfumed. The criteria for medication tapering was apparently nonformal on a clinical basis. Comparing effects of odorant and antidepressant treatment versus antidepressant treatment alone, the odorant had no statistically significant effect on objective measures of depression including the Hamilton Rating Scale for Depression, the Self-Rating Depression Scale, and number of days of hospital treatment. Despite this, the results of the study are difficult to interpret because levels of antidepressant were not kept constant. Furthermore, olfactory ability was never assessed, and because many antidepressants impair olfactory ability, this is particularly important.[223] Also, depression itself is associated with olfactory impairment.[202,224]

Kite et al.[225] suggested that aromatherapy significantly improved depression as determined by the Hospital Anxiety-Depression Scale ($p = 0.001$) and reduced parameters consistent with adjustment disorders or major depressive disorders.

Results of this experiment must be viewed critically for the following reasons:

- Of 89 entrants, only 58 (65%) completed the study, an indication that the dropouts may have been treatment failures.
- The majority of subjects (74%) had breast cancer and were receiving oncologic therapy including radiation therapy or surgery. Olfactory ability was not assessed, yet chemotherapy, radiation therapy, and simply having breast cancer (estrogen receptor positive type)[226] are associated with olfactory impairment. Thus any positive results could be spurious and unrelated to the aromatherapy. The experimental design supports that this may be the case.
- No control group was provided, therefore mood improvement could have been due to coincident improvement of the underlying disease state.
- Aromatherapy was not provided alone, but along with massage and empathic therapeutic sessions, either of which might have been effective.
- One-third of the patients concomitantly received counseling and some were on antidepressants, both of which could improve depression.
- Twenty different essential oils were used, alone or in various combinations. The odors were different for each subject and changed during the course of treatment in more than one-third of the cases.

Thus even though relief of depression was reported, the effects of the odorants are indeterminate.

Depression amongst 14 randomly assigned, mildly to severely depressed patients was significant reduced ($p = 0.01$) when aromas were combined with massage and music, as opposed to the no odor control.[227] To prevent investigator bias, the rating device for depression, the Montgomery-Asberg Depression Rating Scale, was performed by the primary psychiatric nurse or occupational therapist. While intriguing, this study suffers from a primary methodological problem—each of the 14 patients received a different combination of three of nine essential oils, and it is not revealed which ones were used in the depressed treatment group. Thus, it remains unknown which odorant or odorant combination actually acted to help ameliorate depression.

In a study by Wilcock, 46 patients with cancer were randomized into a control group or an aromatherapy and massage group.[228] The Profile of Mood State (POMS) questionnaire was used to determine the mood enhancing effects of the 1% lavender and chamomile aromatherapy. No statistically significant effect was found. On the other hand, the aroma of hiba oil was found to improve depression on the HAMD among 14 women chronic hemodialysis inpatients. On entrance to the study, all met criteria for mild to severe depression, and compared to no-odor baseline ambient room odor, after 1 week of euthenic intervention, statistically significant reduction in depression symptoms occurred ($p = 0.008$). No significant antidepressant effects of lavender were seen.[229] In this same study, anxiolysis was demonstrated on the HAMA in response to both hiba oil and lavender ($P = 0.003$).

While these results are intriguing, skepticism remains given these small sample size and that olfactory ability was never assessed. This is of particular importance since the average age was over 65 years old, in which group approximately one-half have impaired olfactory ability, and they all were in renal failure, a disorder which induces dysfunctional smell.[230] Thus, it is unlikely that even seven of the subjects were normosmic and thus, this sample size became that much more suspect. In the absence of olfactory testing and with such a small sample size, before accepting these results, a study replication is warranted.

At this time, the use of odorants to treat major depression cannot be advocated.

Learning Disabilities, Mild Cognitive Impairment, and Dementia

The odorants that aromatherapists suggest can improve memory, mental function, and learning ability include vanilla,[114] rosemary, basil, cardamom, bergamot, cedarwood, grapefruit, lemon, peppermint, rosemary,[38] clove, coriander, lily of the valley, sage,[231] bay, melissa, ylang-ylang,[41] and juniper.[116] The combined odor of lavender and orange essential oil has been recommended in the management of dementia.[232]

Animal studies support the concept that odorants can improve learning and cognition. Following the logic that if odors improve learning, their lack would impair learning, Sitaras et al induced peripheral anosmia in rats with intranasal infusion of $ZnSO_4$. They found that this markedly impaired the rats conditioned avoidance response ($p = 0.05$).[233] Furthermore, that odors may improve normal learning indicates they may prove therapeutic in disorders of cognition.

Ludvigson and Rottman[99] evaluated the odors of lavender and cloves for their possible impact on learning, using as paradigms the group-embedded figure, word recall, multiple-choice vocabulary, analogies, and arithmetic tasks. They found that these odors did not affect memory or cognition;[234] in fact, the odor of lavender significantly impaired performance of arithmetic tasks ($p = 0.01$).

On the other hand, odors of peppermint and muguet (lily of the valley) improved the performance of stressful visual tasks.[235] Among subjects who found them hedonically positive, these odors improved creativity scores on the remote associates test and increased efficiency in work situations.[236]

Perala demonstrated that the ambient odor of peppermint, rosemary, and lemon improved performance on a memory test in 15- and 16 year-olds with a normal sense of smell as demonstrated on the National Geographic Smell Survey.[237] While a control group was provided, no sample size or statistical significance was reported.

Eucalyptus, lemon, peppermint, and iris root were exposed individually or in combination to 77 seven- to ten year-olds while learning monosyllabic nouns.[238] Those nouns learned in the presence of the aromas were better recalled that those learned in the odor-free environment. Statistical significance and controls were not elaborated upon.

Hirsch and Johnston,[239] in a double-blind, controlled, crossover study found that the presence of a mixed floral odor improved speed of learning on the Halsted-Reitan Test Battery by 17% as compared with an odorless control condition for 10 normosmic adults who found the odor hedonically pleasant ($p = 0.05$). The odors of oriental spice, baked goods, lavender, citrus, parsley, and spearmint, which were tested in a similar manner, showed no effect on learning time even though subjects considered them hedonically positive. Thus positive hedonics alone appear to be insufficient, which argues against the general affective theory of odor.

The neurophysiologic mechanism by which the floral odor mediated the improvement in learning is unclear. The odor may have facilitated deposition of short-term memory, the processing of newly learned material, or the access of these memories for subsequent tasks. Or it could have facilitated the creation of new strategies for solving problems. Because a degree of alertness is necessary for learning, the mixed floral odor may have acted by stimulating the reticular activating system. This system has been shown to be affected by other odors, for example, jasmine and smelling salts.[240,241] The activating effects of inhalation of 1,8-cineol have been demonstrated physiologically through an increase in global cerebral blood flow.[242]

An odor might increase motivation through a classic Pavlovian conditioned response in which a stimulus, in this case the odor, induces recall of a past behavior.[243]

Odors may have a direct physiologic impact on the brain.[244] The anatomy of learning involves multiple structures: Two that are essential are the hippocampus and cortex. These areas are directly influenced by anatomic projections from the olfactory system.

Many of the same neurotransmitters are involved in the processes of learning and of olfaction; modulation of these might explain how an odor enhanced the learning process. The neurotransmitters include the classic norepinephrine, dopamine, serotonin, acetylcholine, and GABA,[245–247] as well as the hypophyseal neuropeptides and nonhypophyseal hormones. Examples of the hypophyseal hormones are methionine-enkephalin and beta endorphin. Examples of the nonhypophyseal hormones include substance P, neurotensin, and cholecystokinin.[245,248]

The floral odor could have induced a positive feeling, which secondarily enhanced cognition. Odors experienced as hedonically positive produce a positive affective state,[236] and positive mood states may directly improve learning.[249] The floral odor may also have acted as an anxiolytic, decreasing anxiety, which inhibits learning. By removing this inhibiting factor, it facilitated learning.

The trail-making test is a paradigm for the learning tasks of spatial analyses, motor control, attention shifting, alertness, concentration, and number sense.[250] Brain damage at any of various locations can impair trail making, so it is logical that intervention at these locations could improve performance. The floral odor may have acted at any of these sites to improve learning. Although the odor may have affected any of these tasks, its effect on improved spatial analysis/orientation is of particular interest. This cognitive process is localized in the nondominant right hemisphere.[251,252] Olfaction also is predominantly processed in the right, nondominant hemisphere.[253] This anatomic overlap may be of such significance that the results of Hirsch and Johnston are not generalizable to learning paradigms that do not involve the right hemisphere.[239]

Possibly the floral odor did not directly affect learning but acted on noncognitive variables mentioned previously to improve hand-eye coordination, cerebellar and basal-ganglia function for coordination of movements, or pyramidal-system function for motor integration of fine movements.

The subjects could have experienced a placebo effect based on preconceived notions that the odor would affect their learning. Another difficulty in generalizing this study is that it was conducted in a relatively isolated environment, unlike a normal classroom where a cacophony of sensory stimuli may be so compelling as to lessen any positive effects of odors on learning.

Inhalation of the essential oils of peppermint, rosemary, and lemon was reported to enhance memory in normosmic 15- and 16-year-old high school students.[254]

Lemon odorant enhanced attention during a simple reaction time test as demonstrated by deceleration of hear rate.[178] The actual attention inducing effect of the aroma of lemon in the study remains suspect since the sample size, statistical significance and results of actual assessment of attention were not provided.

Parasuraman et al[255] and Nelson et al[256] reported that peppermint odor enhanced cognition as measured by inhibition of vigilance decrement, especially in subjects with attention-maintenance difficulties[256] and head injuries.[257] The mechanism of peppermint-enhanced cognition may be that it more efficiently allocates attention. This was demonstrated neurophysiologically; no reduction of amplitude of N160-evoked brain potential occurred in response to peppermint.[255] This seems anatomically reasonable because, as has been demonstrated in PET imaging, odors increase cerebral blood flow to the juncture of the inferior frontal and temporal lobes bilaterally and unilaterally activate the right orbitofrontal cortex.[257] These same areas are essential for vigilance task performance.[257]

Compared to a nonscented control, Felbaum et al found that chocolate scent increased visual motor speed and impulse control, while coffee scent enhanced typing accuracy and speed.[258]

On the other hand, Heuberger[259] found that inhalation of 1,8-cineol and linalool had no effect on human vigilance performance. This contradicts Nagai et al[260] findings of decreased VDT arithmetic workload fatigue in response of inhalation of sweet fennel oil. Of the 12 subjects assessed, this was demonstrated both with the POMS and physiologic parameters of decreased respiratory sinus arrhythmia ($p < 0.05$).[47,261]

Aromatherapy has been advocated for treatment of learning disabilities,[262] including facilitating language acquisition in children with mild language disorders.[263] Among 75 families with a child with attention deficit hyperactivity disorder surveyed, 24% (12) tried aromatherapy for this disorder, but only 5, or 38.5% of these found it helpful.[264] Using a counterbalanced, crossover design, eight adults with profound learning disabilities underwent simple concentration tasks after a combination of massage and aromatherapy with orange flower, lemon grass, and lavender.[2] When compared with the baseline no-treatment condition, aromatherapy demonstrated no effect on concentration.

Shakespeare may have been the first to recommend rosemary for improving the memory: "There's rosemary, that's for rememberance."[265]

Because it contains Cineole, an acetylcholinesterase inhibitor,[266] rosemary has been recommended for treatment of senile dementia of the Alzheimer's type. Rodent studies demonstrated that inhalation of cineole or rosemary enhanced ability to traverse a maze. In human studies, rosemary shortens reaction time. Utilization of aromatherapy in demented patients was encouraged, as a form of sensory stimulation and touted as an effective option for managing behavioral problems in a 2002 editorial in the *British Medical Journal*.[267] However, the issue of the efficacy of aromatherapy in the management of dementia received critical evaluation in a Cochrane Review.[268] Studies of aromatherapy in those with dementia were included with any one of eight outcome measures including cognitive function, function performance, behavior, quality of life, relaxation, wandering, sleep, or mood. They noted, "the great majority of reported research on aroma therapy for people with dementia is of scientifically inadequate quality." The one study included was a double-blind randomized control study of 4 weeks duration. Thirty-six subjects from eight nursing homes with severe dementia and daily agitation causing moderate to severe management problems underwent treatment with either 10% Melissa, applied twice per day for 4 weeks to face and arms or a 10% sunflower oil and base oil control.[200] Based on the Cohen-Mansfield Agitation Inventory and the Neuropsychiatric Inventory, a significant ($p < 0.05$) reduction of both agitation and aberrant motor behavior was seen. These findings remain suspect since no olfactory ability was assessed and myriad primary geriatric dementing illness substantially impairs olfactory ability. The positive effects may have been due to the aroma's impact on the caretakers' affect, to which the subject positively responded. The Cochrane Review concludes, "The one small trial published is insufficient evidence for the efficacy of aroma therapy for dementia." The objective of the absence of olfactory testing was resolved by Snow et al.[269] Each of the seven agitated demented nursing home residents was exposed for 2 weeks each of lavender, thyme oil with control periods with unscented grapeseed oil. Like in Ballard's study, the Cohen-Mansfield Agitation Inventory was the assessment tool. No effect of either aroma was seen to reduce agitation even controlling for poor olfactory ability. Thus it made no difference how well one could smell aroma, lavender and thyme had no effect on agitation.

Upon search of 24 databases, not even including the criteria of double-blinding, only one randomized controlled study met sufficient statistical and scientific validity to be included.[270]

Blindness

Olfactory stimulation may have efficacy in training of the blind through enhancement of tactile sensation.[271]

Risks and Common Susceptibilities

Before using aromatherapy in neurologic conditions, consideration must be given to the potential risks of the treatment. Adverse reactions can occur among patients with diseases that predispose them to the development of side effects, and among the population as a whole as well.

Certain diseases make their sufferers particularly susceptible to adverse effects of aromatherapy. Approximately 40% of migraineurs report osmophobia, whereby an odorant induces a migraine headache.[272] A wide range of odorants can act as such triggers, depending on the individual. These triggers include perfume, cigarette smoke, and food odors.[273]

Asthmatics, upon exposure to common odors, can suffer a worsening of their respiratory status independent of their olfactory ability.[147,261] In a survey of 60 asthmatic patients, 57 (95%) described respiratory symptoms upon exposure to common odors, including insecticide (85%), household cleaning agents (78%), perfume and cologne (72%), cigarette smoke (75%), fresh paint (73%), automobile exhaust or gas fumes (60%), and cooking aromas (37%). Room deodorant and mint candy also could cause respiratory distress.[274] Four subjects who underwent an odor challenge with 4 squirts of a popular cologne all had an immediate decline in 1-second forced expiratory volume (18% to 58% reduction).[274] Even exposure to low levels of perfume, as are found on perfume scented strips in magazines can cause airway obstruction in asthmatic patients.[275] This was seen in 36% of severe asthmatics and even in 8% of those with mild asthma.

Among persons who suffer complaints consistent with multiple chemical sensitivities, 24% of the men and 39% of the women note that odors precipitate their complaints.[276] However, double-blind studies fail to demonstrate odorant-induced multiple chemical sensitivity symptoms.[277]

Inhalation of odorants can produce measurable levels in the blood.[45] And because many common fragrances contain naphthalene-related compounds (including menthol and camphor), persons with G6PD deficiency may be at risk from aromatherapeutic exposures.[278] In neonates, dermal application has demonstrated this, but in adults it remains only a theoretic risk for inhalational aromatherapy. However, even more worrisome is if essential oil fragrances are added to massage oil as part of traditional lay "aromatherapy." This combination can enhance cutaneous absorption such that the blood concentration can exceed inhalational levels by greater than a thousandfold,[279] and these levels can persist in the bloodstream for a considerable period. Lavender oil, for instance, when used as part of a massage treatment was demonstrated at high concentration in the bloodstream 20 minutes after completion of the massage.[280] In those suffering hepatic or renal dysfunction, even greater levels and longer duration of exposure can be anticipated with unexplored toxicological effects.

A variety of essential oils anecdotally have been described to be able to precipitate seizures in epileptics. Whether these effects can occur by inhalation alone as opposed to ingestion or by percutaneous absorption is unclear. Proconvulsant odorants include rosemary,[6,281] fennel, hyssop, sage, and wormwood.[6]

Because aromatherapeutic inhalation of essential oils can produce detectable levels of the oils in the blood, these compounds, like any pharmacologic agents, could induce adverse drug-drug interactions in persons on medication. Such interactions could enhance metabolism of anticonvulsants or pain medications, for example, thus predisposing an epileptic to have a seizure or a chronic pain patient to withdraw from medication. Jori et al[282] demonstrated this potential. Inhalation of eucalyptol by rats increased microsomal enzyme systems, thus decreasing the effect of pentobarbital.

Odorants can produce harmful side effects not only among persons predisposed to disease but among the healthy population as well. Airborne-induced allergic contact dermatitis is a recognized result of aromatherapeutic inhalation of tea tree oil (melaleuca oil).[283] Examples of common melaleuca oil allergens include d-limonene, aromadendrene, alpha-terpinene, 1,8-cineole (eucalyptol), terpinen- 4-ol, p-cymene, and alpha-phellandrene. Because of the highly volatile nature of essential oils, their common constituents and cross-sensitization, DeGroot postulated that the same airborne-induced contact dermatitis could occur with several other essential oils, including lavender and a mixture of eucalyptus, pine, and peppermint.[283] Bridges suggested that if odorants can sensitize the respiratory system as they do the skin, they might not only exacerbate asthma but might actually precipitate asthma.[284]

CONCLUSION

With aromatherapy, just as with any therapeutic tool, practitioners must weigh the relative risk/benefit ratio in deciding upon its use in the treatment of pain and neurologic disorders.

REFERENCES

1. Kaptchuk TJ. Vitalism. In: Micozzi MS, ed. *Fundamentals of Complementary and Integrative Medicine.* 3rd ed. St Louis, MO: Elsevier; 2006:53–66.
2. Lindsay WR, Pitcaithly D, Geelen N. A comparison of the effects of four therapy procedures on concentration and responsiveness in people with profound learning disabilities. *J Intellect Disabil Res.* 1997;41(3):201–207.
3. Roebuck A. Aromatherapy: fact or fiction. *Perfumer & Flavorist.* 1988;13:43–45.
4. Buchbauer G. Biological effects of fragrances and essential oils. *Perfumer & Flavorist.* 1993;18:19–24.
5. Price S, Price L. *Aromatherapy for Health Professionals.* New York, NY: Churchill-Livingstone; 1995.

6. Tisserand R.: *The Art of Aromatherapy.* Rochester, CT: Healing Arts; 1977.
7. Weyers W, Brodbeck R. *Hautdurchdringung atherischer ole* (Skin absorption of volatile oils). *Pharmazie in Unserer Zeit.* 1989;18(3):82–86.
8. King JR. Scientific status of aromatherapy. *Perspect Biol Med.* 1994;37(3):409–415.
9. Brodal A. *Neurological Anatomy in Relation to Clinical Medicine.* Vol. 10. 3rd ed. New York, NY: Oxford University Press; 1969.
10. Freeman WJ. The physiology of perception. *Scientific American.* 1991;February: 78–85.
11. Hirsch AR, Wyse JP. Posttraumatic dysosmia: central vs. peripheral. *J Neurol Orthop Med Surg.* 1993;14:152–155.
12. Acharya V, Acharya J, Luders H. Olfactory epileptic auras. *Neurology.* 1996;46:A446.
13. Hirsch AR. *Scentsational Sex.* Boston, MA: Element Books; 1998.
14. Plaily J, Howard J, Gottfried J. Piriform to orbitofrontal transthalamic pathway involved in olfactory attentional processing. Abstract Book. *AChemS* XXIX. 2007;425:85.
15. Dietz MA, Goetz CJ, Steddings GT. Evaluation of visual cues as a modified inverted walking stick in the treatment of Parkinson's disease freezing episodes. *Mov Disord.* 1990;5:243–247.
16. Gowers WR. Epilepsy and other chronic convulsive diseases. In: Efron R, The effect of olfactory stimuli in arresting uncinate fits. *Brain.* 1957;79:267–281.
17. Efron R. The effect of olfaction stimuli in arresting uncinate fits. *Brain.* 1957;79:267–281.
18. Alaoui-Ismaili O, Vernet-Maury E, Dittmar A, Delhomme G, Chanel J. Odor hedonics: connection with emotional response estimated by autonomic parameters. *Chem Senses.* 1997;22(3):237–248.
19. Dember WD. *The Psychology of Perception.* New York, NY: Rinehart and Winston; 1960:222–223.
20. Dematté ML, Sanabria D, Sugarman R, Spence C. Cross-modal interactions between olfaction and touch. *Chem Senses.* 2006;31:291–300.
21. Hirsch AR, Gruss JJ. Ambient odors in the treatment of claustrophobia: a pilot study. *J Neurol Orthop Med Surg.* 1998;18:98–103.
22. Hirsch AR, Ye Y. The impact of aroma upon the perception of age. *Chem Senses.* 2005;30(5):464.
23. Hirsch AR, Hoogeveen JR, Bussee, AM, Allen ET. The effects of odour on weight perception. *Int J of Essential Oil Ther.* 1:21–28, 2007.
24. Fields H. *Pain.* New York, NY: McGraw-Hill; 1967.
25. Freud S. *Bemerkungen uber einen Fall von Zwangs Neurosa. Ges Schr.* 1908;8:350.
26. MacLean PD. *Triune concept of the brain and behavior.* Toronto, Canada: University of Toronto Press; 1973.
27. Brodal A. *Neurological Anatomy in Relation to Clinical Medicine.* 3rd ed. New York, NY: Oxford University Press; 1981.
28. Ehrlichman H, Halpern JN. Affect and memory: effects of pleasant and unpleasant odors on retrieval of happy and unhappy memories. *J Pers Soc Psychol.* 1988;55:769–779.
29. Hirsch AR. Nostalgia: neuropsychiatric understanding. *Adv Consumer Res.* 1992; 19:390–395.
30. Squire LR. *Memory and brain.* New York, NY: Oxford University Press, 1987.
31. Brown R, Kulik J. Flashbulb memories. *Cognition.* 1977;5:73–99.
32. Proust M. *Remembrance of Things Past.* Vol 1. Scott Moncrieff CK, trans. New York, NY: Random House; 1934.
33. Kline N, Rausch J. Olfactory precipitants of flashbacks in post traumatic stress disorders: case reports. *J Clin Psychiatr.* 1985;46:383–384.

34. Vermetten E, Bremmer JD. Olfaction as a traumatic reminder in posttraumatic stress disorder: case reports and review. *J Clin Psychiatry.* 2003;54(2):202–207.
35. Laird DA. What can you do with your nose? *Scientific Monthly.*
36. Damian P, Damian K. *Aromatherapy scent and psyche.* Rochester, VT: Healing Arts; 1995.
37. Cunningham S. *Magical Aromatherapy: The Power of Scent.* St Paul, MN: Llewellyn Publications; 1995.
38. Feller RM. *Practical Aromatherapy: Understanding and Using Essential Oils to Heal the Mind and Body.* New York, NY: Berkley Books; 1997.
39. Price S. *Aromatherapy for Common Ailments.* New York, NY: Fireside Books; 1991.
40. Schnaubelt K. *Advanced Aromatherapy: The Science of Essential Oil Therapy.* Rochester, VT: Healing Arts; 1995.
41. Keville K, Green M. *Aromatherapy: A Complete Guide to the Healing Art.* Freedom, CA: Crossing Press; 1995.
42. Lorig TS, Huffman E, DeMartino A, DeMarco J. The effects of low concentration odors on EEG activity and behavior. *Journal of Psychophysiology.* 1991;5:69–77.
43. Buchbauer G, et al. Fragrance compounds and essential oils with sedative effects upon inhalation. *J Pharm Sci.* 1993;82(6):660–664.
44. Buchbauer G. Biological effects of fragrances and essential oils *Perfumer & Flavorist.* 1993;18:20.
45. Stimpfl T, et al. Concentration of 1,8- cineol in human blood during prolonged inhalation. *Chem Senses.* 1995;20(3):349–350.
46. Alaoui-Ismaili O, et al. Basic emotions evoked by odorants: comparison between autonomic responses and self-evaluation. *Physiol Behav.* 1997;62:713–720.
47. Vernet-Maury E, Alaoui-Ismaili O, Rousmans S, Olivier R, Georges D, Andre D. Olfaction/emotion connexion: comparison between autonomic and verbal responses [abstract]. *ECRO XIII.* 1998;213:121.
48. Miltner W et al. Emotional qualities of odorants and their influence on the startle reflex in humans, *Psychophysiology* 31:107–110, 1994.
49. Buchbauer G. Aromatherapy: do essential oils have therapeutic properties? *Perfumer & Flavorist.* 1990;15:47–50.
50. Klemm WR, Lutes SD, Hendrix DV, Warrenburg S. Topographical EEG maps of human responses to odors. *Chem Senses.* 1992;17(3):347–361.
51. Lorig TS, Roberts M. Odor and cognitive alteration of the contingent negative variation. *Chem Senses.* 1990;15:537–545.
52. Sano K, Tsuda Y, Sugano H, Aou S, Hatanaka A. Concentration effects of green odor on event-related Potential (P300) and pleasantness. *Chem Senses.* 2002;27: 225–230.
53. Bremner EA, Mainland J, Zelano C, Khan RM, Sobel N. Transformations in odor perception identity as a function of intensity. *Chem Senses.* 2005;30:A237.
54. Sugawara Y, Hino Y, Kawasaki M. Alteration of perceived fragrance of essential oils in relation to type of work: a simple screening test for efficacy of aroma. *Chem Senses.* 1999;24:415–421.
55. Lawless HT, Heymann H. *Sensory Evaluation of Food. Principles and Practices.* New York, NY: Chapman & Hall; 1998.
56. Koenitzer JC, Naqvi F, Dalton PH. Fragrance expectancies and perceived effects: a study of subjective and objective responses. *Chem Senses.* 2003;28:A118.
57. Cameron EL. Effects of pregnancy on olfaction. *Chem Senses.* 2006;31:A34–A35.
58. Satoh S, Morita N, Matsuzaki I, et al. Relationship between odor perception and depression in the Japanese elderly. *Psychiatry and Clinical Neurosciences.* 1996;50: 271–275.

59. Güra E, Roscher S, Kobal. Smell and emotion: emotional conditioning of smell. *Chem Sense*. 2000;25:795.

60. Warm JS, Dember WN, Parasuraman R. Effects of olfactory stimulation on performance and stress in a visual sustained attention task. *J Soc Cosmet Chem*. 1991;42:199–210.

61. American Medical Association. Department of Environmental, Public, and Occupational Health. *The Physician's Guide to Odor Pollution*. Chicago, IL: American Medical Association; 1973.

62. Miner JR. Controlling odors from livestock production facilities: state-of-the-art. In: *Livestock Waste: Renewable Resource*. St Joseph, MI: American Society of Agricultural Engineers, 1980.

63. Hirsch AR, Rankin KM. Trichloroethylene exposure and headache. *Headache*. 1993;33:275.

64. Hirsch AR. Cephalgia as a result of acute nitrogen tetroxide exposure. *Headache*. 1995;35:310.

65. Hirsch AR. *Neurotoxicity as a Result of Acute Nitrogen Tetroxide Exposure*. International Congress on Hazardous Waste: impact on human and ecological health. Atlanta, GA: U.S. Department of Health and Human Services: Public Health Agency for Toxic Substances and Disease Registry; 1995.

66. Hirsch AR. Chronic neurotoxicity of acute chlorine gas exposure. Paper presented at: 13th International Neurotoxicity Conference; 1995; Hot Springs, AR.

67. Neutra R, et al. Hypotheses to explain the higher symptom rates observed around hazardous waste sites. *Environ Health Perspect*. 1991;94:31–38.

68. Shusterman D. Critical review: health significance of environmental odor pollution. *Arch Environ Health*. 1992;47:76–87.

69. Wayne W, Wehrle P, Carroll R. Oxidant air pollution and athletic performance. *JAMA*. 1967;199:901–904.

70. Maruniak JA. Deprivation and the olfactory system. In: Doty RL, ed. *Handbook of Olfaction and Gustation*. New York, NY: Marcel Dekker; 1995.

71. Evans GW. Psychological costs of chronic exposure to ambient air pollution. In: Isaacson RI, Jensen KF, eds. *The Vulnerable Brain and Environmental Risks*. Vol 3, New York, NY: Plenum Press; 1994.

72. Salamon E, Kim M, Beaulleu J, Stefano GB. Sound therapy induced relaxation: down regulating stress processes and pathologies. *Med Sci Monit*. 2003;9(5):RA116-RA121.

73. Tomonobu N, Hagino I, Watanuki S, Yokoyama N, Funada Y. Effect of odor preference on the autonomic nervous system. *Chem Senses*. 2001;26(02):294.

74. Weisse CS. Depression and immunocompetence: review of the literature. *Psychol Bull*. 1992;111:475–489.

75. Alexander M. Aromatherapy & immunity: how the use of essential oils aid immune potentiality. Part 2 Mood-immune correlations, stress and susceptibility to illness and how essential oil odorants raise this threshold. *The Int J of Aromatherapy*. 2001;11(3): 152–156.

76. Hirsch AR. *Chronic Neurotoxicity as a Result of Landfill Exposure in Port Orchard, Washington, International Congress on Hazardous Waste—Impact on Human and Ecological Health*. Atlanta, GA: U.S. Department of Health and Human Services: Public Health Agency for Toxic Substances and Disease Registry; 1995.

77. Izmerov N. Establishment of air quality standards. *Arch Environ Health*. 1971;22: 711–719.

78. Rotton J, et al. Air pollution experience and physical aggression. *J Appl Soc Psychol*. 1979;9:347–412.

79. Ury HK, Perkins MA, Goldsmith JR. Motor vehicle accidents and vehicular pollution in Los Angeles. *Arch Environ Health*. 1972;25:314–322.

80. Shiffman SS, et al. The effect of environmental odors emanating from commercial swine operations on the mood of nearby residents. *Brain Res Bull.* 1995;37:369–375.
81. Rotton J, et al. Air pollution and interpersonal attraction. *J Appl Soc Psychol.* 1978;8:57–71.
82. Brandstatter H, Furhwirth M, Kitchler E. Effects of weather and air pollution on mood: individual difference approach. In: Canter D, et al., eds. *NATO Advanced Research Workshop on Social and Environmental Psychology in the European Context: Environmental Social Psychology.* Boston, MA: G Kluwer; 1988.
83. Bullinger M. Psychological effects of air pollution on healthy residents: a time series approach. *J Environ Psychol.* 1989;9:103–118.
84. Bullinger M. Relationships between air-pollution and well-being. *Z Sozial Praventivmed.* 1989;34:231–238.
85. Zeidner M, Schechter M. Psychological responses to air pollution: some personality and demographic correlates. *J Environ Psychol.* 1988;8:191–208.
86. Rotton J, Frey J. Air pollution, weather, and violent crimes: concomitant time series analysis of archival data. *J Pers Social Psychol.* 1985;49:1207–1220.
87. Briere J, Downes A, Spensley J. Summer in the city: urban weather conditions and psychiatric-emergency room visits. *J Abnorm Psychol.* 1983;92:77–80.
88. Hirsch AR. Negative health effects of malodors in the environment: a brief review. *J Neurol Orthop Med Surg.* 1998;18:43–45.
89. Valentine JH, et al. Human crises and the physical environment. *Man-Environ Sys.* 1975;5(1):23–28.
90. Cunningham M. Weather, mood, and helping behavior: quasi-experiments with the sunshine Samaritan. *J Personal Soc Psychol.* 1979;37:1947–1956.
91. Strahilevitz M, Strahilevitz A, Miller JE. Air pollutants and the admission rate of psychiatric patients. *Am J Psychiatry.* 1979;136(2):205–207.
92. Jones JW, Bogat GA. Air pollution and human aggression. *Psychol Rep.* 1978;43: 721–722.
93. Rotton J. Affective and cognitive consequences of malodorous pollution. *Basic Appl Soc Psychol.* 1983;4:171–191.
94. Robin O, et al. Basic emotions evoked by eugenol odor differ according to the dental experience.: a neurovegetative analysis. *Chem Senses.* 1999;24:327–335.
95. Robin O, et al. Emotional responses evoked by dental odors: an evaluation from autonomic parameters. *J Dent Res.* 1998;77(8):1638–1646.
96. Herz RS. Odor-associative learning and emotion: effects on perception and behavior. *Chem Senses.* 2005;30(1):i250-i251
97. Herz RS. Olfactory cognition and emotion. *Chem Senses.* 2001;26:702.
98. Schiffman SS, Williams CM. Science of odor as a potential health issue. *J Enviorn Qual.* 2005;34:129–138.
99. Ludvigson HW, Rottman TR. Effects of ambient odors of lavender and cloves on cognition, memory, affect and mood. *Chem Senses.* 1989;14:525–536.
100. Distel H, et al. Perception of everyday odors—correlation between intensity, familiarity and strength of hedonic judgement. *Chem Senses.* 1999;24:191–199.
101. White TL, Kurtz DB. The relationship between metacognitive awareness of olfactory ability and age in people reporting chemosensory disturbances. *Am J of Psychol.* 2003;116(1):99–110.
102. Nordin S, Monsch A, Murphy C. Unawareness of smell loss in normal aging and Alzheimer's disease: discrepancy between self-reported and diagnosed smell sensitivity. *J of Gerontol.* 50B(4):187–192.
103. Flaten MA, Simonsen T, Olsen H. Drug-related information generates placebo and nocebo responses that modify the drug response. *Psychosom Med.* 1999;61:250–255.

104. Lieberman MD, Jarcho JM, Berman S, et al. The neural correlates of placebo effects: a disruption account. *NeuroImage.* 2004;22:447–455.
105. Finniss DG, Benedetti F. The neural matrix of pain processing and placebo analgesia: implications for clinical practice. *Headache Currents.* 2005;2(6):132–138.
106. Knasko SC, Gilbert AN, Sabini J. Emotional state, physical well-being, and performance in the presence of feigned ambient odor. *J Appl Soc Psychol.* 1990;20(16): 1345–1357.
107. Deliza R, MacFie HJH. The generation of sensory expectation by external cues and its effect on sensory perception and hedonic ratings: a review. *J of Sensory Stud.* 11: 103–128, 1996.
108. Lorig TS, Roberts M. Odor and cognitive alteration of the contingent negative variation. *Chem Senses.* 1990;15(5):537–545.
109. Visser A. Social desirability in health research. Psychosom Med. 1999;61:106.
110. Holroyd KA, Mauskop A. Complementary and alternative treatments. *Neurology.* 2003;60(2):S58–S62.
111. Keng MK, Martin JH, Wehner S, Birbeck GL. The use of complementary therapies among headache patients newly referred to a neurology clinic. Annual Meeting Program Abstracts. Headache: *The J of Head and Face Pain.* 2004;44(5)(s113):503.
112. Long L, Huntley A, Ernst E. Which complementary and alternative therapies benefit which conditions? A survey of the opinions of 223 professional organizations. *Complement Ther Med.* 2001;9(3):178–185.
113. Buckle S. Aromatherapy and massage: the evidence. *Paediatr Nurs.* 2003;15(6):24–27.
114. Genders R. Perfume through the Ages. New York, NY: G Putnam and Sons; 1972.
115. Gobel H, et al. Essential plant oils and headache mechanisms. *Phytomed.* 1995;2(2):93–102.
116. Walji H. The Healing Power of Aromatherapy. Rocklin, CA: Prima Publishing; 1996.
117. Passant H. A holistic approach in the ward. *Nursing Times.* 1990;86(4):26–28.
118. Price S, Price L. Aromatherapy for Health Professionals. New York, NY: Churchill-Livingstone.
119. Wabner D. Emotional effects of essential oils—the project, art & scent. Proceedings of the World of Aromatherapy II International Conference and Trade Show: September 25–28, 1998. St. Louis, MO:29–35.
120. Saller R, Hellstein A, Hellenbrecht D. Klinische Pharmakologie und therapeutische Anwendung von Cineol (Eukalyptus) und Menthol als Bestandteil atherischer Ole. Internistiche Praxis. 1988;28(2):355–364. Cited by: Gobel H, et al. Essential plant oils and headache mechanisms. Phytomedicine. 1995;2(2):93–102.
121. Hirsch AR, Kang C. The effect of inhaling green apple fragrance to reduce the severity of migraine: a pilot study. *Headache Q.* 1998;9:159–163.
122. Kirk-Smith MD, Van Toller C, Dodd GH. Unconscious odour conditioning in human subjects. *Biol Psychol.* 1983;17:221–231.
123. Halasz N, Shepherd GM. Neurochemistry of the vertebrate olfactory bulb. Neurosci. 1983;10:578–579.
124. Macrides F, Davis BJ. Olfactory bulb. In: Emson PC, ed. Chemical Neuroanatomy. New York, NY; Raven Press; 1983.
125. Haberly LB, Price JL. Association and commissural fiber systems of the olfactory cortex in the rat. II. Systems originating in the olfactory peduncle. *J Comp Neurol.* 1978;178:781–808.
126. Mair RG, Harrison LM. Influence of drugs on smell function. In: Laing DG, Doty RL, Briephol W, eds. Human Sense of Smell. Berlin, Germany: Springer-Verlag; 1991.

127. Zaborsky L, et al. Cholinergic and GABA-ergic projections to the olfactory bulb in the rat. *J Comp Neurol.* 1985;243:468–509.
128. Sjaastad O. Cluster headaches. In: Vinken PJ, Bruyn GW, Klawans HL, eds. *Handbook of Clinical Neurology: Headache.* Vol 48. New York, NY: Elsevier Science; 1986.
129. Gall CM, et al. Events for co-existence of GABA and dopamine in neurons of the rat olfactory bulb. *J Comp Neurol.* 1987;266:307–318.
130. Leston J, et al. Free and conjugated plasma catecholamines in cluster headache. *Cephalalgia.* 1987;7(6):331.
131. Foote S, Bloom F, Aston-Jones G. Nucleus locus coeruleus: new evidence of anatomical and physiological specificity. *Physiol Rev.* 1983;86:844–914.
132. Shipley M, Halloran F, Torre J. Surprisingly rich projection from locus coeruleus to the olfactory bulb in the rat. *Brain Res.* 1985;329:294–299.
133. Igarashi H, et al. Cerebrovascular sympathetic nervous activity during cluster headaches. *Handbook Clin Neurol.* 1987;7(6):87–89.
134. Anselmi B, et al. Endogenous opioids in cerebrospinal fluid and blood in idiopathic headache sufferers. *Headache.* 1980;20:294–299.
135. Nattero G, et al. Serum gastrin levels in cluster headache and migraine attacks. In: Pfaffenrath V, Lundberg PO, Sjaastad O, eds. *Updating in Headache.* Berlin, Germany: Springer-Verlag; 1985.
136. Appenzeller O, Atkinson RA, Standefer JC. Serum beta endorphin in cluster headache and common migraine. In: Rose FC, Zikha E, eds. *Progress in Migraine.* London, England: Pitman; 1981.
137. Hardebo JE, et al. CSF opioid levels in cluster headache. In: Rose FC, ed. *Migraine.* Basel, Switzerland: Karger; 1985.
138. Moskowitz MA. Neurobiology of vascular head pain. *Ann Neurol.* 1984;16:157–158.
139. Gobel H, Schmidt G, Soyka D. Effect of peppermint and eucalyptus oil preparations on neurophysiological and experimental algesimetric headache parameters. *Cephalalgia.* 1994;14:228–234.
140. Gobel H, et al. Effectiveness of peppermint oil and paracetamol in the treatment of tension headache. *Nervenarzt.* 1996;67:672–681.
141. Woolfson A, Hewitt D. Intensive aromacare. *Intl J Aromather.* 1992;4(2):12–13.
142. Aqel MB. Relaxant effect of the volatile oil of Romarinus officinalis on tracheal smooth muscle. *J Ethnopharmacol.* 1991;33:57–62.
143. Kehrl W, Sonnemann U, Dethlefsen U. Therapy for acute nonpurulent rhinosinusitis with cineole: results of a double-blind, randomized, placebo-controlled trial. *Laryngoscope.* 2004;114:738–742.
144. Wilkie J, Prescott J. Sweet odours increase pain tolerance. Abstract Book. AChemS XXVII. 2006;183:46.
145. Bayley R, Matthews L, Street E, Almeida J. Ability of gum flavors to distract participants from painful stimuli: differential effects of retronasal vs. orthonasal scent administration. Abstract Book. AChemS XXIX, 2007;548:115.
146. Gedney JJ, Fillingim RB, Glover TL. Aromatic essential oils produce no direct analgesic effect, but subjects retrospectively report significant benefit. Abstract Book. American Psychsosomatic Society, 62nd Annual Scientific Meeting. 2004;26:1394:33.
147. Opiekun R, Smeets M, Rogers R, Prasad N, Vedula U, Dalton P. Assessment of ocular and nasal irritation in asthmatics resulting from fragrance exposure. *Clin and Exp Allergy.* 2003;33(9):1256–1265.
148. Saeki Y, Tanaka YL. Effect of inhaling fragrances on relieving pricking pain. *The Intl J of Aromather.* 2005;15:74–80.

149. Dale A, Cornwell S. The role of lavender oil in relieving perineal discomfort following childbirth: a blind randomized clinical trial. *J Adv Nurs.* 1994;19:89–96.
150. Burns E, Blamey C. Using aromatherapy in childbirth. *Nurs Times.* 1994;90(9): 54–60.
151. Shirreffs CM. Aromatherapy massage for joint pain and constipation in a patient with Guillian Barré. *Complementary Ther in Nurs & Midwifery.* 2000;7:78–83.
152. Dunning T, James K. Complementary therapies in action—education and outcomes. *Complementary Ther in Nurs & Midwifery.* 2001;7:188–195.
153. Krall B, Krause W. *Efficacy intolerance of mentha arvensis aetheroleum.* In: Proceedings from the 24th International Symposium of Essential Oils; 1993; abstracts.
154. Wang Y, et al. A pilot study of the use of alternative medicine in multiple sclerosis patients with special focus on acupuncture. *Neurology.* 1998;52(2):A550.
155. Doty RL, Shaman P, Dann M. Development of the University of Pennsylvania smell identification test: a standardized microencapsulated test of olfactory function. *Physiol Behav.* 1984;32:489–502.
156. Yamada K, Mimaki Y, Sashida Y. Anticonvulsive effects of inhaling lavender oil vapour. *Biol Pharm Bull.* 1994;17(2):359–360.
157. Betts T, et al. An olfactory countermeasure treatment for epileptic seizures using a conditioned arousal response to specific aromatherapy oils. *Epilepsia.* 1995;36(3): S130–S131.
158. Davies P. *Aromatherapy: An A–Z.* C. W. Daniel. As referenced in: Mantle F. Moving experiences. *Nurs Times.* 1996;92(14):46–48.
159. Markopoulou K, et al. Olfactory dysfunction in familial parkinsonism. *Neurology* 1977;49:1262–1267.
160. Mobert RJ, Doty RL. Olfactory function in Huntington's disease patients and at-risk offspring. *Int J Neurosci.* 1997;89:133–139.
161. Ferry P, Johnson M, Wallis P. Use of complementary therapies and non-prescribed medication in patients with Parkinson's disease. *Postgrad Med J.* 2002;78: 612–614.
162. Plum V. Working with alcoholism. *Intl J Aromather.* 1998;9(1):9–11.
163. Schiffman SS. Taste and smell in disease. *N Engl J Med.* 1983;308:1275–1279.
164. Getchell T, Bartoschuk L, Doty R. *Smell and Taste in Health and Disease.* New York, NY: Raven Press; 1991.
165. Westman EC, Behm FM, Rose JE. Airway sensory replacement combined with nicotine replacement for smoking cessation: a randomized placebo-controlled trial using a citric acid inhaler. *Chest.* 1995;107:1358–1364.
166. Felbaum D, Bloom J, Cessna T, Drake R, Raudenbush B. Effects of peppermint scent on diminishing smoking cravings and withdrawal symptoms. Abstract Book. *AChemS* XXIX 2007;551:116.
167. Macht DI, Ting GC. Experimental inquiry into the sedative properties of some aromatic drugs and fumes. *J Pharmacol Exp Ther.* 1921;18:361–372.
168. Buchbauer G, et al. Aromatherapy: evidence for sedative effects of the essential oil of lavender after inhalation. *J Biosci (Zeitschrift fur Naturforschung).* 1991;Sect C,46 (11–12):1067–1072.
169. Cunningham S. *Magical Aromatherapy: The Power of Scent.* St Paul, MN: Llewellyn Publications; 1995.
170. Buchbauer G, Jirovetz L, Jager W. Passiflora and lime- blossoms: motility effects after inhalation of the essential oils and of some of the main constituents in animal experiment. *Arch Pharm (Weinheim).* 1992;325:247–248.
171. Elisabetsky E, Marschner J, Souza DO. Effects of linalool on glutamatergic system in the rat cerebral cortex. *Neurochem Res.* 1995;20(4):461–465.

172. Schiffman SS, Siebert JM. New frontiers in fragrance use. *Cosmetic & Toiletries.* 1991;106:39–45.

173. Hudson R. The value of lavender for rest and activity in the elderly patient. *Compl Ther Med.* 1996;4:5257.

174. Hirsch AR. Olfaction and aging. *Ann Clin Lab Sci.* 1995;25(1):100.

175. Scott AE. Clinical characteristics of taste and smell disorders. *Ear Nose Throat J.* 1989;68:297–298.

176. Doty R, Reyes P, Gregor T. Presence of both odor identification and detection deficits in Alzheimer's disease. *Brain Res Bull.* 1987;18:598.

177. Karamat E, et al. Excitatory and sedative effects of essential oils on human reaction time performance. Ecro X: Abstracts. *Chem Senses.* 1992;17:847.

178. Kikuchi A, Tanida M, Uenoyama S, Abe T, Yamaguchi H. Effect of odors on cardiac response patterns in a reaction time task. 24th Japanese Symposium on Taste and Smell (JASTS XXIV). *Chem Senses.* 1991;16(2):183.

179. Sugawara Y, Hara C, Tamura K, et al. Sedative effect on humans of inhalation of essential oil of linalool: sensory evaluation and physiological measurements using optically active linalools. *Analytica Chimica Acta.* 1998;365:293–299.

180. Miyake Y, Nakagawa M, Asakura. Effects of odors on humans: effects on sleep latency [abstract]. *JASTS.* 1990;24:183.

181. Klink M, Quan SF, Prevalence of reported sleep disturbances in a general adult population and their relationship to obstructive airways diseases, *Chest, 1987*:91: 540–546.

182. Benton D. The influence of androstenol—a putative human pheromone—on mood throughout the menstrual cycle. *Biol Psychol.* 1982;15:249–256.

183. Miyazaki Y, Motohashi Y, Kobayashi S. Changes in mood by inhalation of essential oils in humans II. *Mokuzai-Gakkaishi.* 1992;38(10):909–913.

184. Inoue N, Kuroda K, Sugimoto A, Kakuda T, Fushiki T. Autonomic nervous responses according to preference for the odor of jasmine tea. *Biosci Biotechnol Biochem.* 2003;67(6):1206–1214.

185. Hirsch AR. Garlic therapy. *Harper's Magazine.* 1999;298(1788):32.

186. Baron RA. The sweet smell of . . . helping: effects of pleasant ambient odors on prosocial behavior in shopping malls. *Per Soc Psychol Bull.* 1997;23:498–504.

187. Baron RA, Kalsher MJ. Effects of a pleasant ambient fragrance on simulated driving performance: the sweet smell of . . . safety? *Environ Behav.* 1998;30:535–552.

188. Hirsch AR. Nostalgia, the odors of childhood and society. *Psychiatr Times.* 1992;9(8):29.

189. Baron RA, Thomley J. A whiff of reality: positive affect as a potential mediator of the effects of pleasant fragrance on task performance and helping. *Environ Behav.* 1994;26:766–784.

190. Dixon JM, Helsel WJ, Rojahn J. Aversive conditioning of visual screening with aromatic ammonia for treating aggressive and disruptive behavior in a developmentally disabled child. *Behav Modif.* 1989;13:91–107.

191. Earls CM, Castonguay LG. The evaluation of olfactory aversion for a bisexual pedophile with a single-case multiple baseline design. *Behav Ther.* 1989;20:137–146. As referenced in: Spector IP, et al. Cue-controlled relaxation and "aromatherapy" in the treatment of speech anxiety. *Behav Cogn Psychother.* 1993;21:239–253.

192. Tanner BA, Zeiler M. Punishment of self-injurious behavior using aromatic ammonia as the aversive stimulus. *J Appl Behav An.* 1975;8:53–57.

193. Baumeister AA, Baumeister AA. Suppression of repetitive self-injurious behavior by contingent inhalation of aromatic ammonia. *J Autism Childhood Schizophr.* 1978; 8(1):71–77.

194. Brooker DJR, Snape M, Johnson E. Single case evaluation of the effects of aromatherapy and massage on disturbed behaviour in severe dementia. *Brit J Clin Psychol.* 1997;36:287–296.

195. Holmes C, Hopkins V, Hensford C, MacLaughlin V, Wilkinson D, Rosenvinge H. Lavender oil as a treatment for agitated behaviour in severe dementia: a placebo controlled study. *Int J of Geriatr Psychiatry.* 2002;17:305–308.

196. Cain WS, Gent JF. Olfactory sensitivity: reliability, generality, and association with aging. *J Exper Psychol.* 1991;17:382–391.

197. Vance D. Considering olfactory stimulation for adults with age-related dementia. *Percep Mot Skills.* 1999;88:398–400.

198. Hawkes C, Fogo A, Shah M. Smell identification declines from age 36 years and mainly affects pleasant odours. *Chem Senses.* 2005;30:A152.

199. Ackerman BH, Kasbekar N. Disturbances of taste and smell induced by drugs. *Pharmacother.* 1997;17(3):482–496.

200. Ballard CG, O'Brien JT, Reicheit K, Perry EK. Aromatherapy as a safe and effective treatment for the management of agitation in severe dementia: the results of a double-blind, placebo-controlled trial with Melissa. *J Clin Psychiatry.* 2002;63(7): 553–558.

201. Beshara MC, Giddings D. Use of plant essential oils in treating agitation in a dementia unit: 10 case studies. *The Int J of Aromather.* 2002;12(4):207–212.

202. Hirsch AR, Trannel TJ. Chemosensory disorders and psychiatric diagnoses. *J Neurol Orthop Med Surg.* 1996;17:25–30.

203. Warren C, Warrenburg S. Mood benefits of fragrance. *Perfumer & Flavorist.* 1993; 18:9–16.

204. Heuberger E, Hongratanaworakit T, Böhm C, Weber R, Buchbauer G. Effects of chiral fragrances on human autonomic nervous system parameters and self-evaluation. *Chem Senses.* 2001;26:281–292.

205. Kuriyama H, Watanabe S, Nakaya T, et al. Immunological and psychological benefits of aromatherapy massage. *ECAM.* 2005;2:2:179–184.

206. Torii S, et al. Contingent negative variation (CNV) and the psychological effects of odour. In: Van Toller S, Dodd G, eds. *Perfumery: The Psychology and Biology of Fragrance.* New York, NY: Chapman and Hall; 1988.

207. Langewitz W, Ruddel H, Von Eiff AW. Influence of perceived level of stress upon ambulatory blood pressure, heart rate, and respiratory frequency. *J Clin Hypertens.* 1987;3:743–748.

208. Allen WF. Effect of various inhaled vapors on respiration and blood pressure in anesthetized, unanesthetized, sleeping and anosmic subjects. *Am J Physiol.* 1929;1988:620–632.

209. Atsumi T, Tonosaki K. Smelling lavender and rosemary increases free radical scavenging activity and decreases cortisol level in saliva. *Psychiatry Res.* 2007;150(1): 89–96.

210. Spector IP, et al. Cue-controlled relaxation and "aromatherapy" in the treatment of speech anxiety. *Behav Cogn Psychother.* 1993;21:239–253.

211. Wiebe E. A randomized trial of aromatherapy to reduce anxiety before abortion. *Eff Clin Pract.* 2000;4:166–169.

212. Evans B. An audit into the effects of aromatherapy massage and the cancer patient in palliative and terminal care. *Compl Ther Med.* 1995;3:239–241.

213. Dunn C. *A Report on a Randomised Controlled Trial to Evaluate the Use of Massage and Aromatherapy in an Intensive Care Unit* [bachelor's thesis]. 1992. As referenced in: Waldman CS, et al. Aromatherapy in the intensive care unit. *Care of the Critically Ill.* 1993;9(4):170–174.

214. Dunn C, Sleep J, Collett D. Sensing an improvement: an experimental study to evaluate the use of aromatherapy, massage and periods of rest in an intensive care unit. *J Adv Nurs*. 1995;21:34–40.

215. Buckle J. Aromatherapy. Does it matter which lavender essential oil is used? *Nurs Times*. 1993;89(20):32–35.

216. Stevensen CJ. The psychophysiological effects of aromatherapy massage following cardiac surgery. *Compl Ther Med*. 1994;2:27–35.

217. Wilkinson S. Aromatherapy and massage in palliative care. *Intl J Palliat Nurs*. 1995;1(1):21–30.

218. Mehta S, Stone DN, Whitehead. Use of essential oil to promote induction of anaesthesia in children. *Anaesthesia*. 1998;53:711–723.

219. DeGroot AC. Airborne allergic contact dermatitis from tea tree oil. *Contact Dermatitis*. 1996;35:101.

220. Lucks BC. Vitex agnus-castus essential oil and menopausal balance: a self-care survey. *The Int J of Aromather*. 2003;13(4):161–168.

221. Kuriyama H, Watanabe, Nakaya T, et al. Immunological and psychological benefits of aromatherapy massage. *eCAM*. 2005;2(2):179–184.

222. Komori T, Fujiwara R, Tanida M. Effects of citrus fragrance on immune function and depressive states. *Neuroimmunomodulation*. 1995;2:174–180.

223. Estrem SA, Renner G. Disorders of smell and taste. *Otolaryngol Clin North Am*. 1987;20:133–147.

224. Pause BM, Miranda A, Göder R, Aldenhoff JB, Ferstl R. Reduced olfactory performance in patients with major depression. *J of Psychiatr Res*. 2001;35:271–277.

225. Kite SM, et al. Development of an aromatherapy service on a cancer centre. *Palliat Med*. 1998;12:171–180.

226. Lehrer S, Levine E, Bloomer W. Abnormally diminished sense of smell in women with estrogen receptor positive breast cancer. *Lancet*. 1985;2:333.

227. Lemon K. An assessment of treating depression and anxiety with aromatherapy. *The Int J of Aromather*. 2004;14:63–69.

228. Wilcock A, Manderson C, Weller R, et al. Does aromatherapy massage benefit patients with cancer attending a specialist palliative care day center? *Palliat Med*. 2004;18:287–290.

229. Itai T, Amayasu H, Kuribayashi M, et al. Psychological effects of aromatherapy on chronic hemodialysis patients. *Psychiatry and Clin Neurosciences*. 2000;54:393–397.

230. Deems RO, Friedman MI, Friedman LS, Maddrey WC. Clinical manifestations of olfactory and gustatory disorders associated with hepatic and renal disease. In: Getchell TV, Doty RL, Bartoshuk LM, Snow JB Jr, eds. *Smell and Taste in Health and Disease*. New York, NY: Raven Press; 1991;805–816.

231. Cunningham S. *Magical Aromatherapy: The Power of Scent*. St Paul, MN: Llewellyn Publications; 1995.

232. Tobin P. Aromatherapy and its application in the management of people with dementia. *Lamp*. 1995;52(5):34.

233. Sitaras N, et al. Olfactory involvement in learning processes. *Rhinology*. 1983;21:273–280.

234. Ehrlichman H, Bastone L. Odor experience as an affective state: effects of odor pleasantness on cognition. *Perfume & Flavorist*. 1991;16:11–12.

235. Ehrlichman H, Bastone L. Olfaction and emotion. In: Serby MJ, Chobor KL, eds. *Science of Olfaction*. New York, NY: Springer-Verlag; 1992;.

236. Baron RA. Environmentally-induced positive affect: its impact on self-efficacy, task performance, negotiation, and conflict. *J Appl Soc Psychol*. 1990;20:368–384.

237. Perala M. Do specific ambient odors enhance long-term memory? [Abstract book]. *The Ohio J of Sci.* 1994;94:2:11.

238. Berg KH. The effect of smell on cognitive processes. *Dragogo Rep.* 1987;39:128–129.

239. Hirsch AR, Johnston LH. Odors and learning. *J Neurol Orthop Med Surg.* 1996; 17(1):119–126.

240. Sugano H. Effects of odors on mental function [abstract]. *JASTS.* 1988;22:8.

241. Arnold MB. *Memory and the Brain.* Hillsdale, NJ: Lawrence Erlbaum Associates; 1984.

242. Nasel C, et al. Functional imaging of effects of fragrances on the human brain after prolonged inhalation. *Chem Senses.* 1994;19(4):359–364.

243. Piaget J. Contributions of the psychosocial sciences to human behavior. In: Kaplan HI, Sadock BJ, eds. *Synopsis of Psychiatry, Behavioral Sciences, Clinical Psychiatry.* 5th ed. Baltimore, MD: Williams & Wilkins; 1988.

244. Long TS, et al. EEG and behavioral responses to low-level galaxolide administration. In: Proceedings from the Associations of Chemoreception Science Annual Meeting (AChemS). 1989; Sarasota, FL; Abstract.

245. Halasz N, Shepherd GM. Neurochemistry of the vertebrate olfactory bulb. *Neurosci.* 1983;10:579–619.

246. Macrides F, Davis BJ. Olfactory bulb. In: Emson PC, ed. *Chemical Neuroanalysis.* New York, NY: Raven Press; 1983.

247. Squire LR. *Memory and the Brain.* New York, NY: Oxford University Press; 1987.

248. Koob GF. Neuropeptides and memory. In: Iversen LL, Iversen SD, Snyder SH, eds. *Handbook of Psychopharmacology.* New York, NY: Plenum Press; 1987.

249. Lauer RE, Giordani B, Boivin MJ, et al. Effects of depression on memory performance and metamemory in children. *J Am Acad Child Adolesc Psychiatry.* 1994;33(5): 679–685.

250. Lishman WA. *Organic Psychiatry: Psychological Consequences of Cerebral Disorder.* Oxford, England: Blackwell Scientific Publications; 1978.

251. Smith ML, Milner B. Role of the right hippocampus in the recall of spatial location, *Neuropsychologia* 19:781–793, 1981.

252. Richardson JTE, Zucco GM. Cognition and olfaction: a review, *Psychol Bull* 105:3: 352–360, 1989.

253. Hirsch AR. Demography of olfaction, *Pro Inst Med Chgo* 45:6, 1992.

254. Perala BT. Do specific ambient odors enhance long-term memory? (Abstract) *Ohio J Sci* 94:2:11, 1994.

255. Parasuraman R, Warm JS, Dember WN. *Effects of Olfactory Stimulation on Skin Conductance and Event-related Brain Potentials During Visual Sustained Attention.* Progress Report No. 6. Submitted to the Fragrance Research Fund, Ltd., 1992. As referenced in: Sullivan TE, et al. Recent advances in the neuropsychology of human olfaction and anosmia. *Brain Inj.* 1995; 9(6):641–646.

256. Nelson WT, et al. *The effects of fragrance administration and attentiveness on vigilance performance.* Paper presented at: the meeting of the Southern Society for Philosophy and Psychology; 1992; Memphis, TN. As referenced in: Sullivan TE, et al. Recent advances in the neuropsychology of human olfaction and anosmia. *Brain Inj.* 1995;9(6):641–646.

257. Sullivan TE, et al. Recent advances in the neuropsychology of human olfaction and anosmia. *Brain Inj.* 1995;9(6):643.

258. Felbaum D, Schmitt J, Koval K, Raudenbush B. Differential effects of chocolate and coffee scents on enhancing cognitive ability and clerical office work performance. *Chem Senses* 2007;32(6):10.

259. Heuberger E, Ilmberger J, Buchbauer G. Fragrance compounds and their influence on human attentional processing. *Chem Senses.* 1999;24:76.

260. Nagai H, Nakagawa M, Nakamura M, Fujii W, Inui T, Asakura Y. Effects of odors on humans (II). Reducing effects of mental stress and fatigue. *Chem Senses.* 1992;16:198.

261. Meynadier JM, Meynadier J, Peyron JL, Peyron L. *Formes cliniques des manifestations cutanées d'allergie aux parfums. Ann Dermatol Venereol.* 1986;113:31–39.

262. Sanderson H, Carter A. Healing hands. *Nurs Times.* 1994;90(11):46–48.

263. Kunieda S, Jingu H, Tokoro. The effect of a scent on the ability to acquire a language. *Chem Senses.* 2005;J25.

264. Sinha D, Efron D. Complementary and alternative medicine use in children with attention deficit hyperactivity disorder. *J Pediatr Child Health.* 2005;41:23–26.

265. Shakespeare W. *Hamlet.* Act 4, scene 6, line.

266. Duke J. Can rosemary save your memory? *Organic Gardening.* 1997;44(8):52

267. Burns A, Byrne J, Ballard C, Holmes C. Sensory stimulation in dementia: an effective option for managing behavioral problems. *BMJ.* 2002;325:1512–1513.

268. Thorgrimsen L, Spector A, Wiles A, Orrell M. Aroma therapy for dementia [review]. *The Cochrane Library, The Cochrane Collaboration.* 2005;3.

269. Snow AL, Hovanec L, Brandt J. A controlled trial of aromatherapy for agitation in nursing home patients with dementia. *The J of Alt and Compl Med.* 2004;10(3): 431–437.

270. Ballard CG, O'Brien JT, Reicheit K, Perry EK. Aromatherapy as a safe and effective treatment for the management of agitation in severe dementia: the results of a double-blind placebo-controlled trial with Melissa. *J of Clin Psychiatry.* 2002;63(7): 553–558.

271. Fox J. Improving tactile discrimination of the blind: a neurophysiological approach. *Am J Occup Ther.* 1965;19:5–7.

272. Blau JN, Solomon F. Smell and other sensory disturbances in migraine. *J Neurol.* 1985;232:275–276.

273. Hirsch AR, Kang C. The effect of inhaling green apple fragrance to reduce the severity of migraine: a pilot study. *Headache Q.* 1998;9:159–163.

274. Shim C, Williams MH Jr. Effect of odors in asthma. *Am J Med.* 1986;80:18–22.

275. Kumar P, Caradonna-Graham VM, Gupta S, Cai X, Rao PN, Thompson J. Inhalation challenge effects of perfume scent strips in patients with asthma. *Ann Allergy Asthma Immunol.* 1995;75(5):429–433.

276. Miller CS. Chemical sensitivity: symptom, syndrome or mechanism for disease? *Toxicology.* 1996;111:69–86.

277. Ross PM, et al. Olfaction and symptoms in the multiple chemical sensitivities syndrome. *Prev Med.* 1999;28:467–480.

278. Olowe SA, Ransome-Kuti O. The risk of jaundice in glucose-6-phosphate dehydrogenase deficient babies exposed to menthol. *Acta Paediatr Scand.* 1980;69:341–345.

279. Buchbauer G, Jirovetz L. Aromatherapy—use of fragrances and essential oils as medicaments. *Flavour and Fragrance J.* 1994;9:217–222.

280. Jäger W, Buchbauer L, Jirovetz L, Fritzer M. Percutaneous absorption of lavender oil from a massage oil. *J Soc Cosmet Chem.* 1992;43:49.

281. Betts T. Sniffing the breeze. *Aromather Quar.* 1994;Spring:19–22.

282. Jori A, Bianchetti A, Prestini PE. Effect of essential oils on drug metabolism. *Biochem Pharmacol.* 1969;18(9):2081–2085.

283. DeGroot AC. Airborne allergic contact dermatitis from tea tree oil. *Contact Dermatitis.* 1996;35:304–305.

284. Bridges B. Fragrances and health. *Environ Health Perspect.* 1999;107(7):A340.

CHAPTER 17

Homeopathy

Ronald Whitmont and Ravinder Mamtani

Homeopathy is a system of medicine that has been in continuous use worldwide for over 200 years. It is based on principles outlined by Samuel Christian Hahnemann, MD, a German physician, in the late 18th century. According to homeopathy (together with much of scientific thinking in the late 18th century) the body has a unifying energy, or "vital force." This vital energy when disordered causes illness and when harmonized, with the gentle assistance of the individualized homeopathic approach, heals the total person. The basic premise of homeopathy is that an illness with symptoms can be treated with a substance that produces similar symptoms in a healthy person. Homeopathic medicines consisting of such substances are given in diluted form to avoid any toxicity associated with these substances. Treatments are patient specific and individualized.

Homeopathy is safe and effective in a wide range of illnesses and conditions. Its acceptance in the United States has been the subject of extensive challenge over the last 200 years due to debate over the healing paradigm.

This chapter describes the history of homeopathy and outlines its fundamental premises. Next, it considers issues of legality and certification. It then examines the scientific evidence concerning effectiveness in the treatment of various health problems and pain management syndromes. Finally, it looks at practical issues including the limits of homeopathic practice.

It is beyond the scope of this chapter to examine all details of the art and science of homeopathy. Discussion of various topics will be brief, giving the reader an overview of the subject matter in the hope of stimulating clinical interest in what is otherwise an unexplored, underutilized, and largely misunderstood field of complementary and alternative medicine (CAM).

HISTORICAL PERSPECTIVES

Global Perspective

A branch of Western medicine, homeopathy has undergone a renaissance in recent years. According to the World Health Organization (WHO), it is the most widely used form of alternative medicine in the world today. The use of homeopathy around the world is widespread and growing. It is practiced in nearly every country in the world. There are active state, national, and international homeopathic medical societies.

Many reports indicate a high level of patient satisfaction and clinical improvement using homeopathy. In one study performed at the Royal London Homeopathic Hospital, over 80% of patients reported an improvement in their well-being and 90% expressed satisfaction with the care they had received from homeopaths.[1]

More than 500 million people worldwide receive homeopathic treatment on an annual basis. Although homeopathy was developed in Germany in the late 18th century, it is most prevalent today on the Indian subcontinent, where an estimated 300,000 homeopathic physicians and more than 300 homeopathic hospitals exist.

Homeopathy is also popular in the United Kingdom and the rest of Europe. In France, an estimated 40% of the population use it on a regular basis. In the Netherlands nearly 50% of physicians consider homeopathy effective. In South America it is highly regarded and utilized by a large percentage of the poplulation.[2] Over 10,000 medical doctors in Latin America are trained in homeopathy and use it in their practices.[3]

In the United States homeopathy is one of the fastest growing forms of CAM. In 1997 alone, there were an estimated 4.8 million visits to homeopathic practitioners in the United States, while sales of homeopathic medicines have increased by 150% over the last decade.[4]

HAHNEMANN'S DISCOVERY OF HOMEOPATHY

Definitions

Homeopathic principles may have been utilized before the 18th century, but it was the German physician Samuel Christian Hahnemann (1755–1843) who was responsible for the first scientific study, systematic investigation, organized development, and documentation of its effects. Hahnemann's work led directly to the definition of homeopathy as an organized medical specialty, its worldwide dissemination, use, and acceptance.

The philosophical and theoretical roots of homeopathy can be traced to the writings of Paracelsus[5] and other alchemical physicians of the Middle Ages. Before that, references to its principles are found in the medical writings of Hippocrates, the ancient Greek Father of Medicine.[6]

Homeo, homion, homoios, and *homoeo* are prefixes derived from the Greek language. They are variations that mean "similar." The suffix *pathos or patheia* means "suffering" in Greek. Thus, homeopathy is the medical specialty that recognizes the relationship between health and illness based upon the healing principle of "similarity with suffering."

Homeopathic physicians select medicines that match individual illnesses and maladies based on the principle of similarity. This means that the medicine whose effects most closely resemble the symptoms of the disease is that which is most capable of alleviating or curing the condition. For example, fevers might be treated with homeopathic preparations of belladonna, a plant containing an atropine like substance capable of producing febrile states. This principle of healing is known as the *law of similars*. It is the fundamental principle underlying the homeopathic method of prescription (see below).

Allopathic medicine, a term also coined by Hahnemann, derives from the Greek words *alloion* and *pathos,* meaning "heterogeneous" (or "unlike") and "suffering." This word describes the orthodox practice of prescribing medicines for illnesses based on the doctrine of contraries. This is the practice of administering pharmaceutical agents whose mode of action is opposite to that of the symptoms of the body. For example, fevers are treated with antipyretics, chemical compounds that act on parts of the brain that lower body temperature.

When homeopathic medicines are administered on the basis of similarity something entirely different from orthodox treatment seems to take place. Instead of the medicine working against the body systems, there appears to be some form of a paradoxical reaction that stimulates the body to heal itself.

Homeopaths match medicines with individuals by comparing the symptom picture of the patient with libraries of data that have been carefully collected and cataloged over the last two centuries. This is information which has been gathered by many clinicians and investigators (homeopathic and allopathic) who have studied the properties of each medicinal substance listed in the pharmacopoeia: the substance's symptom-producing characteristics; how individuals have responded to medical treatment with each of these substances; data pooled from treatment responses in various epidemics; and information gathered from poisonous ingestion and toxic exposures. The data retained on each medicinal substance is only that which has been repeatedly confirmed by clinical experience or scientific report. Sources used include pharmacologic research, toxicologic accounts, and reports made in carefully observed and controlled studies of the medicines with healthy volunteers not suffering from disease.

These latter studies, called *provings,* provide reliable information relating to the disease-promoting and disease-healing effects of each substance. Every medicinal substance in the homeopathic pharmacopoeia has been meticulously studied in this regard to document its ability to both disturb and reestablish health.

The genius in Hahnemann's discovery of homeopathy consists of the finding that each particular medicine has a fundamental relationship with the illness that it treats. This relationship is expressed in the similarity between the symptoms the medicine will cause and those it will cure. The connection does not seem to be related to the physical or chemical characteristics of the medicine itself, or to the pathological changes of the illness. The fundamental bridge appears to reside in its capacity to create a similar state of suffering in the host. This basic principle was first described by Hippocrates more than 2,000 years ago, however, it was not taken up and put into practice until Hahnemann introduced it as the formal practice of homeopathy in 18th century Germany.

Discovery

Hahnemann was a gifted scholar and a master of many languages who translated medical texts to support his growing family. While translating a pharmaceutical treatise by the Scottish physician William Cullen on the properties of Peruvian bark (cinchona, also known in Europe as *Spanish bark* or *Jesuit bark*) in 1789, Hahnemann reached a turning point. He found that he did not agree with the author's statement that Peruvian bark (which was later found to contain quinine) cured intermittent fever because of its "astringent and bitter qualities." Hahnemann believed that successful cure must rest in some other intrinsic relationship between the medicine and the illness.[7] He set out to discover what this was.

To test a hypothesis Hahnemann devised the unique strategy of ingesting small amounts of raw Peruvian bark and observing its effects on his own health. When the bark was taken internally for several days, he began to develop clear symptoms of bark poisoning:

> My feet and finger tips, etc., at first became cold; I became languid and drowsy; then my heart began to palpitate; my pulse became hard

and quick; and intolerable anxiety and trembling (but without rigor); prostration in all the limbs; then pulsation in the head, redness of the cheeks, thirst; briefly, all the symptoms usually associated with intermittent fever, as the stupefaction of the senses, a kind of rigidity of all joints, but above all the numb disagreeable sensation which seems to have its seat in the periosteum over all the bones of the body—all made their appearance. This paroxysm lasted from two to three hours every time, and recurred when I repeated the dose and not otherwise. I discontinued the medicine and I was once again in good health.[8]

Hahnemann observed that the symptoms he experienced from taking the bark were exceedingly similar to the symptoms of the intermittent fever which the bark cured. He recognized this as a demonstration of one of the fundamental laws of healing described by Hippocrates. Because Hahnemann had the mind of a scientist, he knew that a single case was not enough proof. He decided to further test his theory by observing other cases. This would show if his initial finding was a coincidence or if in fact there was some consistent principle at work that governed these phenomena.

After verifying the effects of Peruvian bark on numerous subjects he enlarged the theory by conducting trials on many other drugs and substances. These types of tests were later called *provings*, which was a corruption of the German word *pruefing*, which means "to test." Hahnemann's did not intend to "prove" anything with these tests. His intent was to discover the action and understand the effects of various drugs on healthy subjects so he could later match them with cases of illness whose symptoms resembled these same patterns and thereby effect a cure.

He conducted these drug tests or provings on himself, family members, friends, and colleagues. He was careful to observe and record the findings in meticulous detail. Over his lifetime he studied and cataloged the results of testing nearly 100 medicinal substances in this way. The results of these empirical studies were organized as the *Materia Medica Pura*, published in six volumes beginning in 1830.[9] When he later applied the findings of his provings to the process of treating cases of illness he found that his hypothesis, that like cures like; that the same substance can both cause and cure a disorder, was borne out again and again.

After Hahnemann completed the *provings* of drugs in his early pharmacopoeia, he administered them to the sick. He selected his remedies by comparing the proven symptoms he knew the drugs could produce with the actual symptoms suffered by the patient. He selected those drugs that matched most closely and when he did so he was frequently able to effect a cure.

He had hypothesized that there was a fundamental relationship between medicine and disease observable in the parallel between the effects that a medicinal substance has disordering a healthy body and its ability to stimulate a cure in a diseased body. This principle was repeatedly tested when substances were administered with careful scrutiny and their effects followed with meticulous scientific observation.

He proved that the curative power of a medicine lay in something other than its chemical actions. He found that the essential ability to bring about a cure was linked with a medicines ability to impair health by producing a state of *similar* suffering. Before this time, Hippocrates, Paracelsus, and others had suggested the existence of this unique relationship between medicine and disease, but none had thoroughly worked out the logic or tested the theory scientifically with systematic objective observation and proof in human subjects.

Hahnemann was one of the first physicians to devise and apply the concept of a *drug trial* to study the effects of medicines in healthy individuals. He also used "quantitative and systematic procedures, clinical trials with control groups, and . . . statistics in medicine" for the first time ever in his analytical explorations.[10]

Homeopathy is based on these demonstrated logical principles and on the *clinically observed phenomena* of provings and cure. This means that, at its foundation, homeopathy is rational and empirical, and scientific. It is based upon objective observation and subjective reporting of experience. Explaining the mechanism behind the phenomenon of homeopathy did not concern Hahnemann. He recognized that this task would be left to others. It was enough for him to prove the existence of the relationship and provide a means to apply it to the sick.

United States

Physicians around the world quickly confirmed the soundness of Hahnemann's work. His reputation spread until today the practice of homeopathy extends from Germany throughout Europe, Asia, Australia, and into the Americas.

Homeopathy was first introduced to the United States in 1825, starting in the state of New York. It spread with the movement of German immigrant physicians into Pennsylvania and Virginia, gaining a wide following as they spread out. Homeopathic medical kits even accompanied many early American settlers in their migrations across the continent where there were few regular physicians to be found.

The first homeopathic medical school in the United States was founded in Philadelphia in 1848 (Hahnemann School of Medicine). It grew so rapidly that in 1850 it relocated to a larger facility and the old building was occupied by the first women's' medical school (Women's Medical College of Pennsylvania). The Hahnemann School of Medicine and the Women's Medical College of Pennsylvania merged in the 1990s and shortly thereafter their charter was acquired by Drexel University. After several decades of neglect, homeopathy is once again being taught at Hahnemann Medical College of Pennsylvania in the new Drexel University CAM curriculum. (The original 1848 site is now the location of WHYY public television.)

By the late 19th century there were 110 homeopathic hospitals, 145 homeopathic dispensaries, 62 homeopathic orphanages, over 30 homeopathic nursing homes, and 16 homeopathic insane asylums in the United States[11] In the early days of the 20th century 8% of U.S. physicians used homeopathy. There were 20 homeopathic medical schools and over 140 homeopathic hospitals in the United States, including New York Ophthalmic Hospital and Flower and Fifth Avenue Hospital, which later became New York Medical College.[12] Homeopathy gained further footing through its effectiveness (and the ineffectiveness of regular medical treatments) during epidemic outbreaks, including the yellow fever (1793, 1798) and cholera epidemics in the late 18th to late 19th centuries and the influenza pandemic in the early 20th century (1918–1919; the last yellow fever epidemic in the United States was in 1907 in New Orleans, Charity Hospital). In the United States, homeopathic physicians served on the boards of state and local health agencies in New Jersey, California, Pennsylvania, Indiana, Illinois, Nebraska, Delaware, Florida, Kentucky, and other states.[13]

During the 1930s the only physician serving in the U.S. Senate was S. Royal Copeland, a homeopath. He introduced the U.S. homeopathic pharmacopoeia, which has remained in effect ever since.

Shortly after its introduction into the American medical scene, many able medical practitioners adopted homeopathy. At the same time, there were a great many others who opposed its principles and fought against it. The ensuing battle between homeopathy and allopathy raged for nearly a century. This battle was punctuated by the founding of the American Institute of Homeopathy (AIH) in 1844 and then the American Medical Association (AMA) in 1847. The founding charter of the AMA forbade its members and its member state organizations from including, socializing, or consulting with homeopathic physicians under the threat of expulsion with loss of professional status and licensure.

Each camp was bitterly opposed to the practices and philosophies of the other. Both of these societies remain in existence today, but the overwhelming support of the nation was eventually thrown in behind the AMA. The AIH remains the oldest extant medical society in the United States, predating the AMA by 3 years, but it continues to be dwarfed by the AMA in both budget and membership.

Homeopathy reached its zenith in the United States during the late 19th century and began its decline in the early twentieth century. Some of the reasons why homeopathy faded from the American medical scene in the 20th century included the efforts of the AMA, but other factors including internal conflict within the ranks of homeopathic physicians themselves lead to its demise. Within the field of homeopathy a battle raged between classical Hahnemanian practitioners and those who adopted a more eclectic orientation, which integrated homeopathic treatments with other therapeutic modalities. This internal conflict between homeopaths eventually divided their ranks and weakened their social and political clout, ultimately leading to the dissolution of the profession.

A third factor contributing to the demise of homeopathy in America was the simultaneous rise of the pharmaceutical industry and the emergence of entirely new classes of medications that were increasingly safe and effective.

In 1910, the Flexner report on American medical education, sponsored by the new Rockefeller Foundation, described homeopathy as a medical specialty already in decline. That report further eroded homeopathic medical education and lead to the closing of many homeopathic medical schools and hospitals. This contributed to a trend which allowed homeopathy to nearly disappear from the American medical scene during the 20th century. Homeopathy was barely kept alive in the United States by a small handful of physicians and an emerging group of lay practitioners.

The late 20th century was marked by an expansion of public interest in all forms of alternative medicine. The practice of homeopathy was rediscovered on the American scene and it has since reemerged as a system of medicine that is user-friendly, safe, inexpensive, and effective.

Legal Status of Homeopathy in the United States

Homeopathy has been in continuous use in the United States since 1825 when it was first introduced by Dr. Hans Burch Gram in New York City. These medicines were used safely and effectively throughout the country for more than 100 years before they were incorporated into the U.S. Food, Drug and Cosmetic Act of 1938 (21 U.S.C. Section 301).[13]

Section 201(g)(1) of this Act defines homeopathic medicines or remedies as "drugs." These include articles recognized in the official *United States Pharmacopoeia* (USP), the official *Homeopathic Pharmacopoeia of the United States* (HPUS), or the official *National Formulary* (NF) or any supplement to them.

The Federal Food, Drug, and Cosmetic Act recognizes as official, the drugs and standards in the *Homeopathic Pharmacopoeia of the United States* (HPUS) and its supplements (Sections 201 (g)(1) and 501 (b), respectively). The manufacture of homeopathic medicines accepted by the

HPUS must meet the standards for strength, quality, and purity set forth in the *Homeopathic Pharmacopoeia* according to Section 501(b) of the Act (21 U.S.C. 351). Each new medicine undergoes a thorough clinical proving in a double-blinded setting prior to its acceptance into the HPUS.

Homeopathic drug product labeling must comply with the labeling provisions of Sections 502 and 503 of the Act and Part 201 Title 21 of the Code of Federal Regulations, with certain provisions applicable to extemporaneously compounded over the counter products.

Consumers should look for the USP and HPUS seals when purchasing homeopathic medicines to ensure that they are fully monitored for sanitary manufacturing processes and correct ingredients within these strict guidelines. Manufacturers are required to list all ingredients on their labels.

In the United States, only homeopathic medicines that claim to treat self-limiting conditions may be sold over-the-counter and homeopathic medicines that claim to treat more serious diseases can be sold only by a physicians prescription.[14] Although the production of homeopathic materials is quite inexpensive, the delivery of homeopathic care can be both time and personnel intensive, since individuation of prescription is usually required.

Regulation of the practice of homeopathy is not uniform within the United States but varies somewhat by state. Only four states (Arizona, Connecticut, Nevada, and Washington) currently offer specific medical licensure in homeopathy. Many other states provide legislation that allows physicians to practice it, and some have no measures pertaining to its use. Many states with so-called health freedom legislation allow nonmedically trained lay-persons to practice homeopathy without medical licensure. Questions pertaining to practice guidelines and regulation of homeopathy should be addressed to individual state medical societies and, if applicable, state homeopathic medical societies (see appendices).

The Federation of State Medical Boards has passed model guidelines for practitioners of CAM. These guidelines are not binding, but do reflect a trend toward integration of various CAM disciplines, including homeopathy. These guidelines recognize that "patients have a right to seek any kind of care for their health problems."[15]

Certification of homeopathic training is currently not recognized by the American Board of Medical Specialties of the United States. Certification for physicians is offered by the American Board of Homeotherapeutics, which confers the Diplomate in Homeotherapeutics (DHt) certification in classical homeopathy. Certification is highly recommended but not required by any licensing authorities.[16]

Various state and national professional organizations for physicians who practice homeopathy do exist. These groups are active regionally and nationally promoting legislative action, education, and health care reform.

There is no doubt that the practice of homeopathy requires a thorough knowledge of its principles and methods. Homeopathic practitioners must also be thoroughly grounded in the fundamentals of medicine and have expert clinical training in differential diagnosis and appropriate referral strategies. Experts also recommend that the principles and ethics of informed consent be incorporated, documented, and observed at all times.

Although not expressly required by law, many attorneys specializing in CAM matters recommend that each case receive a thorough discussion (and documentation of this discussion in the medical record) which should include informed consent and assumption of risk.

PRINCIPLES

The basis of homeopathic medicine rests upon its empirically tested clinical effectiveness. The concepts and principles underlying our understanding of homeopathy only evolved after the phenomena were observed.

The key concepts that distinguish homeopathic from allopathic practice include the nature of disease, the nature of medicine, individualization, the psychosomatic totality of symptoms, the law of similars, the single remedy, and the minimum dose.

The Nature of Disease

According to homeopathic principles, all diseases arise as secondary phenomena following a disruption or imbalance of the vital force.

The *vital force* is Hahnemann's designation for the proposed fundamental energy system operating within all living beings. It is a nonphysical, energetic, and spiritually coherent force that underlies all living biological function. The state of the vital force governs health. Disturbances of this energy system are believed to be the fundamental causes of illness. Pathological changes seen in many diseases are believed to be secondary events that take place only *after* the vital force is disturbed.

Hahnemann believed that the vital force acts as a governor, or central directing agency in the balance between health and illness. If this system of energy is disturbed (by either physical, emotional, or energetic events), then the biological machinery can become disturbed, leading to illness or greater susceptibility to illness. Illness is an event that involves the energy of a system before it is apparent as any outward expression or symptoms of sickness.

Since the vital force is not physical, and it can never be directly observed through physical means, its existence can only be inferred through the symptoms and sensations present in an individual. These symptoms are, at best, only an approximation of the vital force, like a shadow cast on the physical plane. Thus, the pattern of symptoms constitutes the closest possible understanding of the fundamental disturbance of the vital force underlying physical illness. These symptoms of illness represent the translation of the vital force into the language of the body. Once the symptoms of the vital force are translated into the language of the body, the homeopath can address the fundamental disturbance of the vital force by utilizing a medicine that acts at the same level.

Hahnemann's study of illness showed him that the dynamics of the body's vital force, that is, the way it energetically changes over time, can be described with the words, *vis medicatrix naturae*. This means that it exhibits a natural tendency for these energies to move toward homeostatic balance and equilibrium; there is an innate drive to restore health. If the physician helps this process along by moving it past the points where it may be "stuck," then the path to restored health will be opened. This process entails using medicines that match symptoms of the illness and stimulates the body at the same level that was initially disturbed, that is, at the level of the vital force.

Homeopathy is not alone in expounding this theory of energy that underlies health. Similar concepts and paradigms can be recognized in many other forms of CAM, non-Western, and prayer-based healing practices. Clinical research into many of these systems suggests that there may be more to health and healthy functioning than just mechanical and biochemical factors.

The Nature of Medicine

The drugs in the *Homeopathic Pharmacopoeia of the United States* are derived from many sources, starting with the three kingdoms of nature: plant, mineral, and animal. In addition, some are derived from diseased tissues, from conventional allopathic medicines and some from so-called imponderable nonphysical sources, such as magnetic fields, electrical currents, electromagnetic radiation, color, and sound.

Homeopathic medicines can be developed from virtually any source. The *Pharmacopoeia Convention of the United States* specifies the manner and method by which these medicines must be prepared and tested prior to use in order to qualify for inclusion.*

Preparation of a homeopathic medicine typically begins by taking one part of a crude substance, then pulverizing, grinding (if it is a solid) or dissolving it (if it is liquid), so it can be diluted in a solvent, whether alcohol, water, or sugar. Immaterial phenomena may be gathered and fixed by other means.

Next, the substance undergoes a process of successive dilutions in the same solvent, until the desired attenuation (*potency*) is obtained. This dilution process frequently reduces the material presence of the substance up to and beyond the point where there may be no mathematical probability of finding even a trace of the original material substance in the homeopathic medicine. In other words, most homeopathic medicines are made so dilute that they contain none or nearly none of the original material substance.** This is called the *infinitesimal dose* or *minimal dose* (see following).

Medicines prepared with only a few dilutions will still have some material amount of the original substance present. These are termed *material doses*. When the dilution process exceeds a certain point, then the potency is considered *nonmaterial* or infinitesimal. Such infinitesimal potencies have been found to have a capacity to cure that is even greater than their material counterparts.

Hahnemann postulated that by preparing a nonmaterial dose a medicine became capable of stimulating the nonmaterial vital force. Material doses, on the other hand, appeared to have less effect, if any, at the level of the vital force. This suggests that homeopathic medicines are energy medicines and their mode of action reside at some energetic level.

Since homeopathic medicines do not appear to act through physical means (because they are so dilute), they are believed to act energetically through means that remain unexplained and unexplored by most physical models. Their mode of action is certainly not a matter of biochemical or biomechanical activity. These substances appear to act at some energetic level through some process, as yet only vaguely understood and largely unexplained by current medical theory.

Hahnemann did not believe that homeopathy could be explained by any mechanistic model known during his lifetime.

> As this natural law of cure manifests itself in every pure experiment and every true observation in the world, the fact is consequently established; it matters little what may be the scientific explanation of how it takes place; and I do not attach much importance to the attempts made to explain it.[17]

Homeopaths have shown that medicines chosen using homeopathic principles and delivered in infinitesimal doses help the body restore healthy functioning. Their theory postulates that the medicines act energetically to assist the vital force of the organism in the process of self-healing, but there is no generally accepted explanation for how this process takes place.

Individualization

Hahnemann considered knowledge of the patient's subjective experience of illness to be a critical element in case analysis leading directly to the determination of the proper medicinal treatment. Using this algorithm, different individuals with the same diagnosis might receive different homeopathic treatments if their subjective experience of illness was different enough. Extending this view further, individuals with different diseases who shared similar subjective experiences of their illnesses might be treated with the same medicine. Successful homeopathic treatment requires the individualization of each case as a unique and particular disturbance of a unique and particular individual. Treatment relies upon matching the unique characteristics of that individual disturbance with the unique characteristics of the correspondingly similar medicine. This process is akin to fitting a key to its corresponding lock and sometimes like searching for a needle in a haystack.

As the example above suggests, homeopaths are only secondarily concerned with differences in disease pathology and the subtleties of different diagnostic categories. Understanding these objective factors may be helpful in tracking the progress of cases, but it does not directly assist in the process of selecting the correct treatment or healing the case. The most important information for the homeopath is the subjective experience of the afflicted individual. The subjective experience provides indirect data on how the vital force has been deranged and how it can be assisted. Understanding of the unique symptoms of the afflicted individual is the primary basis of the homeopathic prescription that allows medicines to be administered in a lock-and-key manner to treat each individual.

Thus, the practice of homeopathy is, by definition, based upon an individualized approach to individuals. The symptoms of illness in each individual constitute the so-called signature of the disease as it is expressed uniquely by that individual's vital force. That signature must be carefully studied so that it can be matched with the unique signature of the corresponding medicine.

The Law of Similars

Hahnemann's initial work uncovered and proved the *Law of Similars*. That law states: *Similia Similibus Curentur.* Translated from Latin this means: "Let likes be cured by likes." This means that an illness may be cured by an agent that is related to the illness by virtue of its ability to produce a *similar* state of suffering when administered to a healthy host.

The *Law of Similars* is the fundamental healing law at the center of homeopathy. It was first mentioned by Hippocrates nearly 2,400 years ago.

This law was suggested by Hahnemann only after its veracity was realized by his painstaking investigation and testing.

The Psychosomatic Totality of Symptoms

Since symptoms are the closest possible description of the disturbance of the vital force, analysis of the entire psychosomatic pattern of symptoms that develop in an individual is necessary to approximate the nature of the disturbance in the vital force.

Hahnemann advised his followers to include all the symptoms of the patient in analysis of the case, a process known as *repertorization*.

> He told the homeopathic physician to take down in writing every single observable symptom of the disease together with anything else the patient could be persuaded to tell. For greater accuracy, this should be written down in the patient's own words whenever possible.[7]

Most substances, not just homeopathically prepared medicines, have demonstrated an ability to produce psychological as well as physical effects in the organism. When substances are proven in healthy individuals, so that they can be used as a homeopathic medicines, a wide spectrum of symptoms are usually elicited. These symptoms range from highly specific to very general; from physical to emotional and cognitive in nature. There is no substance known whose effects are solely limited to one organ system or one local reaction. All medicines of the homeopathic pharmacopoeia have demonstrated physical as well as emotional and mental symptoms in their provings.

Classically trained homeopaths take advantage of these psychosomatic effects when prescribing. The most effective prescriptions are based on physical, emotional, and cognitive symptoms of the individual. As a result, homeopathic treatment is known to be effective in treating a wide range of conditions, encompassing psychological as well as physical disturbances.

The Single Remedy

Homeopathic theory suggests that the vital force is akin to a vibration within the body. It suffuses the entire organism and interconnects the entire system in a unified field effect. The vital force may be acted upon by different factors that disrupt or change its nature, but it only expresses one single frequency pattern at any given point in time. All the combined systems of the healthy body fall under its jurisdiction. All of the symptoms of illness result from a single disturbance of the vital force.

Different illnesses do not reside simultaneously within the same individual at the same time. This theory suggests that if only one disturbance is present, then only one correction, one medicine, is necessary at any corresponding point in time to treat the entire energetic imbalance. For this reason, classically trained homeopaths generally avoid the practice of polypharmacy. They prescribe only one single medicine at a time recognizing that they are treating not just the manifestations of illness but the disturbance of the vital force, which caused the illness.

For this reason Hahnemann strongly cautioned against using more than one medicine at a time. "In no case under treatment is it necessary and therefore not permissible to administer to a patient more than one single, simple medicinal substance at one time."[17] This approach of the "single remedy, single dose" is one of the cornerstones of classical homeopathic prescribing. It persists today among the most authoritative homeopathic practitioners in the world.

The Minimum Dose

The law of the minimum or the infinitesimal dose was not a fundamental principle of early homeopathic practice, as defined by Hahnemann, but it has ascended to this position over time. A rudimentary form of homeopathy could be effectively practiced without this principle, but its inclusion and application enhances not only the safety but also the scope and versatility of homeopathic treatments.

Hahnemann proved that illnesses can be safely and effectively treated by utilizing small amounts of substances prescribed in accordance with the *law of similars*. Through further experimentation he also discovered that the dosage of the medicines could be reduced to surprisingly low levels and still produce the same or even better results. He found that by using infinitesimal doses his treatments were better tolerated, more effective, and accomplished a swifter cure than when the medicines were given in cruder form.

Hahnemann used a method of diluting medicines in serial fashion with repetitive shaking or *sucussing* between dilutions. He discovered that as he did so the toxic effects of these substances were reduced and ultimately eliminated. This was a positive outcome as no practitioner wishes to unwittingly poison a patient.

He further discovered that when dealing with non toxic, so-called inert substances, that diluting and sucussing them resulted in the emergence of unexpected and unforeseen medicinal actions. The study of these properties revealed that even otherwise inert substances had unique and characteristic signatures and symptom pictures, not apparent in crude form:

> The properties of crude medicinal substances gain . . . [by repeated succussion or trituration] . . . such an increase of medicinal power, that when these processes are carried very far, even substances in which for centuries no medicinal power has been observed in their crude state, display under this manipulation a power of acting on the health of man that is quite astonishing.[18]

Hahnemann found that as both the toxic and inert substances were serially diluted and succussed their medicinal actions became more pronounced and more "potent" in a manner inversely related to their material concentration. This surprising finding was laboriously and repeatedly tested until it was no longer surprising but came to be trusted as a reliable fact.

Hahnemann called the process of serial dilution and succussion *potentization* or *dynamization*. The final concentration was termed the *potency* of the medicine. The potency is named based on the number of dilutional steps that had been performed. A 12C potency was one that had been diluted and sucussed 12 times, each dilutional step being at the ratio of 1:99 (centesimal scale). A 30X potency was one that had been diluted and sucussed through 30 different dilutional steps each at a ratio of 1:9 (decimal scale). The result of the dilutional process is known as an *infinitesimal, minimal,* or ultramolecular dose.

A fascinating detail of this process takes place when *potentization* goes beyond a small number of steps (roughly 12C or 30x, depending on scale): the statistical likelihood of encountering even a single molecule of the original chemical substance is reduced to less than zero.

That these ultramolecular preparations should show any effect at all on the biological activity of the organism is somewhat surprising if one's point of view is strictly materialistic. This surprising fact was a controversial topic in its day when homeopathy was introduced and remains so today.

Once Hahnemann carried the dilutional process beyond the point where even a minute trace of the original medicine could be expected to be present in the final medicine, the argument for homeopathy appeared to be absurd to many. Nonetheless, those unbiased physicians who continued to test the practice of homeopathy, learned that the phenomena were indisputably real. They determined that, even though they could find no plausible explanation, the homeopathic medicines reliably worked when used in strict accordance with the law of similars.

The principle of the minimum dose is the most difficult of the homeopathic doctrines to accept on a rational level. Of all the tenets of homeopathy it is the one most frequently ridiculed and parodied. It does not make sense, at the materialistic level of understanding, that smaller quantities of a substance will produce more potent effects than larger quantities. This fact flies against most conventional logic.

PAIN MANAGEMENT

Theory and Application

Homeopathy is rooted in the Hippocratic method of medical therapeutics that emphasizes: (a) rational principles of observation, (b) the study of the patient who is sick is rather than the disease, and (c) assistance to the natural process of healing by strengthening the individual's resistance to illness.

Homeopathy is practiced on a foundation of patient-centered evaluation and observation. It includes careful history-taking, direct and objective observation, and physical examination. Physical pathology and disease classification are of limited use to the homeopath who prescribes on the basis of observable disturbances of an individual's health. Homeopathy does not rely on advanced diagnostic testing, radiographic imaging, or blood chemistry analysis. Although homeopaths may choose to utilize these diagnostic modalities in certain circumstances, the information from these forms of testing is generally not helpful in determining homeopathic treatment. Homeopathic medicines are prescribed on the basis of the directly observed and subjectively reported symptoms of either the individual patient in an individual case or the collectively pooled symptoms of many patients in epidemics and pandemics.

Homeopathic practice is specific to the *individual* rather than the *disease*. Individuals with the same disease diagnosis invariably have differences in their symptoms of illness (the exception may be in epidemics, as noted above). It is these differences, not the similarities, that help the homeopath determine the most appropriate therapeutic intervention.

> Each case of disease that presents itself must be regarded (and treated) as an individual malady that never before occurred in the same manner and under the same circumstances as in the case before us, and will never again happen precisely in the same way.[19(pp441–442)]

Homeopathy is based on the recognition that the entire state of an unwell individual is an expression of illness or disease. Symptoms might arise from physical or psychological areas, but only when considered in totality, do they constitute the particular illness or disturbance of an individual.

While research demonstrating the clinical efficacy of homeopathy may be lacking in many areas, clinical experience demonstrates that there are a wide range of conditions in which homeopathy has demonstrated its utility and effectiveness.

Virtually every organ system has associated pain syndromes that range from acute to chronic. Homeopathy can offer safe nonaddicting pain relief, when symptoms and medicine are correctly matched.

Homeopathic pain management can be a time-intensive procedure on the part of the practitioner because it requires individualization of the prescription based upon the unique features of the individual patient. It does not tend to lend itself to simple so-called cookbook strategies and algorithms. When properly carried out it offers maximal clinical utility and long-term benefit since it often works beyond simple pain management and positively affects the clinical outcome of many disorders which are the source of the pain.

The use of homeopathy in management of pain syndromes also reduces the need for conventional pharmacological analgesia, thereby reducing the risk of drug interactions, side effects, abuse, dependency, and addiction.

The Homeopathic Prescription

The process of selecting a homeopathic medicine begins with the patient interview. Once all the patient's symptoms are determined, the homeopathic practitioner refers to the text of a homeopathic medical repertory. The *repertory* is a catalog of symptoms (organized as *rubrics*) divided, for easy reference, into sections corresponding to each organ system of the body, including the mind. Each *rubric* provides references to the medicines which have been shown to evoke those same symptoms in clinical drug *provings*, toxicity studies, or experience with prior cured cases.

Cross-referencing the medicines corresponding to the symptoms in the complete symptom picture is the process through which the correct medicine can be selected. In the event of confusion or conflict, special emphasis is placed on those key symptoms which are most central in distinguishing an individual case, and the remedies corresponding to them. The initial result of the cross-referencing process, or repertorization of symptoms, is to narrow the field of potential medicines to a short list. Once this is achieved each of these outstanding potential candidate medicines is carefully studied in a homeopathic textbook called the *materia medica*.

The *materia medica* contains a detailed study and compendium of the specifics of each particular medicine and how it affects each organ system in the body. The data is derived from the provings of the substance, records of its toxicity, and the collection of those symptoms found to be relevant in the course of clinical experience with cured cases using this substance as a medicine in homeopathic preparation.

The overall purpose of this study, cross-referencing, and analysis is to find the closest match between the symptoms of the patient and the symptoms elicited from the medicine. The finding of this match is referred to as determining the *simillimum* or "finding the closest matching remedy."

In the system of homeopathy known as classical homeopathy, the desired potency (dilution) of the *simillimum* is administered to the patient, usually as a single oral dose. In other homeopathic system, the *simillimum* might be repeated at more frequent intervals or it might be given in combination with other homeopathic medicines.

Common Remedies for Common Problems

Over the past 200 years homeopathy has been used worldwide in the treatment of nearly every type of medical condition in nearly every branch of human and veterinary medicine. It has been found to be safe and effective in all stages of life from infancy, through childhood, into adolescence, adulthood, and senescence; during pregnancy and lactation; and in the transition to death at the end of life.

Homeopathy is helpful in easing the discomfort due to the changes of pregnancy and childbirth. Complications of these conditions can be handled well with safe, effective but nonpharmacologic, homeopathic means. It is effective in aiding the body recover from a wide range of infectious illnesses and in aiding recovery from injuries. Homeopathy has demonstrated effectiveness in nearly every aspect of human health.

Homeopathy has applications not only as an integrative medical subspecialty but also as a comprehensive medical discipline in its own right. It can even be effectively integrated into surgical settings.

Homeopathy has also shown utility in agricultural applications when used to support the practices of biodynamic farming (a system of organic farming) and in the care of large and small animals in veterinary homeopathy. It is a safe treatment modality for diseased animals that leaves no harmful toxins or residues behind in the food chain or the environment.

Later in this chapter is a list of several homeopathic medicines and some of their common applications in pain management. A full listing with indications would be voluminous and is beyond the scope of this book.

SCIENTIFIC APPRAISAL

Does Homeopathy Work?

This question continues to challenge the scientific community worldwide. In order to better respond to the question and ascertain the usefulness of homeopathy in a conventional health care system, two questions arise: (a) Is homeopathy superior to placebo? (b) What is the evidence that homeopathy helps patients with various medical conditions?

If homeopathy works, what are the mechanisms underlying its beneficial effects? This question presents a significant challenge given the ultra-high dilutional nature of the homeopathic treatments.

Is Homeopathy Superior to Placebo?

A majority of conventional health care providers and various scientific communities attribute most observed health benefits of homeopathy to placebo effects. However, there are many health care practitioners and researchers who refute this argument. They cite many controlled studies and positive clinical outcome data in supporting homeopathy's proven benefit. In these circumstances the question "Is homeopathy a placebo response?" requires a closer examination.

The initial observations made by Dr. David Reilly, a world renowned physician homeopath and researcher, documenting the benefits of homeopathy in the treatment of hay fever received worldwide attention.[20] In three separate randomized controlled trial studies involving the use of homeopathy immunotherapy in the treatment of asthma and hay fever, researchers determined that homeopathy was not a placebo response.[21] Subsequently, a meta-analysis of the three trials published in the *Lancet* "strengthened the evidence that homeopathy does more than placebo (p = 0.0004)." The authors concluded that homeopathy is better than placebo. "Although it's effects are inexplicable, they are reproducible."[21] Reilly's extensive research of two decades, four double blind controlled trials and pooled analysis of the data from the four studies refutes the notion that homeopathy's clinical benefits are due only to its placebo effects.[22]

Several independent reviews or meta-analyses of randomized controlled trials have shown that the positive results of homeopathy are over and above those placebo effects. (See Table 17.1). The quality of homeopathy research, in these reviews, has been found to be rather low by many researchers. However, when only high quality studies have been subjected to analysis, interestingly some show positive results. A review of 17 trials by Cucherat[23] and colleagues demonstrated a low level of positive evidence for homeopathy. But the authors also reported that studies of high quality are likely to be negative. Linde and Melchart in their review of 32 trials, included 19 studies in their meta-analysis. They suggested that individualized homeopathy was more effective than placebo.[24] However, they noted there were methodological problems with several studies. In the systematic review by Linde and colleagues, involving a total of 89 trials, their findings were not consistent with the "null" hypothesis that the clinical effects of homeopathy were completely due to placebo."[25]

TABLE 17.1 Select Systematic Reviews and Meta-Analysis Comparing Homeopathy With Placebo and/or Conventional Treatments

Author (Reference) #	Trials	Results	Conclusions
Cucherat (3)	16 trials representing 17 randomized comparisons.	Pooled p value < 0.0001 in favor of homeopathy; however, for the "best quality" trials; results not significant.	"There is evidence that homeopathic treatments are more effective than placebo, but the strength of this evidence is low because of poor trial quality."
Linde and Melchart (4)	32 RCTs (19 included in meta-analysis)	Results statistically significant in favor of homeopathy; however, results not significant for better-quality trials.	Some evidence; evidence not convincing for "best quality" studies.
Linde et al (5)	89 RCTs	Results statistically significant in favor of homeopathy.	The results "are not compatible with the hypothesis that the clinical effects of homeopathy are completely due to placebo." Further research needed.
Kleijen et al (8)	105 non randomized trials	81 (77%) trials reported positive results for homeopathy.	Results positive, but not definitive.

Adapted from Ernst E. A systematic review of systematic reviews of homeopathy. *Brit J Clin Pharmacol.* 2002;54:577–582; and Jonas BJ, Kapchuk TJ, Linde K. A critical overview of homeopathy. *Ann Intern Med.* 2003;138:393–399. Randomized controlled trial (RCT).

There are some reviews which have failed to demonstrate the superiority of homeopathy to placebo interventions.[26] In a recent comparative study of controlled trials of homeopathy and allopathy, Shang and team concluded that that their finding is compatible with the hypothesis that the clinical effects of homeopathy are due to placebo.[27] It should be mentioned that the authors restricted their main analysis to just eight homeopathy trials and give the impression that their findings are indicative of the entire field of homeopathy, which it is not. Despite these and other findings that support the placebo hypothesis of homeopathy, and the skepticism surrounding its reported beneficial effects, there is some evidence that homeopathy offers more than placebo.[28]

Evidence for Pain, Neurological and Other Conditions

Many randomized trials have documented the usefulness of homeopathy in the treatment of influenza, allergic conditions, childhood diarrhea, post operative ileus, and rheumatoid arthritis (Table 17.2).

TABLE 17.2 Reviews of Select Clinical Trials of Homeopathy for Specific Conditions

Author, Year	Indication	Studies #	Results
Linde and Melchart, 1998	Asthma	3 RCTs	Two trials with positive results; evidence inconclusive.
Earnst, 1999	Headache prophylaxis	4 RCTs	Results are mixed. (Two positive; two negative)
Ludke and Wilkens, 1999	All trauma and post operatively	23 RCTs and 14 non-randomized trials	Evidence suggests that *Arnica homeopathic medication* can be useful.
Vickers and Smith, 2000	Influenza-like syndrome	7 RCTs	*Oscillococcinum* reduces duration of the syndrome
Wiesenauer and Lludke, 1996	Pollinosis	8 RCTs, 1 controlled trial	*Galphia* is more effective than placebo
Barnes, 1997	Post-operative ileus	4 RCTs and 4 uncontrolled trials	Evidence weak
Taylor, 2000	Allergic conditions	4 RCTs	Pooled results in favor of homeopathy
Jacobs, 1993	Childhood diarrhea	3 RCTs	Homeopathy reduces duration of diarrhea.
Jonas et al, 2000	Rheumatoid arthritis	6 RCTs	Four achieved good scores.

Several trials have suggested that homeopathy is ineffective for migraine, and influenza prevention. Randomized controlled trial (RCT)

Adapted from: Jonas BJ, Kapchuk TJ, Linde K. A critical overview of homeopathy. *Ann Internal Med.* 2003;138:393–399.

The number of randomized trials reported in the literature concerning the role of homeopathy in the treatment of pain producing conditions is very small. In a detailed comprehensive review, Kleijen and colleagues examined the role of homeopathy in the treatment of various conditions. Their review included 107 controlled trials involving a wide range of problems including diseases of respiratory, cardiovascular, nervous, and musculoskeletal systems. For rheumatological conditions such as rheumatoid arthritis and myalgia the evidence appears positive. The results for other problems are mixed (Table 17.3). Overall, the evidence of the trials is positive but "not sufficient to draw definitive conclusions."[29] The authors recommend that this is a case "for further evaluation of homeopathy, but only by means of well performed trials."[29]

In a recent review which examined the cumulative research from various randomized trials, Mathie concluded that homeopathy has positive effects in the treatment of conditions such as fibrositis, pain (miscellaneous), sprains, upper respiratory conditions, hay fever, and side effects of radio- or chemotherapy.[30] They also report that homeopathy is unlikely to be effective for conditions such as headache and stroke.

An overview determined that homeopathy may be effective for the treatment of influenza, allergies, postoperative ileus and childhood diarrhea, but added that it may not be effective for muscle soreness and migraine.[24]

The evidence for homeopathy in the treatment of neurological and pain conditions such as rheumatoid arthritis and fibrositis appears encouraging but not conclusive. The effectiveness of homeopathy in the treatment of various neurological and pain syndromes/conditions has not

TABLE 17.3 Clinical Trials of Homeopathy for Rheumatological Trauma or Pain

Author, Year	Indication	Result
Shipley et al, 1983	Osteoarthritis	Negative
Fisher et al, 1987	Fibromyalgia	Positive
Gibson et al, 1980	Rheumatoid arthritis	Positive
Audrarde et al, 1988	Rheumatoid arthitis	Negative
Fisher, 1986	Fibrositis	Positive
Hilderbrand and Eltze, 1983	Myalgia	Positive
Zell et al, 1988	Ankle sprain	Positive
Carlins et al, 1987	Insomnia	Negative

Adapted from: Kleijnen J, Knipschild P, ter Riet G. Clinical trials of homeopathy. *BMJ*. 1991;302:316–23. The list above is not comprehensive. It gives the reader a flavor of evidence for various conditions.

been confirmed. At the same time its benefits cannot be ruled out either. Additional research studies are warranted to better understand its role in neurology and musculoskeletal medicine.

Biological Plausible Mechanisms of Homeopathy

To better understand the mechanisms that underlie the effects of homeopathy from a biomedical standpoint, one must explore several theories. The two main principles behind homeopathy (mentioned above) are the law of similars, or *similia similibus curentur* ("let likes be cured by likes"), and the principle of infinitesimal dose, according to which homeopaths prescribe medicines in extremely high dilutions at which not a single molecule of the original starting substance is present.

That a chemical medicinal substance can have one action (inhibition, toxicity) at a high dose and an opposite action (stimulation, healing) at a low dose has been known to mankind for many years. There are reports, for example, which claim that micro-dilutions of antibiotics and insecticides actually enhance the growth of bacteria and crickets respectively. This mechanism of a seemingly paradoxical and opposite action of pharmacological substances that applies above and/or below their threshold concentrations, or threshold signal strengths, is called *hormesis*.

Conventional treatments of oral immunotherapy and allergen desensitization are considered to be forms of applied hormesis. Therefore, it is possible that homeopathy, by providing an obnoxious stimulus at a low dose, provokes a kind of a defensive response so as to strengthen the host to fight disease and its symptoms. In this respect, homeopathy has frequently been likened to an ultra high dilutional immunization.

The real resistance to the acceptance of homeopathy comes not just from the law of similars, but from its principle of infinitesimal dose. In terms of basic conventional principles of pharmacology, biochemistry, and physics, it is impossible to explain that ultra-molecular dilutions of homeopathic medicines can actually have clinical effects, let alone affects that might be more potent than when given in crude form. In fact, the very suggestion that this is true makes homeopathy appear to be an absurdity and a foolish science.

If it is not the infinitesimal molecules of medicine in the treatments that cause the clinical effects observed in research studies, perhaps it is something else. Several thoughts have been put forward to solve this question. Do homeopathic medicines possess a special form of energy, or biophysical type of information (which cannot be measured with the available tools of medical technology) that can stimulate the body toward healing activities? Does the use of alcohol, water, and other solvents, or the process of rigorous shaking (succussion) required in the preparation of homeopathic medicines generate a biophysically different molecule with encoded biological or energetic information? David Reilly, a world renowned physician researcher wrote that physicists seem more at ease with such ideas than are pharmacologists, considering the possibilities of isotopic stereodiversity, clathrates, or resonance and coherence within water, as possible modes of transmission, while other workers are exploring the idea of electromagnetic changes.

The final answer on how homeopathy works will have to wait until further research is completed and perhaps until the biomedical paradigm is expanded.

Adverse Effects and Safety

Homeopathic medicines are recognized and regulated by the U.S. Food and Drug Administration, are manufactured under strict guidelines, and most can be purchased over the counter from specialty and nutrition stores. Many of the higher potency (greater dilution) preparations and *nosodes* (preparations made from disease and animal sources) are available only by a physician's prescription in the U.S. Homeopathy is considered to be safe, and lacks the potential for life threatening side effects, even though minor side effects have been reported.

Any reported adverse effects are usually mild and transient in nature. Examples of such side effects include headaches, skin rashes, dizziness, diarrhea, and sometimes exacerbation of existing symptoms. The incidence of aggravation of existing symptoms is estimated to occur in 20% cases.[1,31] It should be mentioned that similar side effects are also observed with placebo interventions.[1] Additional studies are warranted to better understand the direct and indirect risks of homeopathy.

Homeopathy Research: Problems and Difficulties

Lack of funding, lack of research and lack of academic infrastructure are common problems facing research in homeopathy. There are methodological problems as well.

Homeopathy, like many other CAM treatments such as ayurveda and acupuncture, are primarily person-specific. Two persons with similar disease patterns could receive two entirely different treatments. Such a treatment approach does not lend itself to a randomized controlled trials (RCT) without significant methodological obstacles. This is because in a RCT all patients in the treatment group must receive the same treatment while those in the control group must receive an indistinguishable placebo. This makes homeopathy incompatible, by definition, with the RCT structure and methodology. This factor has restricted the extent of research in homeopathy and, as a result, most of the information on its efficacy comes from reports of day-to-day practice, and survey reports.

PRACTICAL CONSIDERATIONS

Although there is abundant empirical data from over two centuries of homeopathic practice from around the world supporting the use of homeopathy in the treatment of a wide variety of conditions (See Table 17.4), there is very little data from controlled studies which evaluate its use objectively. The evidence of homeopathy's effectiveness in these conditions is anecdotal, however the case reports are voluminous and compelling.

Empirical data from homeopathic texts demonstrate a wide spectrum of uses of homeopathy (See Table 17.5). What these texts do not offer are scientific explanations of how and why homeopathy works, nor do they offer any insight into statistical analysis of homeopathic treatment when compared with conventional approaches or placebo.

Homeopathy appears to rely on intrinsic, health-restoring functions and self-regulatory responses within the patient. What homeopathy cannot do is to correct a dysfunction that has progressed beyond the healing po-

TABLE 17.4 An Abbreviated Listing of Pain Conditions
Where Homeopathy Has Been Utilized

Cardiovascular: Myocarditis, Pericarditis.

ENT: Otalgia, Sinusitis, Glossodynia.

Gastroenterologic: Anal Fissure, Colic, Gastritis, Hemorrhoids, Pancreatitis, Proctitis.

Neurologic: Migraine Headache, Post Herpetic Neuralgia, Raynaud's Phenomena, Reflex Sympathetic Dystrophy, Trigeminal Neuralgia.

Opthalmologic: Eye pain.

Orthopedic: Back Pain, Bone and Joint Pain, Plantar Fasciitis, Sciatica, Sprains, Strains.

Rheumatologic: Arthritis, Chronic Fatigue Syndrome, Fibromyalgia.

Surgery: Post Operative Pain Syndromes, Traumatic Injuries.

Urology: Cystitis, Dysuria, Epididymitis, Prostatitis, Renal Colic.

Women's Health Issues: Dysmenorrhea, Endometriosis, Menopause, PMS, Vulvodynia, Vulvitis.

From: Eizayaga, FX, Eizayaga's Repertory, From MacRepertory, Kent Homeopathic Associates, San Rafael, CA.

TABLE 17.5 Several Homeopathic Medicines and Some of Their Indications in Certain Pain Syndromes

---

Aconite—Acute, sudden violent pains. Anxiety, fright, and shock, Asthma, bronchitis, dysmenorrhea, headache, muscle pain, myelitis, nephritis, otitis, peritonitis, pleurisy, toothache.

Arnica montana—Acute and chronic affects of trauma, bruising, and injury. Back pain, pleurodynia, gout, headache, rheumatism.

Bryonia alba—Pains worse from motion. Apthous ulcers, asthma, bronchitis, cancer, constipation, dyspepsia, eczema, hernia, migraine headache, nephritis, pericarditis, ovarian cysts, pleurisy, pleurodynia, pyuria, rheumatism, toothache.

Calendula officinalis—Abrasions, corneal abrasions, gunshot wounds, lacerations, mastitis, muscle tears, paronychia, post operative pain, puncture wounds, ruptured tympanic membrane, soft tissue injuries, varicose veins.

Chamomilla matricaria—Intolerable pains, unendurable pains, oversensitive tissue. Asthma, blepharitis, dysmenorrhea, dyspepsia, gout, headache, intestinal colic, labor pains, neuralgia, otalgia, rheumatism, sciatica, seizures, toothache.

Colocynthis—Cutting pains better from hard pressure. Abdominal pain, arthritis, coxalgia, cramps, facial neuralgia, headache, peritonitis, sciatica.

Eupatorium perfoliatum—Violent deep aching pains. Back pain, bone pains, headache, HSV, opthalmia, rheumatism.

Hepar sulpuris calcareum—Splinter-like pains. Angina pectoris, asthma, blepharitis, constipation, corneal pain, diaphrapmitis, eczema, headache, hemorrhoids, hepatitis, labial abscess, otalgia, laryngitis, menorrhagia, pleurisy, rheumatism, SLE.

Hypericum perforatum—Asthma, brachial neuralgia, coccyx injury, crush injuries, headache, herpes zoster, hemorrhoids, lacerated wounds, neuralgia, neuritis, nerve injury, painful scars and keloids, post concussive syndrome, reflex sympathetic dystrophy, rheumatism.

Staphisagria—Back injury and backaches, blepharitis, cystitis, crural neuralgia, dyspareunia, epididymitis, gastralgia, irritable bladder, lacerations, post operative pains, posttraumatic pains, PID, rheumatism, salpingitis, sciatica, testicular pain, throat pain.

---

tential of the body. It will not reverse congenital malformations or birth defects, severe pathological deteriorations, amputations, Type I Diabetes, or deficiency states. The use of homeopathy in serious, life threatening conditions in place of proven conventional treatments is imprudent.

For patients with chronic conditions including chronic pain, arthritis, and myalgias who wish to be treated homeopathically, the adjunctive and supportive use of homeopathic treatments is certainly worth exploring.

Examples of situations in which homeopathy could be explored include those in which (a) conventional treatments for the condition being treated do not exist, (b) conventional treatments have produced maximal benefit, and (c) patients are unwilling to accept side effects of the conventional treatments.

It is imperative that physicians utilizing homeopathy fully explain the benefits, limitations and risks associated with it before making any recommendation concerning its use. Homeopathy must be practiced only within the framework of evidence-based medicine and with informed patient consent.

CONCLUSION

The use of homeopathy is widespread, worldwide, and growing. Its use by those with chronic problems such as chronic pain, arthritis, and neurodegenerative diseases is extensive. Its safety profile is outstanding. The practice of homeopathy lends itself to an integrated medical approach so long as the standards of conventional care and the fundamental principles of homeopathy are observed and respected.

Homeopathic medicines are recognized and regulated by the United States FDA and manufactured under strict guidelines. When practiced according to homeopathic principles, observing the standards of care and rules of informed consent, it is safe, and lacks the potential for life-threatening side effects or addiction. Only mild and transient side affects have been reported. The most dangerous effect of homeopathy might be its use in place of other proven conventional treatments and lifesaving measures.

Research indicates that there is positive evidence for the effectiveness of homeopathy in influenza, allergies (hay fever), postoperative ileus, childhood diarrhea, and rheumatic conditions.[28,31] For many other conditions the evidence is either weak or lacking. No good scientific explanation for the mechanism of action of homeopathy currently exists. However, current evidence seems to suggest that the beneficial effects of homeopathy may not be entirely due to placebo actions.

Based on the available scientific information, the evidence concerning homeopathy can neither be confirmed nor refuted. It should be reiterated that the absence of compelling evidence should not be viewed as lack of effectiveness. The absence of evidence should be balanced against over 200 years of clinical experience, patient satisfaction, and homeopathy's extensive use worldwide. Rather than stressing its implausibility, or the notion that its practice fits the definition of quackery or represents a cult, a productive way forward is to do rigorous research until the truth is found. We should keep an open mind and remember that a treatment might work although we may fail to understand why it does.[10]

Homeopathy appears to provide a unique and a refreshing approach to disease management and its role in pain management merits further investigation.

Sincere thanks to Andrew D. Whitmont, Ph.D., clinical psychologist, in Yakima, Washington, for his keen and insightful editorial assistance.

APPENDIX

Homeopathic Resources

The following is a list of professional homeopathic organizations currently active in the United States.

American Institute of Homeopathy
801 North Fairfax Street
Alexandria, VA 22314–1757
(888) 445–9988
www.homeopathyusa.org

The American Institute of Homeopathy, a 501(C)6 trade association whose membership comprises medical and osteopathic physicians, dentists, advanced practice nurses, and physician assistants, has as its purposes the promotion and improvement of homeopathic medicine and the dissemination of medical knowledge pertaining thereto. It strives to elevate and improve the standards of homeopathic medical education while safeguarding the interests of the profession and attaining general recognition and public acceptance of homeopathy.

National Center for Homeopathy.
801 North Fairfax Street, Suite 306
Alexandria, VA 22314
(703) 548–7790
www.homeopathic.org

The National Center for Homeopathy is an open-membership organization whose mission is to promote health through homeopathy. By providing general education to the public about homeopathy, and specific education to homeopaths, we help to make homeopathy available throughout the United States.

Homeopathic Medical Society of the State of New York.
6250 Route 9
Rhinebeck, NY 12572
(845) 876–6323
www.hmssny.org

The Homeopathic Medical Society of the State of New York was established in 1862 as a professional organization open to MDs and DOs formed for the advancement of homeopathic therapeutics. The society meets twice annually and distributes a newsletter to its members.

American Board of Homeotherapeutics
801 N Fairfax Street, Suite 306
Alexandria, VA 22314
TEL: (703) 548–7790
FAX: (703) 548–7792
Contact Person:
Sandra Chase, MD, DHt, President
10418 Whitehead Street
Fairfax, VA 22030
TEL: (703) 273–5250
www.homeopathyusa.org/ABHt

The ABHt was founded in 1959 and incorporated in 1960 (New York) for the purpose of promoting the science of homeopathy, and demonstrating its effectiveness to the medical profession, and insuring homeopathy's growth as a viable medical specialty in the United States. The ABHt grants Diplomate (advanced specialty) status (DHt) to those medical and osteopathic physician applicants who meet the prerequisites and successfully pass a written and an oral examination.

Council on Homeopathic Education
801 North Fairfax Street, Suite 306
Alexandria, VA 22314
(212) 560–7136
www.chedu.org

The Council on Homeopathic Education (CHE) was founded in 1982 as an independent agency to assess homeopathic training programs in the United States and Canada. The Council is comprised of representatives of the founding nationally recognized homeopathic organizations, accredited school designees, and homeopathic education professionals.

NOTES

* Homeopathic medicines are derived from many sources. Before they are accepted into the Homeopathic Pharmacopoeia of the United States they must be tested (or proven) on healthy individuals, and their characteristic symptoms must be clearly identified. Because almost any substance can be made into a homeopathic medicine, the determining factor that makes a medicine homeopathic is the manner in which is prescribed for use. If this prescription process follows the principles of the *Law of Similars*, then they may be considered homeopathic to the case (regardless of the source of the medicine). If these medicines are selected randomly, by a machine, or on some basis other than the *law of similars*, then they are not, by definition, homeopathic.

** The dilutional process (termed "potentization") involves taking one part of the raw medicinal substance and diluting it in either 9 or 99 parts of diluent to produce a 1X or 1C (from the system of Roman numerals designating the total number of parts X = 10 and C = 100); taking one part of the new concentration (1X or 1C) and adding one part of it to another 9 or 99 more parts of fresh diluent to produce a 2X or 2C dilution. This process is repeated serially as many times as desired to create 3X or 3C; 4X or 4C; 5X or 5C, and so forth, ad infinitum. This process of dilution, or potentization, frequently goes on into the hundreds and even thousands of steps of dilutions!

When this process of dilution is carried out with a specified number of shakes (termed "succussions") at each level then the vial containing the new mixture is called a "potentized" homeopathic medicine. The potency is assigned a number depending upon the number of steps of dilution used, that is, 30 steps make 30x or 30c, and so forth.

REFERENCES

1. *The Evidence Base of Complementary Medicine.* 2nd ed. The Royal London Homeopathic Hospital; 1999.
2. Ridley K. ODE. January/February 22–29, 2006.
3. Reilly DT. The puzzle of homeopathy. *J of Alt and Comp Med.* 2001;7(2):S2103–2109.
4. D'Epiro NW. CAM Spotlight: a focus on complementary and alternative medicine, based on research and expert commentary. Homeopathy: can like cure like? *Patient Care.* 1999;16–27.
5. Coulter. HL *Divided Legacy.* Vol. 1. Berkeley, CA: North Atlantic Books; 1982.
6. Lyons AS, Petrucelli RJ. *Medicine An Illustrated History.* New York, NY: Harry N. Abrams Inc; 1987.
7. Coulter HL. *Divided Legacy.* Vol. 3. Berkeley, CA: North Atlantic Books; 1973:22.
8. Haehl R. *Samuel Hahnemann: His Life and Work.* London: Homeopathic Publishing Co; 1922.
9. Hahnemann HCF. *Materia Medica Pura.* Dresden, Germany: Arnoldischen Buchhandlung; 1830.
10. Ernst E, Kaptchuk TJ. Homeopathy revisited. *Arch Int Med.* 1996;156:2162–2164.
11. Bradford TL. *Homeopathic Bibliography.* 483–536.
12. Rothstein WG. *American Physicians in the 19th Century.* Baltimore MD: The Johns Hopkins University Press; 1992.
13. Chase S, Borneman JA, Borneman JP. Legal status of homeopathy in The United States of America. *Am Inst Hom.* 2003;1.
14. U.S. Food and Drug Administration, Office of Regulatory Affairs. *Compliance Section 400.400 Conditions Under Which Homeopathic Drugs May Be Marketed.* CPG 7132.15.

15. Federation of State Medical Boards. Model guidelines for physicians use of complementary and alternative therapies in medical practice. http://www.fsmb.org. Accessed February 29, 2008.

16. Milan F. An overview of complementary and alternative medicine for the primary care provider. *Primary Care Rep.* 2001;7:17–28.

17. Boericke W. *Organon of Medicine by Samuel Hahnemann.* 6th ed. New Delhi, India: B. Jain Publishers, 1988.

18. Tyler ML. *Homoeopathic Drug Pictures.* 5th ed. Saffron Walden, Essex, England: The C. W. Daniel Company LTD; 1982.

19. Hahnemann, SC. *The Lesser Writings of Samuel Hahnemann.* Dudgeon RE, trans. Radde, NY: 1852

20. Reilly DT, Taylor MA, Beatle N, Campbell JH, McSahrry C, Stevenson RD. Is evidence for homeopathy reproducible? *Lancet.* 1994; 344:1601–1606.

21. Reilly DT, Taylor MA, McSahrry C, Aitchison T. Is homeopathy placebo response? Controlled trial of homeopathic potency, with pollen in hay fever as model. *Lancet.* 1986;ii:881–886.

22. Taylor MA, Reilly D, Llewellyn-Jones RH, McSharry C, Aitchison T. Randomized controlled trial of homeopathy versus placebo in perennial allergic rhinitis with overview of four trials series. *BMJ.* 2000;321:471–476.

23. Cucerat M, Haugh MC, Gooch M, Boissel JP. Evidence of clinical efficacy of homeopathy. A meta-analysis of clinical trials. Homeopathic Medicines Research Advisory Group (HMRAG). *Eur J Clin Pharmacol.* 2000;56:27–33.

24. Linde K, Melchart D. Randomized controlled trials of individualized homeopathy: a state of the art review. *J Alt Comp Med.* 1998;4:371–88.

25. Linde K, Clausius N, Ramirez G, Melchart D, Eitel F, Hedges LV. Are the clinical effects of homeopathy placebo effects? A meta-analysis of placebo controlled trials. *Lancet.* 1997;350:834–43.

26. Ernst E. A systematic review of systematic reviews of homeopathy. *Brit J Clin Pharmacol.* 2002;54:577–582.

27. Shang A, Huwiler K, Nartey L, et al. Are the clinical effects of homeopathy placebo effects? Comparative study of placebo-controlled trials of homeopathy and allopathy. *Lancet.* 2005;366 (9487):726–32.

28. Jonas BJ, Kapchuk TJ, Linde K. A critical overview of homeopathy. *Ann Intern Med.* 2003;138:393–399.

29. Kleijnen J, Knipschild P, ter Riet G. Clinical trials of homeopathy. *BMJ.* 1991;302: 316–23.

30. Mathie RT. The research evidence base for homeopathy: a fresh assessment of the literature. *Homeopathy.* 2003;92,84–91.

31. Ernst E, ed. *The Desktop Guide to Complementary and Alternative Medicine: An Evidence Based Approach.* St. Louis, MO: Mosby Elsevier; 2006.

CHAPTER 18

Prolotherapy

Donna Alderman

Prolotherapy is a method of injection treatment designed to stimulate healing.[1] This evidence-based treatment is used for musculoskeletal pain that has gone on longer than 8 weeks such as low back pain, sciatica, disc disease, neck pain, some types of headaches, chronic sprains and/or strains, whiplash injuries, tennis and golfer's elbow, knee, ankle, shoulder or other joint pain, chronic tendonitis/tendonosis, and musculoskeletal pain related to osteoarthritis. Prolotherapy works by raising growth factor levels or effectiveness to promote tissue repair or growth.[2] It can be used years after the initial pain or problem began, as long as the patient is healthy. Prolotherapy works to repair weak and painful joint areas and is a long-term solution rather than a palliative measure such as drug therapy.

Prolotherapy has been practiced in the United States since the 1930s, is endorsed by former U.S. Surgeon (1981–1989) General C. Everett Koop,[3] and has made its way into major medical centers. In the April 2005 issue of the *Mayo Clinic Health Letter*, the authors wrote that in the case of chronic ligament or tendon pain that has not responded to prescribed exercise and physical therapy, prolotherapy may be helpful.[4] Lloyd Saberski, MD, former Medical Director of Yale University School of Medicine Center for Pain Management, wrote that prolotherapy is the only methodology with limited risk yet potential for significant benefit."[5] Prolotherapy has also made its way into the professional sports world.[5] One sports medicine journal reports:

> Prolotherapy, considered an alternative therapy, is quietly establishing itself in mainstream medicine because of its almost irresistible draw for both physicians and patients: nonsurgical treatment for musculoskeletal conditions.[6]

The subject of prolotherapy has also been discussed in *The New York Times,* Personal Health column, where this author states: "Since prolotherapy is a nonsurgical technique, patients who are now facing surgery because all else has failed might consider it before having an operation."[7] Yet many individuals, even physicians, may still know little about this treatment. The purpose of this chapter is to provide an introduction to prolotherapy, how and why it works, and indications for its use.

BACKGROUND AND HISTORY

Prolotherapy is based on the premise that chronic musculoskeletal pain is due to inadequate repair of fibrous connective tissue, resulting in ligament and tendon weakness or relaxation (laxity),[1] also known as connective tissue insufficiency.[8] Ligament and tendon tissues have a poor blood supply, and therefore take longer to heal than other tissues. In fact, incomplete healing is common after an injury to those structures.[9(p42),10] It has been estimated that the usual best result of a completed connective tissue repair process is a return to normal connective tissue length, but only 50% to 60% of preinjury tensile strength.[11] Over time, and multiple injuries, this can result in laxity and connective tissue insufficiency.[2] When the connective tissue is weak, there is insufficient tensile strength or tightness.[12] Load bearing then stimulates pain mechanoreceptors.[6] As long as connective tissue remains functionally insufficient, these pain mechanoreceptors continue to fire with use.[13] If laxity or tensile strength deficit is not corrected sufficiently to stop pain mechanoreceptor stimulation, chronic sprain or strain results.[2]

   This is the problem that prolotherapy addresses, by stimulating growth factors to resume or initiate a connective tissue repair sequence that is incomplete or never started, repairing and strengthening lax ligaments and/or tendons, reducing or eliminating pain.

   Historically, the use of concept of prolotherapy dates back to Hippocrates, who treated dislocated shoulders of soldiers on the battlefields with red-hot needle cautery to stabilize the joint. From 1835 to 1935, injection of sclerosing type agents was used for hernias to proliferate new fibrous tissue. It was during the 1930s that George Hackett, a general surgeon, made an observation, while doing hernia surgery on patients previously treated with proliferant type therapy, that injections made (usually in error) at the junction of ligament and bone resulted in profuse proliferation of new tissue at this union.[14] Hackett then spent many years developing and refining injection therapy for tendons and ligaments, publishing his research and text in 1956. He defined prolotherapy as the rehabilitation of an incompetent structure [ligament or tendon] by the generation of new cellular tissue and concluded that a joint is only as strong as its weakest ligament.[1] Prolotherapy is sometimes called "Regenerative Injection Therapy" (RIT), "Reconstructive Therapy," "Non-Surgical Tendon, Ligament and Joint Reconstruction, or Growth Factor Stimulation Injection."[15]

Sclerotherapy is an older, inaccurate term for prolotherapy, based on the original theory that scar formation was the treatment mechanism. However biopsy studies have not demonstrated scar formation with mechanical, inflammatory, or growth factor prolotherapy with the agents and concentrations currently in use.[2] Rather, studies have shown a proliferation of new, normal, thicker, and stronger connective tissue after prolotherapy injections.[16]

SOFT TISSUE HEALING

In addition to the inherent paucity of blood supply in ligament and tendon areas, interfering factors may decrease the body's healing response to injury. It is well known that smoking slows repair of collagen in connective tissue.[17] Sleep issues are also important in healing as growth hormone, important for rebuilding of tissue, peaks during a normal sleep cycle. Poor nutrition can also be an issue with tissue repair. It is well known that vitamin C is necessary for the body to produce healthy collagen, a major component of connective tissues such as joint ligaments and tendons. Vitamin C is so important that prolonged deficiency causes scurvy, a disease where collagen production is defective and connective tissue breaks down.[18] However, other micronutrients also play a role in tissue repair, and deficiencies may be involved in poor tissue repair. In repetitive trauma, another problem exists in that each individual trauma may be insufficient to provide enough stimulus to prompt complete healing, so that even minor injury may be enough to accumulate damage to the point of initiating chronic pain.[2] Another reason that has been suggested for incomplete healing is the use of anti-inflammatory medications immediately after an injury.[19] Inflammation is a necessary component of soft tissue healing and the use of anti-inflammatory medication for sports injuries has been questioned and remains controversial. In the January 2003 issue of *The Physician and Sportsmedicine*, a review article examined the physiology and healing of soft tissue injuries and concluded that the use of NSAIDs may interfere with healing and is questionable in treatment of musculoskeletal injuries.[20]

MECHANISM OF ACTION AND RESEARCH STUDIES

Prolotherapy works by causing a temporary, low-grade inflammation at the site of ligament or tendon weakness (fibro-osseous junction), "tricking" the body into initialing a new healing cascade. Inflammation activates fibroblasts to the area, which synthesize precursors to mature collagen, reinforcing connective tissue.[2] It has been well-documented that direct exposure of fibroblasts to growth factors causes new cell growth and collagen deposition.[21-25] Inflammation creates secondary growth factor elevation.[2] This inflammatory stimulus raises the level of growth factors to resume or initiate a new connective tissue repair sequence to complete one which had prematurely aborted or never started.[2] Animal biopsy studies show ligament thickening, enlargement of the tendinosseous junction, and strengthening of the tendon or ligament after prolotherapy injections.[26,27]

Over the years since the 1930s, studies and reports have demonstrated the effectiveness of injection prolotherapy for musculoskeletal complaints, including case reports, pilot, retrospective, open face prospective, and double-blind placebo controlled studies.[28-51]

These studies have clearly indicated the effectiveness of prolotherapy in the treatment of chronic musculoskeletal pain arising from posttraumatic and degenerative changes in connective tissue such as ligaments, tendons, fascia, and intervertebral discs.[51]

Several studies are noteworthy. In a study of chronic low back patients treated with prolotherapy, biopsies of sacroiliac ligaments 3 months after treatment demonstrated a 60% increase in collagen fibril diameter, as well as decrease in pain and increased range of motion in subjects tested.[50] A double-blind animal study done at the University of Iowa showed significant increase in rabbit bone-ligament-bone junction strength and increase of collagen fibrils after proliferant injections.[17]

A 2005 study of elite rugby and soccer athletes with chronic groin pain preventing full sports participation showed the marked efficacy of prolotherapy. After an average of 2.8 treatments, 20 of 24 athletes reported no pain, and 22 were unrestricted with sports.[52]

Knee injuries have been studied and shown to be successfully treated with prolotherapy. A study involving patients with signficiant knee ligament laxity and instability showed highly significant tightening of the cruciate and collateral ligaments measured by standard electrogoniometer measurements, as well as subjective improvement in pain and increased activity level 9 months after treatment start.[53] A double-blind study by Reeves showed that injection prolotherapy resulted in elimination of ACL laxity by machine measurement in over 60% of patients with statistically significant improvement at 3-year follow-up, with a larger percentage experiencing reduction in pain, including improvement in symptoms of osteoarthritis even in those who tested loose.[54]

The largest follow-up studies to date on the pain reducing effects of prolotherapy treatment involved 1,800 patients followed-up for more than 2 years and showed marked reduction in upper or lower body pain in 80% of subjects.[55] A review of the medical literature by the Florida Academy of Pain Medicine in 2001 analyzed the medical literature from 1937 to 2000, including case studies, retrospective, prospective, and animal studies. The calculated number of patients reported in those studied exceeded 530,000. Improvement in terms of return to work and previous functional/occupational activities was reported in 48 to 82% of patients, with reduction of pain up to 100%. The academy concluded that this injection treatment was effective as a type-specific treatment for posttraumatic degenerative, overuse, and painful conditions of the musculoskeletal system related to pathology of the connective tissue.[39]

APPROPRIATE CANDIDATES FOR PROLOTHERAPY

In the Hackett, Hemwall, and Montgomery book on prolotherapy, which was one of the first texts on the subject, the authors write:

Criteria for Injection Therapy in New Patients:

1. Appropriate medical problem.
2. Desire for recovery.
3. No underlying medical conditions which would significantly interfere with healing.
4. Ability and willingness to follow instructions.
5. Willingness to report progress.
6. Willingness to receive painful injections in an effort to recover from injury.[1]

These criteria are still true today. The problem must be an appropriate musculoskeletal problem. The patient needs to have the desire to get better, no known illness which could prevent healing, and willingness to follow instructions and to undergo injections. Illnesses that would prevent healing include autoimmune or immunodeficiency disorders, or active cancers, for example. Also, the patient should not be taking drugs that lower the immune system such as systemic corticosteroids or immune suppressants. And because prolotherapy works to stimulate inflammation, patients should not be taking anti-inflammatory medication during treatment. In fact, as mentioned above, although frequently prescribed for musculoskeletal pain, use of NSAIDs may interfere with healing and is questionable in treatment of musculoskeletal injuries.[56]

Age is not a factor, as long as the individual is healthy. It also does not matter how long the person has been in pain, or how long ago they injured themselves, again, as long as the person is in good, general health.

MRI STUDIES CAN BE MISLEADING IN DIAGNOSING MUSCULOSKELETAL PAIN

The Ombregt and ter Veer *Textbook of Orthopedic Medicine* states that the results of radiographic examinations should never be given as a diagnosis."[57(p739)] As many health care practitioners know, an MRI may show nothing wrong and yet the patient is still in pain. And, because MRIs may also show abnormalities not related to a patient's current pain complaint, these MRI findings should always be correlated to the individual patient. Many studies have documented the fact that abnormal MRI findings exist in large groups of pain-free individuals.[57(p59),58–63] A study published in the *New England Journal of Medicine* showed that out of 98 pain-free people, 64% had abnormal back scans.[64] Many other studies have also shown abnormal neck MRI scans in asymptomatic subjects,[65–67] and the finding of asymptomatic changes in knee joints during surgery is not uncommon.[68,69] One study looked at the value of MRIs in the treatment of knee injuries and concluded that, overall, magnetic resonance imaging diagnoses add little guidance to patient management and at times provide spurious [false] information. However, many surgeons base their decisions to operate primarily on the outcome of these investigations.[57(p700)] It is inevitable, then, that some of the surgeries done are unnecessary and will not resolve the pain for which they are intended. So an MRI alone should not be used to determine a treatment course. The MRI should be used in combination with a history of the complaint, precipitating factors or trauma, and a physical exam.

PAIN REFERRAL PATTERNS

The concept of pain referral is not new in medicine. A tooth infection may cause ear pain; a heart attack may produce arm or jaw pain. Referral patterns also exist for injured joints, ligaments, and tendons. An important concept in musculoskeletal medicine is that of ligament referral patterns. Injury in one part of the body can affect distant body parts.[9(p46)] Ligament injury may cause severe pain because ligaments are full of nerve endings[70] and may refer nerve-like pain, making diagnosis difficult. Pain from sciatica, for instance, may actually be coming from injured sacroiliac or sacrospinous ligaments rather than the sciatic nerve (Figure 18.1), or musculoskeletal

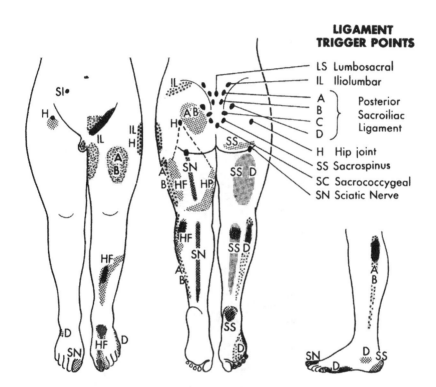

LIGAMENT TRIGGER POINTS

LS Lumbosacral
IL Iliolumbar
A ⎫
B ⎬ Posterior Sacroiliac Ligament
C ⎪
D ⎭
H   Hip joint
SS Sacrospinus
SC Sacrococcygeal
SN Sciatic Nerve

PAIN REFERRAL PATTERNS
FROM LUMBOSACRAL AND PELVIC JOINT LIGAMENTS

ABBREVIATION	LIGAMENT	REFERRAL PATTERN
IL:	ILIOLUMBAR	GROIN, TESTICLES, VAGINA, INNER THIGH
AB:	POSTERIOR SACROILIAC (UPPER TWO-THIRDS)	BUTTOCK, THIGH, LEG (OUTER SURFACE)
D:	POSTERIOR SACROILIAC (LOWER OUTER FIBERS)	THIGH, LEG (OUTER CALF) FOOT (LATERAL TOES)— ACCOMPANIED BY SCIATICA
HP:	HIP—PELVIC ATTACHMENT	THIGH—POSTERIOR & MEDIAL
HF:	HIP—FEMORAL ATTACHMENT	THIGH—POSTERIOR & LATERAL LOWER LEG—ANTERIOR & INTO THE BIG TOE & SECOND TOE
SS:	SACROSPINUS & SACROTUBERUS	THIGH—POSTERIOR LOWER LEG—POSTERIOR TO THE HEEL
SN:	SCIATIC NERVE	CAN RADIATE PAIN DOWN THE LEG

FIGURE 18.1   Ligament referral pain patterns.

headaches, which may be referring from weak cervical ligaments or occipital attachments (Figure 18.2). If the ligaments from which the pain is being referred are treated with prolotherapy, the ligaments heal, pain receptors stop firing, and this type of pain resolves. Therefore, knowledge of areas in which individual ligaments may produce referred pain is extremely valuable in diagnosis and treatment with prolotherapy.[9(p38)]

TENDONITIS/TENDONOSIS

Tendonitis is defined as "an inflammatory condition of a tendon, usually resulting from strain."[71] If the condition has gone on longer than 6 weeks, it is sometimes called chronic tendonitis. However, biopsies of so-called

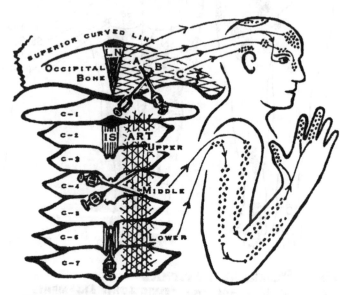

HEAD AND NECK REFERRAL PAIN PATTERNS
LIGAMENT AND TENDON RELAXATION

AREA OF WEAKNESS	REFERRAL PATTERN
OCCIPUT AREA A	FOREHEAD AND EYE
OCCIPUT AREA B	TEMPLE, EYEBROW AND NOSE
OCCIPUT AREA C	ABOVE THE EAR
CERVICAL VERTEBRAE 1-3 (UPPER)	BACK OF NECK AND POSTERIOR SCAPULAR REGION (NOT SHOWN)
CERVICAL VERTEBRAE 4-5 (MIDDLE)	LATERAL ARM AND FOREARM INTO THE THUMB, INDEX AND MIDDLE FINGER
CERVICAL VERTEBRAE 6-7 (LOWER)	MEDIAL ARM AND FOREARM INTO THE LATERAL HAND, RING AND LITTLE FINGER

FIGURE 18.2   Head and neck ligament referral pain patterns.

chronic tendonitis tissue has shown lack of inflammatory cells and repair but rather collagen degeneration occuring.[72-74] For this reason, in recent years the word *tendonosis* (*osis* meaning "diseased or abnormal condition") is being used in the medical literature to describe what has previously been known as chronic tendonitis, which some authors believe may be a more accurate diagnosis. In this type of tendonopathy, inflammation is no longer occurring and collagen breakdown is the primary problem. Traditional treatments include NSAIDs and corticosteroids; however, studies provide little evidence that these treatments are helpful.[75] Therefore, treatment should target the stimulation of collagen production rather than the elimination of inflammation, which may not even be present.[76] Prolotherapy is a more reasonable treatment option in that the focus is to stimulate the proliferation of fibroblasts which then stimulate collagen repair and proliferation. The tendonosis is turned into a tendonitis (on purpose) in order to stimulate the repair process to start again.[77(p92)]

LOW BACK PAIN

Low back is a common medical complaint. In the United States alone, more than 5 million people are disabled by low back pain, half of these permanently.[78] Low back pain affects most people at some point during their lifetimes. It is the second most frequently reported illness in industrialized countries, next to the common cold.[78] In fact, it has been reported that 80% of the general U.S. population will at some time suffer from low back pain, and 20% are suffering at any given time.[79,80] It is the subject of numerous books, articles, and media reports. A variety of sports activities, such as gymnastics, football, weight lifting, rowing, golf, dance, tennis, baseball, basketball, and cycling, have been linked to low back pain.[81] Nonathletes and athletes alike, however, can suffer from this condition.

CAUSES OF MUSCULOSKELETAL LOW BACK PAIN

Ninety percent of low back pain is mechanical. This type of low back pain is the result of overuse or straining, spraining, lifting, or bending that results in ligament sprains, muscle pulls, or disc herniations.[82] Mechanical low back pain is the most common cause of work-related disability in persons under 45 years old.[83] While disc problems have gotten much of the credit for low back pain, ligament injury is a more important source of back pain.[57(p775)] In fact, it has been reported that *only 4% of low back pain is due to a herniated disc.*[83]

To understand why the disc has been given so much credit for low back pain, one has to understand some medical history. In 1934 researchers named Mixter and Barr became popular.[84] They focused attention on the disc, giving root to a popular theory; from that time forward, so-called disc disease has overshadowed ligaments' importance. Then, with the introduction of cat scanners (CT) in the 1970s, and the popularity of MRIs in the 1980s and 1990s, further attention was focused on the disc as the cause of low back pain—because discs are easily seen in these types of studies. On the other hand, ligament injury which involves very small micro-tears usually does not show up well on these investigations so have been largely overlooked.

Low back prolotherapy studies have shown improvement in treated groups[38,85–87] including a randomized double-blind trial which showed statistically significant improvement in the treated group after 6 months.[88] A 2004 study showed improvement in two groups of chronic low back patients, treated with dextrose or saline injections (both can be used as proliferants). Both groups showed a statistically significant decrease in pain and disability scores at both 12 and 24 months follow-up.[89] Hackett himself reported on 543 chronic low back patients with ages ranging from 15 to 88, with duration of disability before treatment from 4 to 56 years. Hackett reported that 82% of these patients considered themselves cured over periods ranging up to 12 years of follow-up.[28] A recent study by Ross Hauser also shows statistically significant improvement in low back pain patients treated with prolotherapy.[90]

WEAK SPINAL LIGAMENTS PRECEDE DISC HERNIATION

Weakening of the spinal ligaments precedes disc herniations.[91] For a disc to herniate, there must first be a primary ligament weakness and a deteriorating disc.[1(p9)] Disc degeneration has become so common that it is considered part of the normal aging process.[57(p729)] In the natural course of aging a disc loses pliability and is less able to withstand normal pressures. Thus, it is more prone to having its outside edges become cracked or torn.[92] If the pressure goes high enough, the fluid in the disc's center can leak through these cracks or fissures. This also leads to decreased disc height. In addition, the ligament that holds the disc in place becomes weakened. As a result, the joint becomes even more unstable and more likely to herniate (Figure 18.3). Ligaments hold the disc in place, so if the ligament weakens, the disc can more easily herniate through it. In fact, increased pressure in the disc together with increased ligament laxity is the perfect recipe for disc herniation.[57(p745),93]

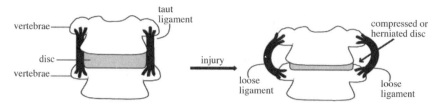

FIGURE 18.3   What happens to the ligament when the disc flattens.

SPINAL DISC DISEASE

Although initial onset of disc herniations is usually extremely painful and acute, in a few days to a few weeks the protruding disc segment slowly shrivels away.[57(pp747,765)] In fact, with or without treatment, most disc herniations reabsorb and resolve within 2 to 6 weeks, with up to 90% back-to-normal activity within 1 month regardless of treatment.[94,95] However, it has been estimated that 10% of people who suffer a disc herniation continue to have pain and go on to experience chronic back pain that includes muscle pain, spasm, and stiffness (a sign of a ligament laxity and a weak joint), sometimes with pain going down the legs. These symptoms may persist long after the disc herniation itself has shriveled away because of weakened back ligaments and connective tissue support which has not healed. Even after someone has "recovered" from a back injury or disc herniation to the point that he or she is out of severe pain, where ligaments are weak there still exists a predisposition to further injury. In addition to that, the change in biomechanics when a ligament weakens can contribute towards osteoarthritis in that joint as well as stress on other joints. Prolotherapy can help stabilize and strengthen the ligaments around these weakened joints and reduce or eliminate pain.

SCIATICA

Sciatica is defined as "pain emerging from the lower back that is felt along the distribution of the sciatic nerve in the lower extremity."[96(p1851)] A diagnosis of sciatica describes a symptom and is not specific in terms of cause. Frequently, the cause of sciatica is attributed to a finding on an MRI such as a disc herniation. However, for the majority of people who experience this type of pain, even in cases when numbness is present, the cause of the problem is not a disc but rather sacroiliac ligament weakness.[9] In fact, it has been stated that ligament laxity in the sacroiliac joint is the number one reason for sciatica and is one of the most common reasons for chronic low back pain.[97]

As discussed above, ligament referral patterns overlap nerve pathways. Note that the referral pattern for the sacroiliac ligaments are similar to those of the sciatic nerve (see Figure 18.1).

Piriformis syndrome is another often overlooked reason for sciatica, leg, or buttock pain.[98] The piriformis muscle tendon attaches directly over the exiting sciatic nerve. Injury, straining, or micro-tears to the piriformis tendon or other surrounding ligamentous structures result in inflammation and swelling, which puts pressure on the sciatic nerve, causing pain and referral.

A study by Merriman compared prolotherapy to fusion for sciatic pain, evaluating patients treated during his 40 years as a general and industrial surgeon. His conclusion was that conservative physiologic treatment by prolotherapy after a confirmed diagnosis of ligamental and tendinous laxity was successful in 80% to 90% of more than 15,000 patients treated with prolotherapy, with fewer side effects than with fusion.[99]

LIGAMENT INJURIES LEAD TO DEGENERATIVE ARTHRITIS

Osteoarthritis almost always begins as ligament weakness.[77] Unresolved ligament sprains (overstretching) results in ligament relaxation and weakness. Relaxation of the ligament results in joint instability and a change in joint biomechanics, which eventually results in osteoarthritis of that joint as bones glide over each other unevenly. The observation that bones remodel and grow in response to their mechanical environment is best explained in Wolff's Law which states: "Bones respond to stress by making new bone."[100(p8)] Tendon injuries, if unresolved, over a long period of time also have an influence on joint biomechanics and can contribute to the development of osteoarthritis. In fact, *Postgraduate Medicine* reports in its investigation of the causes of arthritis: "There is no question that trauma and mechanical stress on the joint lead to the development of osteoarthritis."[101]

In veterinary medicine, it is well-established that ligament sprains also favor the development of osteoarthritis in animals.[102] This has also been demonstrated in the human medical literature. One study of female soccer players who had sustained knee ligament injury showed a very high percentage with knee osteoarthritis 12 years later.[103] Another study, published in *Sports Medicine*, observed the increased incidence of arthritis with individuals who engaged in certain sports, for instance wrestlers, boxers, baseball pitchers, football players, ballet dancers, soccer players, weight lifters, cricket players, and gymnasts.[104]

OSTEOARTHRITIS

In a recent double-blind placebo controlled study, there was clinically and statistically significant improvement in knee osteoarthritis symptoms at 1- and 3-year follow-up after prolotherapy injections, with radiographic readings also noting improvement in several measures of osteoarthritis severity. When present, ACL laxity also improved.[105] Another study showed improvement in finger and thumb osteoarthritis after prolotherapy injections, with 42% improvement in pain and 8 degree improvement in flexibility after 6 months.[106]

If ligament and tendon injuries are stimulated to heal, this downward progression of degenerative changes can be prevented or stopped. Prolotherapy can, therefore, be seen as a method to prevent or stop the arthritic process because it strengthens the joint, thus ending the need for the knee or other treated joint, to grow bone or form bone spurs (Figure 18.4).[77]

KNEE PAIN WHEN MRI SHOWS MENISCAL INJURY

Meniscal tears are a common diagnosis with knee pain, in part because MRIs clearly show these tears. However, as noted above, MRIs can be misleading, and this is especially true with the meniscus. A knee MRI study addressed this issue. The authors looked for meniscal abnormalities in asymptomatic, pain-free individuals aged 20s to 80s and found Grade 1, 2, and 3 changes present in essentially all decades, with an increase in prevalence with increasing age. 62% of individuals as young as their 20s had abnormal medial meniscal scans while 90% of these scans were abnormal for pain-free individuals in their 70s.[107]

Another interesting note is that the medial meniscus firmly adheres to the deep surface of the medial collateral ligament (MCL), an important stabilizing ligament.[108] Therefore injury to the medial meniscus will very often also result in injury and sprain to the MCL. The cause of the knee pain may be the MCL sprain; however, MCL sprains are usually not addressed, especially if the MRI shows a meniscal tear. This could explain pain persisting after meniscal surgery. Clearly, the presence of meniscal tears on MRI needs to be correlated to an individual's pain complaint. Pain may not be related to the abnormal findings on an MRI but rather ligament or tendon injury or sprain/strain. In fact, individuals with abnormal MRIs showing meniscal tears have successfully been treated with prolotherapy. It is unclear whether prolotherapy has any direct effect on meniscal tissue, and this has not been specifically studied. However, even when patients have these meniscal abnormalties on MRI, they often improve after prolotherapy treatment.

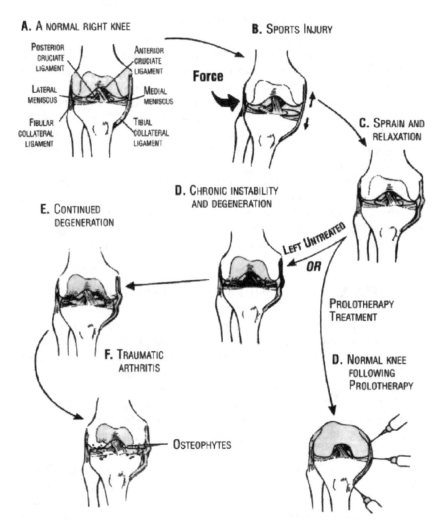

FIGURE 18.4   How soft tissue injury leads to degenerative arthritis. Ligaments become sprained following trauma. When healing does not occur, the ligaments become relaxed, resulting in chronic instability and degeneration from meniscal and articular cartilage degeneration. When left untreated, posttraumatic "arthritis" or degenerative osteoarthritis follows. This degenerative process can be prevented with appropriate intervention through prolotherapy.

CARTILAGE REGENERATION

An important issue in joint diseases is the difficulty in regenerating damaged articular cartilage, and therefore cartilage regeneration is one of the most preferred subjects for medical research investigation.[109] It has been suggested that prolotherapy may help in cartilage regeneration, however no specific controlled studies have yet been done to confirm this. Laboratory studies demonstrate cartilage cells respond to injury (inflammation) by changing into chondroblasts, cells capable of cell proliferation, growth, and healing.[110] And although not studied in humans, cartilage effects of growth factor stimulation in animals has shown healing of full thickness cartilage defects and improvement of osteoarthritis lesions in injection studies.[111-113] Therefore, it has been suggested that prolotherapy might help in cartilage regeneration because of its ability to raise growth factor levels. A case report by Dr. Ross Hauser in Oak Park, Illinois, shows clinical evidence of such a change. X-rays were taken of a patient with severe arthritic degeneration were done before and after prolotherapy treatment, 1 year apart. Please note that it is difficult, if not impossible, to take two X-rays of the same joint and have them be exactly the same view and beam penetration, and this was not a formal study. However, it does raise an interesting question. The patient was a 62-year-old female who when first seen was unable to ambulate without a cane. After 12 prolotherapy sessions approximately 1 month apart, this patient was pain free with full mobility. Clearly, more clinical trials need to be done on the question of prolotherapy and cartilage regeneration, and this would be a good future area of investigation.

NECK PAIN AND MUSCULOSKELETAL HEADACHES

The optimal long-term, symptomatic therapy for chronic neck pain has been investigated for unresolved neck pain at a charity clinic in rural Illinois. Ninety-eight patients were followed on an average of 18 months after prolotherapy treatment. Prior to treatment, these patients had suffered with pain an average of 59 months. Some of the patients had been told by their doctors that there were no other treatment options or that surgery was their only answer for their chronic pain. Ninety-seven percent of patients reported some pain relief with prolotherapy. Ninety-one percent considered the prolotherapy treatment on them to be very successful (greater than 50% pain relief), and 90% of patients who were on medications at the start of prolotherapy treatment were able to curb their pain medication usage by 50% or more.[90]

Headaches can have many different causes. In addition to musculoskeletal causes, there may be neurological, hormonal, allergic, or pathological causes for headaches that need to be addressed. If the cause of a headache is musculoskeletal, prolotherapy may be helpful since upper cervical ligament dysfunction may refer pain to the head (see Figure 18.2).

OTHER PAIN CONDITIONS

Prolotherapy has been used to successfully treat a large variety of musculoskeletal syndromes, including cervical, thoracic, and lumbar pain syndromes, patients diagnosed with disc disease, mechanical low back pain, plantar fascitis, foot or ankle pain, chronic rotator cuff or bicipital tendonitis/tendonsis, lateral and medial epicondylitis, TMJ dysfunction, musculoskeletal pain related to osteoarthritis, and even finger or toe joint pain including so-called turf toe. It is important to rule out a systemic or nonmusculoskeletal origin for the complaints, confirm no underlying illness which would prevent healing, and also to ensure there are no contraindications to treatment (see section below).

The Florida Academy of Pain Management laid out indications for prolotherapy (regenerative injection therapy or RIT) based on their review of the literature:

1. Chronic pain from ligaments or tendons secondary to sprains or strains.
2. Pain from overuse or occupational conditions known as "Repetitive Motion Disorders," i.e., neck and wrist pain in typists and computer operators, "tennis" and "golfers" elbows and chronic supraspinatous tendinosis.
3. Chronic postural pain of the cervical, thoracic, lumbar and lumbosacral regions.
4. Painful recurrent somatic dysfunctions secondary to ligament laxity that improves temporarily with manipulation. Painful hypermobility and subluxation at given peripheral or spinal articulation(s) or mobile segment(s) accompanied by a restricted range of motion at reciprocal segment(s).
5. Thoraic and lumbar vertebral compression fractures with a wedge deformity that exert additional stress on the posterior ligamento-tendinous complex.
6. Recurrent painful subluxations of ribs at the costotransverse, costovertebral and/or costosternal articulations.
7. Osteoarthritis of axial and peripheral joints, spondylosis, spondylosis and spondylolisthesis.

8. Painful cervical, thoracic, lumbar, lumbosacral and sacroiliac instability secondary to ligament laxity.
9. Intolerance to NSAIDs, steroids or opiates. RIT (Prolotherapy)
   may be the treatment of choice if the patient fails to improve
   after physical therapy, chiropractic or osteopathic manipulations,
   steroid injections or radiofrequency denervation or surgical interventions in the aforementioned conditions, or if such modalities
   are contraindicated.[51]

PROLIFERANT SOLUTIONS

The most common proliferant used in prolotherapy injections is hyper-
tonic dextrose, 12.5% to 25%, with 15% being the most used. This
is a safe solution which works by creating an osmotic gradient in the
area of injection, dessicating the local connective tissue cells, initiating
an injury response, and activating the inflammatory cascade. Once the
cell fluid is able to dilute the dextrose, the inflammation ceases, however
growth factor activation continues.[16] A local anesthetic such as lidocaine
or procaine is also used. Sarapin (extract of pitcher plant) is added in the
Hackett-Hemwall-Hauser formula. A saline, rather than dextrose, based
formula may also be used as a proliferant. Other solutions in use include noninflammatory dextrose (10% or less), which has been shown in
two double-blind studies to be effective in both finger and knee arthritis
and also improve knee ACL laxity and pain. Other, more inflammatory
formulas in use are phenol-containing-solutions, such as P2G (phenol,
glycerin, and dextrose).

CONTRAINDICATIONS

Active infection or cancer is a contraindication to treatment, as is any
underlying illness that could interfere with healing. Immunodeficiency
conditions, acute gout or rheumatoid arthritis, complete rupture of a tendon or ligament, nonreduced dislocations, or severe, unstable spondy-
lolithesis are also contraindications. Other contraindications are allergy
to any of the ingredients in the prolotherapy formula or unwillingness
to experience possible after-treatment discomfort. Patients should understand the course of the prolotherapy treatment and be participants in
their treatment plan.

   Relative contraindications include current and long-term use of
high doses of narcotics as these medications can lower the immune response. Current use of systemic corticosteroids or NSAIDs are also relative

contraindications as these are counter-productive to the inflammatory process. Other relative contraindications include central canal spinal stenosis and severe degenerative hip osteoarthritis with loss of range of motion.

RISKS

The most common risk is soreness after treatment. However, prolotherapy is a medical procedure, and as such there are risks. While prolotherapy is a low-risk procedure, any possible risk should always be fully discussed with a patient prior to treatment and a medical consent signed. Typical risks include bruising around the injected area and the risk of being in more pain, typically for 1 or 2 days after treatment because of the intended inflammation. However there is a risk that the pain after treatment will continue longer than expected. Other more rare risks include infection, headache, nerve irritation, allergy, puncture of an organ (such as the lungs) if injecting around that region, epidural puncture, or other unexpected risk. There is also the risk that the procedure will not work.

TYPICAL TREATMENT COURSE

Treatment intervals are spaced according to how that individual heals. On the average, the treatment interval is usually 3 to 4 weeks between treatments. In some people it is shorter, in others it is longer. The average number of treatments for any given area is usually between 4 and 6 total treatments, each treatment involving multiple injections to a particular area. Improvement is sometimes noticed after the initial treatment, however more often noticed by the second or third treatment. Some individuals require more than six treatments, and in some cases less treatments are needed. Individuals with hypermobility often take longer.

CONCLUSION

Prolotherapy is a reasonable and conservative approach to many different types of musculoskeletal pain, including back and neck pain; disc disease; headaches; chronic sprains and/or strains; whiplash injuries; tennis and golfer's elbow; knee pain including meniscal injuries; ankle, shoulder, or other joint pain; chronic tendonitis. It also may work in some aspects of cartilage regeneration. Prolotherapy is a treatment modality that provides a long-term solution rather than just palliation, and therefore should be considered in appropriate patients prior to long-term narcotic therapy or surgery in most cases.

REFERENCES

1. Hackett GS, Hemwall GA, Montgomery GA. *Ligament and Tendon Relaxation Treated by Prolotherapy.* 5th ed. Oak Brook, IL: Gustav A. Hemwall, Publisher, Institute in Basic Life Principles; 1991.
2. Reeves KD. Prolotherapy: basic science, clinical studies, and technique. In: Lennard TA, ed. *Pain Procedures in Clinical Practice.* 2nd ed. Philadelphia, PA: Hanley and Belfus; 2000:172–190.
3. Koop CE. Forward. In: Hauser, R. *Prolo Your Pain Away!* 1st ed. Oak Park, IL: Beulah Land Press; 1998:forward.
4. Alternative treatments: Dealing with chronic pain. *Mayo Clinic Health Letter.* April 2005;23(4).
5. Hauser R, et al. *Prolo Your Sports Injuries Away!* Oak Park, IL: Beulah Land Press; 2001.
6. Schnirring L. "News Brief: Are your patients asking about Prolotherapy?" *The Physician and Sportsmed.* August 2000;28(8):15–17.
7. Brody JE. Injections to kick-start tissue repair. *The New York Times.* August 7, 2007: D8.
8. Leadbetter W. Soft tissue athletic injuries. In Fu FH, ed.: *Sports Injuries: Mechanisms, Prevention, Treatment.* Baltimore, MD: Williams & Wilkins; 1994;736–737.
9. Hauser R, Hauser M. *Prolo Your Pain Away!* 2nd ed. Oak Park, IL: Beulah Land Press; 2004.
10. Browner B. *Skeletal Trauma.* Vol. 1. Philadelphia, PA: WB Saunders; 1992:87–88.
11. Andriacchi T, Sabiston P, DeHaven K, et al. Ligament: injury and repair. *Acta Rheum Scand.* 1956;2:109–116.
12. Frank C, Amiel D, Woo SL-Y, et al. Normal ligament properties and ligament healing. *Clin Orthop Res.* 1985;196:15–25.
13. Biedert RM, Stauffer E, Friederich NF. Occurrence of free nerve endings in the soft tissue of the knee joint. A histologic investigation. *Am J of Sports Med.* 1992;20(4):430–433.
14. Pomery KL. Sclerotherapy, prolotherapy and orthopedic medicine, a historical review. Presented at: American College of Osteopathic Sclerotherapeutic Pain Management seminar; April 2002.
15. Dagenais S, Haldeman S, Wooley JR. Intraligamentous injection of sclerosing solutions (prolotherapy) for spinal pain: a critical review of the literature. *The Spine J.* 2005;5:310–328.
16. Reeves KD. Prolotherapy: present and future applications in soft-tissue pain and disability. injection techniques: principles and practice. *Phys Med and Rehabil Clinics of North Am.* 1995;(6)4:917–923.
17. Gill CS, Sandell LJ, El-Zawawy HB, et al. Effects of cigarette smoking in early medial collateral ligament healing in a mouse model. *J Orthop Res.* 2006;24:1–9.
18. Laumann A. Scurvy, Article excerpt on emedicine.com. http://www.emedicine.com/derm/byname/scurvy.htm. Accessed on [[date]].
19. Banks AR. A Rationale for Prolotherapy. *J of Orthopaedic Med* 1991;13(3).
20. Stovitz SD, Johnson RJ. NSAIDs and musculoskeletal treatment—what is the clinical evidence? *The Physician and Sportsmedicine.* 2003;31:1.
21. Des Rosiers E, Yahia L, Rivard C. Proliferative and matrix synthesis response of canine anterior cruciate ligament fibroblasts submitted to combined growth factors. *J Orthop Res.* 1996;14:200–208.
22. Kang H, Kang ED. Ideal concentration of growth factors in rabbit's flexor tendon culture. *Yonsei Med J* 1999;40:26–29.

23. Lee J, Harwood F, Akeson W, et al. Growth factor expression in healing rabbit medial collateral and anterior cruciate ligaments. *Iowa Orthop J.* 1998;18:19–25.

24. Marui T, Niyibizi C, Georgescu HI, et al. Effect of growth factors on matrix synthesis by ligament fibroblasts. *J Orthop Res.* 1997;15:18–27.

25. Spindler KP, Imro AK, Mayes CE. Patellar tendon and anterior cruciate ligament have different mitogenic responses to platelet-derived growth factor and transforming growth factor beta. *J Orthop Res.* 1996;14:542–546.

26. Liu Y. An in situ study of the influence of a sclerosing solution in rabbit medical collateral ligaments and its junction strength. *Connect Tissue Res.* 1983;11(2): 95–102.

27. Maynard JA, Pedrini VA, Pedrini-Mille A, Romanus B, Ohlerking F. Morphological and biochemical effects of sodium morrhuate on tendons. *J of Orthop Res.* 1983.3: 236– 248.

28. Bahme, B. Observations on the treatment of hypermobile joints by injections. *The J of the Am Osteopath Assoc.* 1945;45(3):101–109.

29. Barbor R. A treatment for chronic low back pain. Proceedings from: the IV International Congress of Physical Medicine. September 6–11, 1964; Paris, France.

30. Bourdeau Y. Five-year follow-up on sclerotherapy/prolotherapy for low back pain. *Manual Med.* 1988;3:155–157.

31. Chase R. Basic sclerotherapy. *Osteop Ann.* 1978;6(12).

32. Dorman T. *Prolotherapy in the Lumbar Spine and Pelvis.* Philadelphia, PA: Hanley and Belfus Inc; 1995.

33. Gedney E. Use of sclerosing solution may change therapy in vertebral disk problem. *The Osteop Profession.* 1952;34(38,39):1113.

34. Gedney E. Progress report on use of sclerosing solutions in low back syndromes. *The Osteop Profession.* 1954;18–21,40–44.

35. Gedney E. The application of sclerotherapy in spondylolisthesis and spondylolysis. *The Osteop Profession.* 1964:66–69,102–105.

36. Hackett G. Joint stabilization through induced ligament sclerosis. *Ohio State Me. J.* 1953;49:877–884.

37. Hackett G, Henderson D. Joint stabilization: an experimental, histologic study with comments on the clinical application in ligament proliferation. *Am J of Surgery.* 1955; 89:968–973.

38. Hackett G. Ligament relaxation and osteoarthritis, loose jointed vs. closed jointed. *Rheum (London).* 1959;15(2):28–33.

39. Hackett G. Low back pain. *Indust Med Surg.* 1959;28:416–419.

40. Hackett G. Prolotherapy in whiplash and low back pain. *Postgraduate Med.* 1960; 27:214–219.

41. Hackett G. Prolotherapy for sciatic from weak pelvic ligament and bone dystrophy. *Clin Med.* 1961;8:2301–2316.

42. Hackett G et al. Prolotherapy for headache: pain in the head and neck, and neuritis. *Headache.* 1962. 2:20–28.

43. Leedy R et al. Analysis of 50 low back cases 6 years after treatment by joint ligament sclerotherapy. *Osteo Med.* 1976;6.

44. Linetsky F et al. Regenerative injection therapy: history of application in pain management, part I 1930s–1950s and part II 1930s–1950s. *The Pain Clinic.* 2000;2(2):8–13; and 2001;3(2):32–36.

45. Matthews J. A new approach to the treatment of osteoarthritis of the knee: prolotherapy of the ipsilateral sacroiliac ligaments. *Am J of Pain Manage.* 1995;5(3): 91–93.

46. Myers A. Prolotherapy treatment of low back pain and sciatica. *Bull Hosp Joint Disease*. 1961;22:48–55.
47. Schultz L. A treatment for subluxation of the temporomandibular joint. *JAMA*. 1937.
48. Schultz L. Twenty years' experience in treating hypermobility of the temporomandibular joints. *Am J of Surg*. 1956;92.
49. Klein RG, Dorman TA, Johnson CE. Proliferant injection for low back pain: histologic changes of injected ligaments and objective measurements of lumbar spine mobility before and after treatment. *The J of Neurol and Orthop Med & Surg*. 1989;10(2).
50. Linetsky FS, Botwin K, Gorfine, L, et al. Regenerative injection therapy (RIT) effectiveness and appropriate usage. The Florida Academy of Pain Medicine Position Paper. http://www.aaomed.org/library/documents/RIT_Position_Paper_052301.pdf, May 24, 2001.
51. Topol GA, Reeves KD, Hassanein K. Efficacy of dextrose prolotherapy in elite male kicking-sport athletes with chronic groin pain. *Arch of Phys Med and Rehabil*. 2005;86:697–702.
52. Ongley MJ, Dorman TA, Eek BC, Lundgren D, Klein RG. Ligament instability of knees: a new approach to treatment. *Manual Med*. 1988;3:152–154.
53. Reeves KD, Hassanein K. Long term effects of dextrose prolotherapy for anterior cruciate ligament laxity: A prospective and consecutive patient study. *Alt Ther*. 2003;9(3):58–62.
54. Reeves KD. Prolotherapy: present and future applications in soft-tissue pain and disability. Injection techniques: principles and practice. *Phys Med and Rehabil Clin of North Am*. 1995;(6)4:917–923.
55. Stovitz SD, Johnson RJ. NSAIDs and musculoskeletal treatment—what is the clinical evidence? *The Physician and Sportsmed*. 2003;31:1.
56. Ombregt, Bisschop, ter Veer. *A System of Orthopaedic Medicine*. 2nd ed. Churchill Livingstone; 2003.
57. MacRae DL. Asymptomatic intervertebral disc protrusion. *Acta Radiologica*. 1956; 46–49.
58. Hitselberger WE, Whitten RM. Abnormal myelograms in asymptomatic patients. *J of Neurosurgery*. 1968;28:204.
59. Wiesel SW, et al. A study of computer-assisted tomography: the incidence of positive CAT scans in an asymptomatic group of patients. *Spine*. 1984;9:549–551.
60. Powell MC, et al. Prevalence of lumbar disc degeneration observed by magnetic resonance in symptomless woman. *Lancet*. 1986;13:1366–1367.
61. Boden SD, et al., Abnormal magnetic resonance scans of the lumbar spine in asymptomatic subjects. *J of. Bone and Joint Surgery*. 1990;72A:503–408.
62. Kaplan PA. MR imaging of the normal shoulder: variants and pitfalls. *Radiol*. 1992; 184:519–524.
63. Deyo R. Magnetic resonance imagaing of the lumbar spine—terrific test or tar baby? *New England J of Med*. 1994;331:115–116.
64. Matsumoto M, et al. MRI of the cervical intervertebral discs in asymptomatic subjects. *J of Bone and Joint Surgery* (Br). 1998;80(1):19–24.
65. Humphreys SC, et al. Reliability of magnetic resonance imaging in predicting disc material posterior to the posterior longitudinal ligament in the cervical spine, a prospective study. *Spine*. 1998;23(22):2468–2471.
66. Kaiser JA, Holland BA, Imaging of the cervical spine. *Spine*. 1998;23(24):2701–2712.

67. Jerosch J, Castro WH, Assheuer J. Age related magnetic resonance imagaing morphology of the menisci in asymptomatic individuals. *Arch of Orthop Trauma Surg.* 1996;115(3–4):199–202.
68. LaPrade RF, et al. The prevalence of abnormal magnetic resonance imaging findings in asymptomatic knees. With correlation of magnetic resonance imaging to arthroscopic findings in symptomatic knees. *Am J of Sports Med.* 1994;22(6):739–745.
69. Rhalmi S. Immunohistochemical study of nerves in lumbar spine ligaments. *Spine.* 1993;18:264–267.
70. *Mosby's Medical Dictionary.* Elsevier/Saunders; 2006.
71. Astrom M, Rausing A. Chronic Achilles tendinopathy: a survey of surgical and histopathologic findings. *Clin Orthop.* 1995;316:151–164.
72. Khan KM, Bonar F, Desmond PM, et al. Patellar tendinosis (jumper's knee); findings at histopathologic examination, US and MR imaging. Victorian Institute of Sport Tendon Study Group. *Radiol.* 1996;200(3):821–827.
73. Khan KM, Cook JL, Bonar F, et al. Histopathology of common teninopathies: update and implications for clinical managements. *Sports Med.* 1999;27(6):393–408.
74. Almekinders, Temple. Etiology, diagnosis and treatment of tendonosis: an analysis of the literature. *Med & Science in Sports and Exercise.* 1998;30(8).
75. Khan et al., Overuse tendonosis, not tendonitis. *The Physician and Sportsmed.* 2000;28(5).
76. Hauser, R. Prolotherapy: *An Alternative to Knee Surgery.* Beulah Land Press, Oak Park, IL, 2004.
77. Frymoyer JW, Cats-Baril WL. An overview of the incidences and costs of low back pain. *Orthop Clin of North Am.* 1991;22:263–271.
78. Valkenburg HA, Haanen HCN. The epidemiology of low back pain. In: White AA, Gordon SL, eds. *Idiopathic Low Back Pain.* St. Louis, MO: Mosby; 1982.
79. Biering-Sorensen F. A prospective study of low back pain in general population. I. Occurrence, recurrence and aetiology. *Scand J of Rehabil Med.* 1983;15:71.
80. Drezner J, Herring S. Managing low-back pain. *The Physician and Sportsmed.* 2001;29:8.
81. Borenstein DG. Chronic low back pain. *Rheumatological Dis Clin of North Am.* 1996;22:439–456.
82. Hills EC, Wieting JM, et al., eds. Mechanical low back pain. From: http://www.emedicine.com/pmr/topic73.htm. Updated November 21, 2004.
83. Mixter WJ, Barr JS. Rupture of the intervertebral disc with involvement of the spinal canal. *N Engl J of Med.* 1934;211, 210.
84. Ongley MJ, Klein RG, Eek BC, Dorman TA, Hubert LJ. A new approach to the treatment of chronic low back pain. *The Lancet.* 1987:143–146.
85. Dechow E, et al. A randomized, double-blind, placebo-controlled trial of sclerosing injections in patients with chronic low back pain. *Rheumatol (Oxford).* 1999;38(12):1255–1259.
86. Matthews JA, et al. Back pain and sciatica: controlled trials of manipulation, traction, sclerosant and epidural injections. *Br J of Rheumatol.* 1987;26(6):416–423.
87. Klein RG, Eek BC, DeLong WB, Mooney V. A randomized double-blind trial of dextrose-glycerine-phenol injections for chronic, low back pain. *J of Spinal Disord.* 1993;6(1):23–33.
88. Yelland MJ, et al. Proltoherapy injections, saline injections, and exercises for chronic low back pain: a randomized trial. *Spine.* 2004;29(1):9–16.
89. Hauser R, Hauser M. An observational study on dextrose prolotherapy for unresolved low back pain at an outpatient charity clinic in rural Illinois. *J of Spinal Disord.* In press.

90. Alpers BJ. The problem of sciatica. *Med Clin of North Am.* 1953;37:503.

91. Acarpglu ER, et al. Degeneration and aging affect the tensile behavior of human lumbar annulus fibrosus. *Spine.* 1995;20:2690–2701.

92. Krag MH, et al. Thoracic and lumbar internal disc displacement distribution from in vitro loading of human spinal motion segments: experimental results and theoretical predictions. *Spine.* 1987;12:1001–1007.

93. Nachemson A. Advances in low back pain. *Clin Orthop.* 1985;200:266.

94. Paster RZ. Nonpharmacologic management of low back pain. *Family Practice Recertification Management of Chronic Low Back Pain Special Supplement.* 1999;21(7):9–21.

95. *Taber's Cyclopedic Medical Dictionary.* 19th ed. Philadelphia, PA: F. A. Davis Company; 1997.

96. Schwarzer A. The sacroiliac joint in chronic low back pain. *Spine.* 1995;20:31–37.

97. Parziale JR, Hudgins TH, Fishman LM. The piriformis syndrome. *Am J of Orthop.* 1996;25(12):819–823.

98. Merriman J. Prolotherapy versus operative fusion in the treatment of joint instability of the spine and pelvis. *J of the Int College of Surgeons.* 1964;42(2):150–159.

99. Cervoni TD, et al. Recognizing upper-extremity stress lesions. *The Physician and Sportsmed.* 1997;(25):8.

100. Morehead K, Sack K. Osteoarthritis: What therapies for this disease of many causes? *Postgraduate Med.* 2003:12–17.

101. Farrow CS, Newton CD. Ligamentous injury (sprain). *Textbook of Small Animal Orthopaedics.* Ithaca, NY: International Veterinary Information Service; 1985.

102. Lohmander LS, Ostenberg A, Englund M, Roos H. High prevalence of knee osteoarthritis, pain and functional limitations in female soccer players twelve years after anterior cruciate ligament injury. *Arthritis & Rheum.* 2004;50(10):3142–3152.

103. Panush R. Recreational activities and degenerative joint disease. *Sports Med.* 1994;17:1–5.

104. Reeves KD, Hassanein K. Randomized prospective double-blind placebo-controlled study of dextrose prolotherapy for knee osteoarthritis with or without ACL laxity. *Alt Thera.* 2000;6(2):68–79.

105. Reeves KD, Hassanein K. Randomized prospective placebo controlled double blind study of dextrose prolotherapy for osteoarthritic thumbs and finger (DIP, PIP and Trapeziometacarpal) joints: evidence of clinical efficacy. *J of Alt and Complementary Med.* 2000;6(4):311–320.

106. Kormick J, Trefelner E, McCarthy S, et al. Meniscal abnormalities in the asymptomatic population at MR Imaging. *Radiol.* 1990;177:463–465.

107. Moore K, Dalley A. *Clinically Oriented Anatomy.* 5th ed. Lippincott Williams & Wilkins; 2006.

108. Moritani NH, Kubota S, Sugahara T, et al. Comparable response of ccn1 and ccn2 genes upon arthritis: an in vitro evaluation with a human chondrocytic cell line stimulated by a set of cytokines. *Cell Communication and Signaling.* 2005;1478–1481.

109. Mankin H. The response of articular cartilage to mechanical injury. *J of Bone and Joint Surgery.* 1982;64A:460.

110. Otsuka Y, Mizuta H, Takagi K, et al. Requirement of fibroblast growth factor signaling for regeneration of epiphyseal morphology in rabbit full-thickness defects of articular cartilage. *Dev Growth Differ.* 1997;39:143–156.

111. Van Beuningen H, Glansbeek H, van der Kraan P, et al. Differential effects of local application of BMP-2 or TGF-beta 1 on both articular cartilage composition and osteophyte formation. *Osteoarthritis Cartilage.* 1998;6:306–317.

112. Nishida T, Kubota S., Kojima S, et al. Regeneration of defectsin articular cartilage in rat knee joints by CCN2 (connective tissue growth factor). *J of Bone and Mineral Research*. 2004;19:1308–1319.
113. Reeves KD, Hassanein K. Randomized prospective double-blind placebo-controlled study of dextrose prolotherapy for knee osteoarthritis with or without ACL laxity. *Alt Thera*. 2000;6(2).

CHAPTER 19

Ethical and Legal Implications

Michael Cohen and Marc S. Micozzi

Complementary and alternative medical (CAM) therapies are moving into the mainstream of American medicine.[1,2] Indeed, for some conditions, patients may resort to CAM therapies more than conventional treatments.[3] The innovative nature of these treatments does not free them from the medical-legal issues that affect conventional medical practice. As CAM providers venture into traditional areas of medicine, they may expose themselves to liability issues previously limited to practitioners practicing standard forms of Western medicine.[4,5] In this chapter, we review basic medical-legal issues as they apply to the application of CAM therapies by physicians as well as steps that might be taken to reduce potential liability risk.

MEDICAL MALPRACTICE

Malpractice Generally

The threat of being sued for malpractice poses an ongoing concern for health care professionals generally. Approximately once a decade, there is a so-called crisis in medical malpractice, marked either by skyrocketing malpractice insurance premiums, increased incidence of claims, large damage awards, or some combination of these.[6] In the 1990s, increasing damage awards and declining investment income for insurers set the stage for increasingly burdensome malpractice insurance premiums.[7] In the current decade efforts at medical malpractice reform have focused on alterations in mandatory insurance coverage ceilings and on limiting awards for noneconomic damages (the infamous "pain and suffering" awards). However, sufficient attention has not been given to the two major underlying causes of harm due to medical therapies: (1) the invasiveness and inherent riskiness of standard medical procedures,[8] together with (2) the high rate of medical errors, as documented by the Institute of Medicine of the National Academy of Sciences in their landmark report, "To Err is Human." These two factors set the stage for establishing (1) harm or damages and (2) liability in medical malpractice tort law. With damages but no liability, or with liability but no damages, there is no case. Unfortunately from this perspective, the practice of modern mainstream medicine inherently contains circumstances for both conditions. Insofar as alternative/complementary therapies emphasize the use of the least invasive therapy that is effective, appropriate approaches to integrating CAM therapies into medical practice carries with it the promise of fewer and lower malpractice problems and costs, since damages are inherently limited.

Physicians have been the traditional objects of malpractice claims. There are a number of possible reasons for this, including the relatively high-risk conditions addressed and the more invasive treatments. Because of the increased risk of suit, physicians have carried mandatory substantial insurance coverage, providing so-called deep pockets that likely have the double effect of encouraging litigation. Malpractice insurance serves dual purposes: It protects the practitioner from personal liability for acts of negligence and ensures that compensation is available for patients injured by negligent acts of physicians. Whether malpractice insurance should be regarded as personal protection for practitioners or as a fund to compensate injured patients is the subject of lengthy debate that is outside the scope of this chapter. Regardless, it is unwise for a physician to practice without malpractice insurance or go bare; most, if not all, states require that practicing physicians carry malpractice insurance.

Malpractice is a subset of personal injury or tort law. A tort is defined as a civil (as opposed to criminal) wrong that gives rise to a right to sue for damages. The purpose of awarding damages is two-fold. First, it provides compensation to those injured by the acts of others will be compensated. Second, the imposition of liability for negligent behavior serves as a disincentive for negligence and an inducement to exercise reasonable care.

There are two basic types of torts: intentional and unintentional. Intentional torts arise when one person purposefully engages in an act that is likely to cause harm to another person. Unintentional torts arise when an injury results from negligence in the pursuit of an activity that is not intended to cause harm, such as medical treatment.[9,10]

Malpractice insurance is intended to protect practitioners from liability for medical negligence and not for liability from intentional acts.[8,11] Certain intentional torts are covered by malpractice policies, however. Battery (the intentional touching of another person without consent or justification) is an intentional tort that may fall within the realm of malpractice coverage if the touching occurred in the course of medical treatment, such as where a patient is injured following a treatment for which full informed consent was not obtained. This circumstance results because battery was a theory of recovery that later morphed, in many states, into treatment with inadequate informed consent. Further, the nonconsensual touching itself may be the negligent act. A battery by a practitioner that is unrelated to treatment would not fall within malpractice coverage, however. For example, injury to a patient in the course of spinal manipulation by a chiropractor might be covered—as the battery, negligence, and failed informed consent are related—whereas injury to a patient in the course of an altercation in the waiting area would not be. In addition to battery, malpractice coverage may be afforded in some cases for certain intentional acts such as abandonment and, on a limited basis, for inappropriate sexual involvement with a patient.[12,13] These two areas will be discussed specifically below. It should be noted that while malpractice insurance may cover these arenas, courts are reluctant to allow physicians to disclaim liability or to have patients waive their right to sue for damages, in these arenas.

Elements of a Malpractice Claim

For a claim of malpractice to succeed, the plaintiff (the injured party making the claim) must establish four elements: The defendant had a duty towards the plaintiff to use reasonable care, the defendant was derelict in that duty, that dereliction directly led to harm, and that harm can be measured in the form of damages that are provable.[14]

Duty. Every practitioner has a duty to possess the skills and knowledge of the average, reasonable practitioner in his or her field of practice. Pursuant to the "School Rule," each practitioner is judged according to the standards of practice of his or her field.[15] Thus, in general, physicians are held to a medical standard of practice, but CAM providers are each held to the standard of care in their own profession (e.g., acupuncture, chiropractic, massage therapy, etc.).[16] However, there is a general standard of practice applied to all those who hold themselves out to the public as being able to diagnose and treat illness.[17] Thus, when

CAM providers offer treatment that overlaps with medical diagnosis and treatment (for example, a chiropractor ordering an X-ray), that provider could be held to a medical standard.[16(pp66-67)] Similarly, when a physician incorporates CAM therapies, it is unclear whether that physician will be held to a mixed standard of care that includes medical and CAM practice standards—that is, the physician might be compared to that of similarly situated physicians incorporating CAM therapies in like fashion; physicians in this situation may, however, be able to use as a potential defense to malpractice the respectable minority argument, which suggests that practice is legitimate if followed by a significant number of similarly situated clinicians.[16(p58)]

The locality rule, which calls for practitioners to be judged according to the standard of practice in their community,[17,18] has been in decline with the wide availability of medical information in publications, at conferences, and online. Instead, courts tend to judge practitioners according to national standards of care. In addition, those who represent that they have specific expertise in a given area are held to a higher standard of knowledge and skill. Thus, a primary care physician who represents having special expertise in treating heart ailments will be judged according to the standard of practice of cardiologists, not of other primary care physicians or CAM practitioners who treat general ailments.

The number of schools of CAM poses a challenge in terms of identifying specific schools of practice and determining what standards of practice might apply to CAM practices not clearly defined by any one profession. Statutory recognition, specialized education, and distinctive treatment can all be considered in determining whether a type of practice represents a distinct school.[17] In any event, practitioners of all types, licensed or unlicensed, have a duty to refer when the condition they are attempting to treat is outside the range of their knowledge and experience.[19,20] CAM providers, therefore, have a duty to refer the patient to a medical doctor when the condition exceeds the CAM provider's knowledge, skill and expertise, although no court yet has found such a reverse duty back from the medical doctor to the CAM provider.[16(pp68-70)]

Dereliction (Breach of Duty). Dereliction (or breach of duty) refers to negligent failure to comply with the standard of care. This may occur when the practitioner fails to take routine steps in the course of evaluation and treatment—for example, treating chest pain with spinal manipulation without taking a thorough history and obtaining appropriate testing, such as an ECG. It can also arise if the appropriate workup is done, but the information is handled in a negligent fashion, for example, ignoring key elements of the history or misinterpreting the ECG.

Direct Causation. The negligent departure from the standard of care must have a direct connection with some injury to the plaintiff.[21]

This has two aspects to it. The first is direct causation in the mechanical sense, as measured by the so-called but for rule: But for the negligent behavior, the injury would not have occurred. The second aspect is proximate or legal cause. This refers to the principle that liability will only be imposed for harm that was reasonably foreseeable from any negligent action.[22] Foreseeability is broadly interpreted, and physical injury following medical treatment is easy to establish through the testimony of a medical expert that, to a "reasonable degree of medical certainty," the alleged negligence is the cause of the harm in question.[23]

Damages. Finally, to recover on a claim of negligence, the plaintiff must prove that damages have been suffered. Damages can be financial (e.g., lost earning capacity, medical costs), physical (e.g., loss of a body part or function), or emotional, that is, pain and suffering (e.g., depression or anxiety following an injury.)[24(pp39–49)] Damages, like the other elements of a malpractice claim, are established through the testimony of expert witnesses. For example, an economist is typically called to testify about the lost value of future earnings and a psychiatrist or psychologist to testify about emotional damages.

Where the negligent behavior results in a missed opportunity to prevent harm, a plaintiff may recover under the loss of chance doctrine. For example, a physician who does not perform a physical examination on his patient, and thus misses a cancerous breast tumor that ultimately leads to the patient's death, may be held liable for her wrongful death under the loss of chance rule. Clearly, the lack of examination did not cause the cancer, but it represented a lost opportunity for the cancer to be detected.[25,26] *Loss of chance is a potent legal theory with regard to negligence in the field of CAM.* Failure to diagnose or treat, or prescription of ineffective treatment techniques in the absence of full informed consent or use of the wrong treatment could all serve as bases for such claims.

BURDEN OF PROOF

In any personal injury litigation, the plaintiff has the burden of establishing his or her case by a preponderance of the evidence, that is, it is more likely than not that the facts are as the plaintiff alleges and so the plaintiff is entitled to judgment. This should be contrasted with the burden of proof in criminal cases, which is beyond a reasonable doubt. Thus, the plaintiff must present testimony that establishes each of the elements of a malpractice claim outlined above. The testimony of an expert witness must be introduced on the subjects of standard of care and proximate cause.[14]

Under the doctrine of *res ipsa loquitur* (the thing speaks for itself), the burden of proof shifts to the defendant who then has to prove compliance with the standard of care or lack of proximate cause. This doctrine applies where the procedure, instrument, or medication was under the sole control of the defendant and the defendant alone has knowledge of the events leading up to the injury. For example, if a patient has complications from a surgical sponge discovered in the abdomen, the surgeon who performed the prior surgery has the burden of proving compliance with the standard of care, a lack of relationship between the sponge and the new injury, or that the sponge got there by some other means.[14]

Selected Malpractice Issues in CAM

To date, CAM has been light on malpractice claims relative to medicine. Studdert et al found that malpractice claims against chiropractors, acupuncturists, and massage therapists were fewer in number and involved less serious injuries than those against traditional practitioners.[27] As the CAM field grows, expands the range of conditions it treats, and makes greater claims for efficacy, it may come to greater attention by the plaintiff's personal injury bar and become subjected to the same malpractice rules as other areas of medicine.[4,5,27,28]

In this section, we review some of the specific areas of CAM in which claims for malpractice may arise. Consider the following case and its variations.

C is a board-certified physician who is well-versed in mind-body therapies and in herbal medicine and nutrition, and has taken sufficient weekend courses in acupuncture and traditional oriental medicine to receive certification appropriate to the state law requirements. C also has a referral network consisting of a licensed chiropractor, a licensed naturopathic physician, and a clinical psychologist who has staff privileges at the same hospital as C. P, the patient, visits C complaining of chest pain. C takes a medical history and learns that P is 2 weeks away from taking a state exam to become a licensed stockbroker.

CASE A

C determines that P is suffering from anxiety over the coming exam and refers P to the clinical psychologist for a mental health check-up and some relaxation techniques. On the drive to the clinical psychologist, P suffers a heart attack. An autopsy reveals that the heart attack easily could have been prevented had C, instead of referring P, simply followed conventional diagnostic and monitoring techniques.

CASE B

Part 1. C, summarily concludes that P is simply suffering from anxiety, fails to treat P with necessary medication for P's heart, and does not refer him to anyone. The next day, P has a heart attack that could have been prevented by conventional diagnosis and treatment.

Part 2. C applies regular diagnostic methods and concludes that P is at risk of a heart attack if P continues to neglect diet and exercise, and continues to pile up stressors. C recommends the Ornish diet, a regimen of light yoga, and various stress reduction methods. "I want you to come back in 2 weeks and let's test you again," C says. "In the meanwhile, try these methods and call me if your chest pain worsens or you feel any other symptoms. And try to ease off on your hours at the firm."

CASE C

C applies regular diagnostic methods and concludes that P is at risk of an impending heart attack. C applies magnets to P's chest wall, telling P: "This treatment will reverse your cardiovascular disease." The next day, P has a heart attack that could have been prevented by conventional diagnosis and treatment.

CASE D

C tells P: "With your lifestyle and emotional constitution, your heart's in danger." C recommends that P adopt a nutritional protocol and seek counseling for anger management. P yells back: "But I love my salami for breakfast, lunch, and dinner and I refuse to change. Stop trying to control me!" C replies: "You're a lost cause. I refuse to see you anymore. Good luck finding someone who can handle your temper tantrums." The next day, P has a heart attack that could have been prevented by conventional diagnosis and treatment.

CASE E

Part 1. In Case D above, C goes to his chief and reports the stormy encounter with P. The chief replies: "That's okay, our patient volume is up and your research grant just came through. You don't have to deal with an obstreperous personality like that; why get yourself all stressed out? Walk the talk and take some deep breaths, and let that one go." C goes for a long walk and determines never to speak to P again.

Part 2. Assume instead that after speaking with the chief, C goes for a walk, takes some deep breaths, and, feeling responsible for P, calls and suggests that P make an appointment with the clinical psychologist affiliated with the hospital. P does so. C fails to mention P's angry blow-ups, and, during P's visit, P is in a mild and charming state, and the psychologist fails to do an adequate assessment. The next day, P is involved in a minor traffic accident but in an act of road rage, severely injures the other driver in a physical confrontation. P is arrested and is prevented from getting his broker's license.

CASE F

C describes P's case (and discloses P's name) to the licensed chiropractor, a licensed naturopathic physician, and a clinical psychologist without receiving an appropriate, signed consent form from P. P receives a phone call from one of these providers, offering services, and is embarrassed and irate.

CASE G

C diagnoses P conventionally and determines that P must schedule bypass surgery to avoid a possible myocardial infarction. P has the bypass surgery, and later learns that there is some evidence in the medical literature, albeit conflicting, that chelation therapy might have been a preferred alternative. P is angry at C for not disclosing the possibility of chelation therapy and claims that if he had been properly informed, he would have elected to try this treatment instead of bypass surgery.

CASE H

C diagnoses P conventionally and determines that P might have to schedule bypass surgery to avoid a possible myocardial infarction; C also discloses to P that there is some evidence in the medical literature, albeit conflicting, that chelation therapy might be a preferred alternative. P wants to try the therapy. "We'll schedule you for follow-up," C tells P. "If chelation therapy doesn't work, we'll have to do the bypass surgery." P receives chelation therapy and, delighted by the results, tells his clinical psychologist, who promptly reports C to the state medical board for engaging in professional misconduct by using an off-label therapy that is not supported by medical evidence.

CASE I

C continues to treat P over a number of years, and during one visit, attempts to console P for a family tragedy by giving him a hug. P mistakes the gesture for an uninvited sexual intimacy.

Misdiagnosis. Misdiagnosis refers to both a failure to diagnose a condition as well as inaccurate diagnosis. It is important to emphasize the fact that an error alone is not sufficient to establish negligence. The error must result from a departure from the standard of care in order to provide a basis for a successful claim.[29,30] For CAM practitioners, misdiagnosis may be an issue where adherence to a particular school of practice leads to a failure to detect a condition. Thus, both the physician who fails to diagnose ischemic cardiovascular disease and the chiropractor that misdiagnoses intermittent chest pain as the product of subluxation of the thoracic spine, rather than angina, could both be held liable for misdiagnosis.

In Case A, the cardiologist misdiagnosed the patient's impending heart attack by failing to implement standard conventional diagnostic techniques. C's referral without conventional diagnosis is inexcusable, as is the diagnosis of P as simply a case of anxiety. C's inclusion of CAM therapies does not relieve the obligation to practice in accordance with the standard of care as regards conventional medical diagnosis.

Failure to Treat. Most malpractice cases arise from an act of misfeasance, that is, failure to act in an appropriate manner. Generally speaking, there is no obligation to act to help another person in distress. However, once a person undertakes to provide such assistance, a duty arises to exercise reasonable care. Ironically, this "undertaking to treat" is that which establishes liability for the therapeutic encounter. However, in terms of the healer-patient relationship, undertaking to treat is a powerful part of the healing dynamic. For the patient to feel they are being treated (cared for) by an ethical healer who is there to help is a very potent component of the therapeutic encounter. In the contemporary world of medical malpractice, a positive feature of healing has taken on a negative connotation.

Once a condition is diagnosed, or should have been diagnosed by the reasonable practitioner practicing in accordance with the standard of care, there is an obligation to offer treatment or transfer care to another clinician. Claims that a necessary treatment is not offered by the practitioner do not alleviate the duty to treat or refer for treatment. This can be an issue when newer treatments with demonstrated efficacy have not been adopted by a particular practitioner who continues to offer treatments that were previously state-of-the-art but no longer retain that status.[31,32]

In Case B, Part 1, the physician compounds the initial misdiagnosis with failure to treat, thus presenting an additional and alternate theory of malpractice liability. Case B is egregious, and represents one end of a possible spectrum, in which overreliance on CAM therapies or on the mind-body connection leads to ignoring tested, conventional methods of diagnosis and treatment.

In Case B, Part 2, the physician is offering CAM therapies that have some reasonable evidence of safety and efficacy in the medical literature, without neglecting conventional monitoring and diagnosis.[33,34] In such a scenario, malpractice liability is unlikely. Where a CAM therapy has significant evidence of safety and efficacy, physicians should recommend that therapy to patients and know that liability is highly unlikely; where a CAM therapy has significant evidence of safety but not efficacy, or efficacy but not safety, physicians should allow fully informed and consenting patients to try such a therapy, while continuing to monitor conventionally, and to intervene conventionally when necessary, as liability is possible but again unlikely; and where a CAM therapy has significant evidence of either serious danger or inefficacy, physicians should avoid and actively discourage patients from using such a therapy, as liability here would be highly likely.

Fraud and Misrepresentation. The tort of fraud and misrepresentation is defined as the knowing inducement of reliance on inaccurate or false information for the benefit of the person committing the fraud and to the detriment of the victim. In order to prove fraud and misrepresentation by a practitioner of any type, the following elements must be established.

A false representation by the practitioner.

1. Knowledge or belief on the part of the practitioner that the representation is false or an insufficient basis in fact to make the representation.
2. Intent to induce the patient to rely upon the false representation either by accepting the offered treatment or foregoing other treatment.
3. Reliance upon the representation by the patient that is reasonable and justified under the circumstances. The reasonableness of the reliance is determined by a number of factors, including the credentials of the person recommending the treatment, the sophistication and educational level of the patient, and the nature of the representation. The more outlandish the claim of efficacy, the more persuasive the misrepresentation must be in order to establish reasonable reliance.

4. Damage to the patient as a result of relying upon the false representation.[14(pp725-728)] As mentioned above, this damage may take the form of injury resulting from the patient being induced to rely on a fraudulent treatment, preventing the patient from pursuing care that is more likely to have a positive result.

In Case C, all five elements are present: the physician falsely represented to the patient that applying magnets to the chest wall would reverse the patient's condition; the cardiologist knew this representation was false (or recklessly believed it to be true)—it would be sufficient if he either knew the claim is false or lacked a scientific basis for making the claim. The physician induced the patient to rely on the magnet claim and thereby forego necessary, conventional care; the patient reasonably relied on the advice, and thereby was injured. This physician therefore would be liable for fraud—a higher level of culpability than negligence, and one that would likely trigger punitive (as well as compensatory) damages.

Abandonment. Abandonment in the context of malpractice liability is defined as the unilateral and unjustified termination of the treatment relationship by the treater that results in damage to the patient. As the term *unjustified* indicates, there are situations in which it is reasonable and appropriate for treaters to unilaterally terminate the treatment relationship. These include threatening or violent patients, patients who repeatedly fail to keep appointments, and patients who are noncompliant to the point where the clinician can no longer justify seeing them.[35-37]

Even where termination of the relationship may seem justified to the clinician, however, it is advisable: (a) to consult with one or more colleagues to see how they assess the situation, (b) make arrangements for emergency coverage until the patient can find another treater, and (c) wherever possible, help facilitate the identification of a new treater and transfer of patient care. When the treater needs to withdraw, for whatever reason, reasonable time must be allowed to enable the patient to obtain substitute treatment.[38]

Case D certainly presents a patient who may be difficult to manage. The patient's anger, refusal to comply with medical advice, and even, one might argue, tendency to lash out against the provider, may (in the physician's mind) justify terminating treatment. As mentioned, however, the physician has a legal and ethical duty not to abandon the patient who needs conventional medical care. C in this hypothetical would be wise to refer the patient to a provider that is a better match, where P can receive the necessary conventional care, augmented by any psychological intervention that may be necessary.

Vicarious Liability/Referral. Clinicians may be held liable for the harm caused by employees or others under their direction (as may institutions in which those clinicians are employed) under the doctrine of vicarious liability or *respondeat superior* ("Let the master answer").[39] This legal principle holds that an employer may be vicariously liable for the acts of employees, performed within the scope of their duties, where the employer has the right to control the employee in the performance of those duties.[14(pp501–509)] The liability may arise as a result of negligent hiring (employment of someone who is known, or should be known, to pose a risk of negligent or inappropriate behavior). For example, a clinician who hires an assistant with a history of sexual misconduct with patients may be held liable for such misconduct if it is again repeated with the employing clinician's patients.[40]

Vicarious liability may be imposed on physicians who supervise residents and other trainees or nonphysicians treating the physician's patients. Whether or not liability will be imposed in these situations is determined by the degree to which the defendant has actual or potential control over the supervisee's clinical decision-making and performance of other duties. Liability is unlikely to be imposed if it is primarily a consulting relationship, in which the defendant provides recommendations but does not control whether or not those recommendations are accepted.[41–43]

Vicarious liability may be imposed in CAM in connection with employees, cotreaters, and clinicians to whom patients are referred.[44,45] An arms-length referral to a specialist, without more, however, rarely generates liability; but in "integrative care," when conventional providers closely collaborate with CAM providers to comanage patient diagnosis, monitoring, and treatment, shared liability is more likely.[46]

In Case E, Part 1, the hospital would be vicariously liable for any negligence on C's part, under *respondeat superior.* In addition, the Chief may be directly negligent for failing to properly supervise C and for encouraging C to engage in patient abandonment.

In Part 2, C would not necessarily be liable simply for referring P to the clinical psychologist. If, however, the physician and clinical psychologist were actively working together and thus engaged in "joint treatment" of the patient, each may have liability for the other's negligent acts.[46] When referring to a CAM provider, the physician should take reasonable care to ensure that the CAM provider does not have a significant history of malpractice liability or professional discipline and does not include practices that are marginal to or outside the CAM profession itself. These reasonable steps will help protect against a claim of negligent referral and/or vicarious liability for the CAM provider's negligence. Some basic information is available to help physicians reasonably assess a CAM provider's credentials and qualifications.[47]

Confidentiality. Medical information is highly personal and society, through case law and statutes, recognizes that the privacy of that information is entitled to protection. This is true regardless of the discipline of the person providing the treatment. Unauthorized breach of that privacy can cause personal embarrassment and have implications for personal and professional relationships. For those reasons, the decision to disclose personal medical information is left to the patient, except under limited circumstances. The law protects the privacy of medical information by imposing a duty of confidentiality on clinicians.[48,49]

Confidentiality is the ongoing obligation of physicians and other clinicians to keep private the information shared with them by patients in the course of treatment. It is an obligation that exists until the patient grants permission for confidentiality to be breached or a situation arises that falls within one of the exceptions to confidentiality. Signed release of information forms, granting the clinician permission to release information to a specific party or parties, have become routine, although many clinicians have traditionally felt comfortable obtaining verbal permission and recording it in the patient's record. State and Federal statutes, including the Health Insurance Portability and Accountability Act (HIPAA, originally known as the Kennedy-Kassebaum bill), have increased the requirements for signed releases. HIPAA formalizes many of the preexisting protections of medical information, which it refers to as Protected Health Information (PHI).[50,51] It is important to note, however, that HIPAA is aimed, in part, at facilitating the disclosure of information in order to increase the efficiency of health care. For example, HIPAA would allow the sharing of information between cotreaters, without the patient's permission. Physicians should be aware that HIPAA regulations set the minimum standard for protection of confidentiality. If state law provides greater protection for confidentiality, the state law governs.[52]

The duty of confidentiality imposed by case law and statutes applies to all medical information, including that related to CAM. While it is an evolving field, these obligations will be applied to nonphysician practitioners who treat various ailments, as the focus of confidentiality is the privacy of the information and not the discipline of the practitioner. Thus, a physician who offers CAM therapy and discloses the identity of a patient at a conference or in an article will be as subject to liability for breach of confidentiality as a physician offering more widely accepted treatments.[4,51,53] In case F, disclosure of P's confidential health information to the licensed chiropractor, a licensed naturopathic physician, and a clinical psychologist without receiving an appropriate, signed consent form likely would result in liability.

There are exceptions to the duty of confidentiality that allow information to be disclosed without a patient's express permission. The exceptions to confidentiality include emergency, implied or express waiver, incompetence, and imminent danger to self or others. Even under these exceptions, however, confidentiality should be breached to the least extent necessary to accomplish the necessary goal. For example, under the emergency exception, the identity of a patient brought unconscious to the emergency room could be revealed in the course of telephone calls to numbers found in the patient's address book. Such calls are permissible as they have the goal of gathering medical information necessary to provide emergency care, and the potential risk of harm from releasing the patient's identity is outweighed by the risk of having inadequate information. In a nonemergent situation, with a stable patient, such a call without the patient's permission, would not be considered permissible and might lead to a legitimate complaint of breach of confidentiality.

Clinicians may also have a duty to breach confidentiality where it is necessary to protect third parties from potential violence, other risks posed by a patient, such as infection, or genetic predisposition to serious diseases. A detailed discussion of this exception is beyond the scope of this chapter, but readers are advised to familiarize themselves with the law on this topic in their jurisdictions.[54-56]

Informed Consent. The doctrine of informed consent was one of the most important developments in law, medicine, and ethics of the 20th century. It is grounded in the fundamental ethical and legal notions that every person of adult age and sound mind has a right to determine what shall be done with his or her body.[57] Informed consent has evolved from an ethical to a medical-legal construct, with an unfortunate focus on the latter. Freed from such legalistic thinking, informed consent is an essential element of good patient care, improved compliance, and risk management. As a matter of medical ethics, it promotes the autonomy of individuals with regard to making individual medical decisions.[58] In CAM, informed consent issues are of utmost importance, as patients must be given an opportunity to weight the risks and benefits of choosing a CAM approach rather than a more conventional approach.[59] While the doctrine of informed consent emphasizes that the choice belongs to the patient, it in no way discourages the age-old practice of the patient looking to the physician for advice, and the physician providing it.[60]

Informed consent is the process through which a clinician proposing treatment provides information to a current or prospective patient, who then voluntarily consents to the treatment. It is this process of exchanging information that constitutes informed consent. The signing of a form, required by various hospital, administrative, and governmental regulations, is merely evidence that the informed consent process has taken place.[61]

All three elements of informed consent—information, voluntariness, and competence—must be present for consent to be valid. Informed consent, standing alone, is infrequently the subject of malpractice claims. The proximate cause element of malpractice, discussed above, requires that "but for" the failure to obtain proper informed consent, that harm would not have occurred, that is, the patient would not have accepted the treatment.[14(pp173–193)] As a result, a patient from whom proper informed consent was not obtained would have to argue that he would have foregone the treatment in question. This is potentially a greater risk issue for CAM than for traditional medical treatments, as the patient could more easily argue that, had he known that more widely accepted treatments with established efficacy were available, he would have chosen one of those as opposed to the CAM treatment offered.

Information. Questions are often raised about the amount of information that needs to be provided in order for consent to be valid. Does every risk and side effects have to be described? As a rule of thumb, patients should be advised of risks and side effects along a continuum, from those that are common but not very serious to those that are infrequent but are potentially significant. It is the materiality of risks that govern whether or not they need to be discussed specifically.[14(pp45–48),62]

As a legal requirement, the amount and type of information that must be provided depends upon the jurisdiction in which the physician is practicing. In jurisdictions that apply a physician-oriented or community standard, the physician must provide the information that the average, respectable physician in the community would provide under similar circumstances. The patient-oriented or materiality standard applied in other jurisdictions requires that all the information that an average patient (or in some states, the specific patient) would find material in making a decision.[63]

In *Harnish* v. *Children's Hospital Medical Center,*[64] the Massachusetts Supreme Judicial Court set out requirements for information sharing that satisfy legal and ethical requirements in virtually all jurisdictions. They include:

- The diagnosis and nature of the condition being treated
- The benefits the patient can reasonably expect from the proposed treatment
- The nature and probability of material risks
- The inability to predict results
- The potential irreversibility of the procedure
- The likely results, risks, and benefits associated with CAM treatments and no treatment.

The last element of the *Harnish* requirements is of particular relevance in CAM. Clinicians need not inform their patients of all available CAM therapies, only those that would be offered by the average, reasonable physician in the community. Thus, in *Moore* v. *Baker,* a Federal Court held that a physician had not breached a statutory duty to obtain informed consent by failing to inform a patient of chelation therapy as an alternative to carotid endarterectomy. The court held that the physician was obligated to inform the patient only about those treatments that are practical and generally recognized and accepted by reasonably prudent physicians.[65]

While such an approach does not help promote CAM therapies, it does not prevent them from being offered. Rather, it remains true to the reasonableness standard with regard to the imposition of duties on physicians. If, over time, chelation therapy were to be established as an accepted and reasonable treatment option, the court noted, same case might be decided differently. On the other hand, the CAM practitioner who fails to advise the patient of more widely accepted treatment as another option to CAM therapies may be breaching the duty to provide adequate information. In Case G, P would not likely succeed without offering convincing evidence that of general medical acceptance of the CAM therapy proposed.

Voluntariness. The consent to treatment must be voluntary, meaning that it cannot be the result of coercion by the person offering the treatment. The largely elective nature of CAM treatments and the conditions treated make it unlikely that overt coercion would be used. More subtle forms of coercion, such as denying access to requested treatment unless other treatments or supplements are also accepted, can also render consent invalid.

While the voluntariness requirement speaks to coercion by the clinician, questions sometimes arise about coercion by family members. This could arise, for example, with an elderly parent whose child insists that she accept alternative treatment modalities that are the preference of the child but not the parent, on pain of losing a place to live or other support. While such coercion does not automatically violate the legal acceptability of the consent, it does raise significant ethical and clinical compliance issues. In such situations, it is advisable for the treating clinician to focus the consent process on the patient while including concerned family members, in order to reach a clinical resolution. Similar problems arise in the treatment of children and adolescents.[66]

Competence. Competence is the threshold element of informed consent; only a competent person can give valid consent to treatment or treatment refusal. The law presumes that all adults are legally competent to make their own medical treatment decisions; that legal status remains intact until a court declares the person legally incompetent. In medical care, questions frequently arise about an individual patient's capacity to make treatment decisions. While a clinical determination of lack of decision-making capacity does not strip the patient of competency in the eyes of the law, clinicians are obligated to take note of this potential lack of capacity before accepting a patient's consent (or refusal) as being informed.[65,67] The fact that a patient disagrees with the physician's recommendations, or even chooses a course of treatment that most others would reject, does not mean that he lacks capacity. Competent individuals are well within their rights to make decisions that are incompetent in the eyes of others.[68,69]

As with other rules, there are exceptions to informed consent. Full informed consent does not need to be obtained in emergencies, where the patient waives the consent process, where the patient is incompetent, or in very limited cases where the informed consent process would worsen the patient's condition.[70-72]

If the emergency exception is to be invoked, there must first be an assessment of the patient's capacity to participate in the decision making process. If the patient lacks capacity, the physician acting in an emergency should turn to a family member for consent, if time and circumstances permit. The emergency exception does not allow the treating physician to override the patient's refusal of care expressed prior to the emergency.[73]

Just as patients have the right to make their own decisions, they have the right to leave the decision making to others, including their physicians. The key inquiry here, as with other aspects of informed consent, is whether the decision to waive is being made by someone who has the capacity to do so. If the patient from whom consent is sought lacks the capacity to engage in the decision-making process, then an alternative decision maker should be sought. The decision to seek a substitute decision maker turns on the degree of impairment and the risk-benefit balance of the proposed treatment. A sliding scale approach, with less capacity required for consent to low risk/high benefit treatments and refusal of high risk/low benefit treatments; and more capacity required for consent to high risk/low benefit treatments and refusal of low risk/high benefit treatments, is widely endorsed as an acceptable and practical approach to the competency issue.[74,75] In many jurisdictions, judicial involvement is required for treatments that are considered to be extraordinarily intrusive or dangerous.[76]

The doctrine of therapeutic privilege allows informed consent from the patient to be deferred, and consent obtained from another decision maker, where the consent process itself would have a deleterious effect on the patient's condition. Such situations are rare, and this exception must be invoked only with great care. Even when it may be justified, there is an obligation to seek an alternate decision maker.[77,78]

Off-Label Use of FDA-Approved Medications. The Food and Drug Act of 1936 was enacted to protect public health and safety by ensuring that food and medications offered to the public would not pose inherent risks. It was not intended to interfere with the doctor-patient relationship or the ability of physicians to exercise clinical judgment in treating patients. Once a medication receives FDA approval, physicians are free to use it for any treatment purpose based on their clinical judgment. Use of medications for nonapproved or off-label purposes exposes the physician to potential liability if an injury results. While the lack of FDA approval may not be considered a material risk for informed consent purposes, it is advisable to discuss the lack of FDA approval, and its implications, along with other information as part of the informed consent process.[79-81]

While the FDA cannot regulate the practice of medicine, state licensing boards can discipline physicians for professional misconduct. Most state statutes contain a number of defined categories for such misconduct, including such matters as practicing while under the influence of alcohol or drugs, sexual misconduct and malpractice liability. In addition, most state medical boards can discipline physicians for using therapies that are not generally medically accepted.[16(pp87-92)] Unfortunately, such a broad mandate leaves medical boards free to discipline physicians who include CAM therapies, since many such therapies may not be medically accepted. In response to this conundrum, many states have enacted medical freedom laws, providing that medical boards may not discipline physicians *solely* based on inclusion of CAM therapies.[16(92-95)] The Federation of State Medical Boards recently has issued Model Guidelines on Physician Use of Complementary and Alternative Therapies in Medical Practice that reiterate this principle.[82] In Case H, C may or may not be subject to discipline, depending on the medical board's view of chelation therapy and the applicable state licensing rules; physicians should investigate the law in the state in which they practice.

Sexual Involvement With Patients. In the 1980s and 1990s, sexual contact between physicians and therapists and their patients came to be recognized as a significant problem. It has been the basis for numerous ethics complaints against physicians and nonphysician treaters alike and has been addressed by the American Medical Association[83] and specialty societies.[84]

Sexual involvement with patients, also referred to as sexual misconduct and boundary violations, has been the subject of malpractice suits.[85,86] These suits have a number of bases, depending upon the specialty of the clinician and the nature of the relationship. Among the allegations are negligent handling of the doctor-patient relationship, as fraud and misrepresentation, breach of fiduciary duty, undue influence, and lack of valid consent due to disparity in the levels of power relationships within the relationship.[87] In addition, a number of states have made sexual contact with a current patient a criminal offense, with physicians being sentenced to prison time for such activity.[88]

Traditionally, the issue of sexual involvement with patients has been viewed as a problem for mental health professionals. This relates, in part, to the level of emotional intimacy that occurs in the course of psychotherapy and the emotional vulnerability of many patients (often due to previous sexual abuse or exploitation). Similar problems are encountered in obstetrics and gynecology and parishioner-clergy relationships.[89] The sexual relationships between attorneys and clients have also received increasing criticism.[90] The basis for recovery in psychotherapy cases has been on negligent handling of the transference (the emotional reaction of the patient to the therapist) and countertransference (the emotional reaction of the therapist to the patient).

It should be expected that a similar analysis would apply to other treaters who endeavor to treat the emotional problems of their patients and have close physical and emotional contact with them. For example, those who practice in the field of mind-body medicine, which acknowledges the essential interplay between psychological and physical states, would be expected to understand and properly handle the emotional and physical feelings that arise in the course of the treatment.

In Case I, the issue of physical touch has always been a 'hot button' for mental health professions, but supportive gestures such as this are rarely problematic, even in mental health. As hands-on treatments such as chiropractic and massage therapy enter conventional settings, the boundaries around physical contact with patients will change, and new emphasis is being given to how psychic boundaries are defined.[91] If C had treated P for many years, it is possible that a sensitive and engaged relationship would have arisen in which such a gesture would be well within professional boundaries. Indeed, integrative care emphasizes the power of the therapeutic relationship, including the closeness of provider and patient in the shared aligning of therapeutic intentionality.[92] In the absence of such a relationship, a gesture like this could be misinterpreted as being unduly familiar and experienced by the patient as inappropriate. Crossing of those boundaries, either in the form of treatment using physical contact or a supportive hug, needs to be done with consideration and with the patient's consent. Boundary violations, such as sex with patients, is outside the realm of treatment, and as noted above, may be considered inherently nonconsensual.

Risk Management

The experience of being sued for malpractice, charged with regulatory violations, or being brought up on ethics charges are universally acknowledged to be unpleasant. Such allegations disrupt the defendant's relationships with friends, family, patients, and colleagues. They cause tremendous personal sadness, often accompanied by anger and self-doubt.[93,94] The goal of risk management involves taking steps to decrease the likelihood of becoming the subject of malpractice or other litigation.

Relationship Matters. Liability risk management efforts often focus on the technical aspect of medicine. Only a small percentage of medical errors lead to allegations of malpractice; however, the percentage suggests that there are other factors that account for the decision of a patient or family member to pursue a malpractice claim.[95,96]

The prevailing view is that the relationship between the treater and the patient and his or her family plays the greatest role in determining whether a given adverse event will give rise to litigation. It has been widely suggested that malpractice cases arise from the combination of bad outcomes plus bad feelings.[97] A more sophisticated, but less widely publicized, formulation hones in on how some physicians may behave or be regarded by their patients. This formulation, known as Russell's Rule of Risk (after its creator, statistician A. Russell Localio) posits that the probability of a malpractice suit is directly proportional to a physician's arrogance (real or perceived) divided by physician's competence.[98]

Much can be done to improve the doctor-patient relationship, including the perception of arrogance. Good communication with patients, which includes tailoring the communication content and style to the needs of the individual patient, has been shown to enhance the perception of the physician's competence and decrease the risk of malpractice.[99,100] Scheduling enough time to talk with patients, taking telephone calls directly (rather than having a staff member return them), self-awareness of the physician's own stress level, and general satisfaction with one's own professional practice all seem to be associated with decreased risk.[101] One study suggested that characteristics of the relationship had a greater effect for primary care physicians than for surgeons.[102]

These communication skills, along with respect for patients' time, appreciation of the validity of their concerns, and honest sharing of what we know and do not know, humanize the doctor-patient relationship. By disabusing patients and their families of the myths that physicians know and can control everything, and that outcomes are guaranteed, we can manage expectations in a way that limits the risk of unnecessary disappointments and surprises. That, in turn, can decrease the risk of litigation.[103]

If this prevailing view of the role of relationships in risk management is valid, it may explain why CAM practitioners have experienced fewer malpractice claims. It may also bode well for the future. Attention to the whole patient, a focus on the person rather than the procedure, and a willingness to listen to patient concerns should all have a positive impact on risk reduction. It is the context and not the substance of the treatment that is protective, however. As CAM becomes part of mainstream medicine, and the treatments are offered during rushed office visits with little time for communication, we should expect the risk of litigation to approach that of conventional treatment.

An often-overlooked risk reduction measure is the practice of apologizing for adverse or unexpected outcomes. This does not mean that the clinician should engage in self-blame and assume all fault for every adverse event; there are no guarantees in any field of medicine, and the ultimate adverse outcome is preordained for every human being. Rather, this is the very simple practice of saying "I'm sorry" and offering support when things go badly. Genuine sympathy can do much to decrease the anger, frustration, and perception of indifference that may lead to litigation.[104] Beyond risk management, acknowledgment of errors and apology may be seen as ethical obligations.[97,105]

Good Clinical Care. Beyond attention to the doctor-patient relationship, there are a number of steps that can be taken to decrease the likelihood of a suit and increase the chances of prevailing should one occur.[106] First among these is consistently good clinical care, which includes ongoing education and management of clinical information.[107] Good clinical care includes monitoring for potential adverse reactions between conventional and CAM therapies—such as, for example, monitoring for adverse herb-drug interactions. Recent literature has suggested that not all herbal products are safe (or natural, for that matter), and that significant adverse interactions can result from their use.[108–110]

The case examples have emphasized the importance of conventional diagnosis and monitoring when CAM therapies are recommended or allowed. This is probably the most important means of ensuring that patients do not receive substandard care. Continuing to monitor conventionally and intervene conventionally when medically necessary means that the standard of care will have been met, and the possibility of patient injury minimized. For example, the physician and patient may wish to try a CAM therapy for a predefined period of time instead of conventional care (e.g., a combination of lifestyle changes) and return to conventional care (e.g., surgery) when it becomes necessary.

Another risk reduction measure is the practice of obtaining consultation. Ongoing supervision, as well as occasional curbside consultations regarding a specific case should be documented in the patient's record. These serve to establish the standard of care in the community, can provide valuable input into clinical decision making, and show that the clinician is willing to take extra steps for the benefit of the patient.[97]

Documentation. Good clinical care is not sufficient if the medical record does not adequately document that care. The record should reflect the diagnosis and the proposed treatment, the bases for them, the informed consent process, and the treatment plan, including follow-up.[111,112] In the absence of documentation, the litigation may come down to the word of the injured patient versus the memory and reputation of the defendant clinician. Poor medical records can suggest negligence to a jury. In general, it is advisable to keep complete and accurate medical records that include documentation of the patient's medical history concerning use of CAM therapies, and of conversations with patients concerning potential inclusion of such therapies. Such thorough documentation can help physicians prove that informed consent requirements were satisfied, and also may help protect against undue disciplinary action by state medical boards concerned with use of CAM therapies.[4]

If the physician recommends or allows use of a CAM therapy based on the medical literature, it is a good idea to keep a back-up file of the medical literature supporting the specific medical recommendation.[4] On the other hand, if the physician believes that, based on the medical literature, the patient's continued use of one or more CAM therapies is medically inadvisable, and the patient insists on using such therapies against medical advice, this event should be documented in the medical record. Such a record may help show the patient's involvement in selection and use of such therapies. Physicians should familiarize themselves with documentation standards suggested by the Federation of State Medical Board Guidelines, and whether these are applicable in their state or home institution.

Assumption of Risk. As noted above, competent patients have the right to make decisions that others consider ill-advised. Under the doctrine of voluntary assumption of risk, a patient who requests or consents to a novel or high-risk procedure may do so, so long as the decision is voluntary and based on adequate information. For assumption of risk to apply as a defense to a malpractice claim, it must be shown that the injured party knew that there was a risk, understood the nature of the risk, and voluntarily agreed to undertake it.[14(pp480–498)]

Assumption of risk has been allowed in at least one case involving patient election of a CAM therapy instead of conventional care (i.e., of a nutritional protocol in lieu of conventional oncology care).[113] In this case, the court allowed the patient's signing of an appropriate consent form to serve as an "express" assumption of risk and therefore a complete defense to the claim of medical malpractice. In another case, a New York court found that the patient had "impliedly" assumed the risk because she was aware of and voluntarily chose a CAM protocol for cancer care, even without signing the requisite form.[114] Most courts, however, disfavor waivers of negligence,[115] and many might not allow either express or implied assumption of risk as a defense to a malpractice claim involving CAM therapies. It has been said in terms of consent, that "the patient can not sign away their constitutional rights." Physicians should, nonetheless, engage in clear conversations with patients concerning options involving CAM therapies, since such an approach is likely to satisfy informed consent concerns, respect an ideal of shared decision making, and encourage positive relationships that can help mitigate the prospect of litigation.

ETHICAL ISSUES

The dominant ethical principles in medicine are nonmaleficence (doing no harm), beneficence (acting for the good of the patient), and autonomy (promoting the patient's independence and freedom of choice regarding treatment).[116-119] Conventional medicine and CAM share these same ethical principles and the same clinical goals of curing disease, relieving suffering, and promoting the quality of life.

Ethical issues in CAM may arise when a patient requests an alternative treatment that the physician does not endorse, or when the patient refuses a treatment that the physician feels is best. Others relate to the dissemination of information, that is, does a conventional physician have an obligation to inform a patient with back pain that chiropractic or acupuncture may help the condition? Courts by and large have not explicitly imposed a legal obligation on conventional physicians to provide information about CAM therapies, although as individual CAM therapies become more widely used and accepted, such an obligation may be imposed.[120]

While the legal obligation to provide such information is not well-established, it should be kept in mind that legal and ethical obligations are not always the same. Patient autonomy and risk management arguments can be made for providing that information. As discussed in the section on informed consent, patients have a right to information as to the risks and benefits of proposed treatments, CAM therapies, and no treatment. That includes treatments that the clinician does not offer or even fully endorse. An important part of this obligation is the provision of information about the risks of CAM therapies,[121,122] the extent to which their efficacy has been demonstrated,[123] and their risks and benefits, relative to conventional treatments. Clinical experience and research evidence show that patients want to hear the options, but they also want to hear what their physician recommends and frequently base their decisions upon it.[124] The sharing of information about CAM therapies strengthens, rather than dilutes, the physician-patient relationship. Physicians who disagree with patient choices may choose not to treat those patients, but preferably will see whether they can engage their patients in shared decision making while continuing to monitor and treat conventionally when necessary. If this fails, referral can be made to a provider who can fulfill these functions.[125]

Finally, as a matter of nonmaleficence and beneficence, as well as good clinical practice, physicians should maintain an ongoing record of what medications, herbal and mineral supplements, and other treatments a patient may be utilizing. This provides an opportunity to review and discuss the relative risks and benefits of these treatments, and, as suggested earlier, to assess for possible drug interactions.[126]

For a complete, book-length review of all the ethical and legal issues relevant to the practice of CAM in integrative medicine please see the current text by Cohen, Ruggie, and Micozzi, *Practice of Integrative Medicine: A Legal and Operational Guide*.[127]

CONCLUSION

Generally, physicians should inform and engage patients in shared decision making about the option of trying CAM therapies that have reasonable support in the medical literature concerning safety and efficacy. Nutritional, exercise and lifestyle, and mind-body approaches may be viable ways to help patients empower themselves and augment conventional medical care with self-care. At the same time, physicians should monitor patients conventionally and be prepared to intervene conventionally when medically necessary. On the other hand, physicians should discourage patients from CAM therapies that the literature suggests may be unsafe or inefficacious. Such an approach respects patient interest in autonomy and choice, expands the repertoire of medical alternatives, incorporates health and wellness concepts, yet preserves the duty to do no harm. The suggested approach also makes sense from the standpoint of trying to minimize risk of potential malpractice liability.

REFERENCES

1. Barnes PM, Powell-Griner E, McFann K, et al. Trends in alternative medicine use in the United States: results of a follow-up national survey. U.S. National Center for Health Statistics and Centers for Disease Control. 2004
2. Ruggie M. *Marginal to Mainstream: Alternative Medicine in America*. Cambridge, MA: Cambridge University Press; 2004.
3. Kessler RC, Soukup J, Davis RB, et al. The use of complementary and alternative therapies to treat anxiety and depression in the United States. *Am J Psychiatry.* 2001;12:289–294.
4. Cohen MH, Eisenberg DM. Potential physician malpractice liability associated with complementary and integrative medical therapies. *Ann Intern Med.* 2002;596–603.

5. Doyle A. Alternative medicine and medical malpractice. *J Leg Med.* 2001;169:533–552.
6. Studdert DM, Mello MM, Brennan TA. Medical malpractice. *N Engl J Med.* 2004; 7:283–292.
7. GAO. Medical Malpractice Insurance: Multiple Factors Have Contributed to Increased Premium Rates. 2003.
8. Cassidy C. Social and cultural factors In: Micozzi MS, ed. *Fundamentals of Complementary and Integrative Medicine.* 3rd ed. St Louis, MO: Elsevier, 2006:27–52.
9. Studdert DM, Mello MM, Brennan TA. Medical malpractice. *N Engl J Med.* 2004;283–292.
10. Gittler GJ, Goldstein EJ. The elements of medical malpractice: an overview. *Clin Infect Dis.* 1996;8:1152–1155.
11. Schwartz WB, Komesar NK. Doctors, damages and deterrence. An economic view of medical malpractice. *N Engl J Med.* 1978;37:1282–1289.
12. Lang DM. Sexual malpractice and professional liability: some things they don't teach in medical school—a critical examination of the formative case law. *Conn Insur Law J.* 1999;151–186.
13. Rice WE. Article: insurance contracts and judicial discord over whether liability insurers must defend insureds' allegedly intentional and immoral conduct: a historical and empirical review of federal and state courts' declaratory judgments—1900–1997. *Am University Law Rev.* 1998;1131–1219.
14. Keeton WP. Prosser and Keeton on torts. In: Prosser, F, and Keeton,WP, eds. *Prosser and Keeton on the Law of Torts.* St. Paul, MN: West Publishing; 1984;239–242.
15. *Dolan v. Galluzo.* [379 N.E. 2d 795 (Ill. Ct. App. 1978, aff'd 396 N.E. 2d 13 (Ill. 1979)]. 1978. N.E.2d, Illinois Court of Appeals.
16. Cohen MH. *Complementary and Alternative Medicine: Legal Boundaries and Regulatory Perspectives.* Baltimore, MD, and London, England: Johns Hopkins University Press; 1998.
17. Feasby C. Determining standard of care in alternative contexts. *Health Law J.* 1997; 45–65.
18. Karlson HC, Erwin RD. Medical malpractice: informed consent to the locality rule. *Indiana Law Rev.* 1979;181:653–685.
19. *Mackey v. Greenview Hospital, Inc.* 249[587]. 1979. S.W.2d, Kentucky Court of Appeals.
20. *Keir v. United States.* 398[853]. 1988. F.2d, Sixth Circuit Court of Appeals.
21. *Rivera v. E.L.A.* 890[99]. 1971. D.P.R.
22. Wright RW. Causation, responsibility, risk, probability, naked statistics, and proof: pruning the bramble bush by clarifying the concepts. *Iowa Law Rev.* 1988;1001–1077.
23. Lewin JL. The genesis and evolution of legal uncertainty about "reasonable medical certainty." *University Of Maryland Law Rev.* 1998;380–502.
24. Cole CA, McCoy LA. Health care litigation: a common theory of noneconomic damages compensation. *Med Staff Couns.* 1991.
25. Garwin MJ. Risk creation, loss of chance, and legal liability. *Hematol Oncol Clin North Am.* 2002;1351–1363.
26. *Brown v Willington.* Negligence—Failure to carry out physical examination and biopsy—Damages for loss of chance of extended lifespan. [2001] ACTSC 100. *J Law Med.* 2002;397–398.
27. Studdert D, Eisenberg D, Miller F, et al. Medical malpractice implications of alternative medicine. *JAMA.* 1998;1620–1625.
28. Silverstein D, Spiegel A. Are physicians aware of the risks of alternative medicine? *J Community Health.* 2001;159–161.

29. Tracy TF Jr, Crawford LS, Krizek TJ, Kern KA. When medical error becomes medical malpractice: the victims and the circumstances. *Arch Surg.* 2003;447–454.

30. Perez Torres v. Dr. Wallace Balduell Ramos. 88[88], 4. 1988. J.T.S., Puerto Rico Perez Torres v. Dr. Wallace Balduell Ramos.

31. Klerman GL. The psychiatric patient's right to effective treatment: implications of Osheroff v. Chestnut Lodge. *Am J Psychiatry.* 1990;6:409–418.

32. Stone AA. Law, science, and psychiatric malpractice: a response to Klerman's indictment of psychoanalytic psychiatry. *Am J Psychiatry.* 1990;16:419–427.

33. Koertge J, Weidner G, Elliott-Eller M, et al. Improvement in medical risk factors and quality of life in women and men with coronary artery disease in the Multicenter Lifestyle Demonstration Project. *Am J Cardiol.* 2003;1316–1322.

34. Ornish D, Scherwitz LW, Billings JH, et al. Intensive lifestyle changes for reversal of coronary heart disease. *JAMA.* 1998;2001–2007.

35. Fentiman LC, Kaufman G, Merton V, Teitell EF, Zonana H. Current issues in the psychiatrist-patient relationship: outpatient civil commitment, psychiatric abandonment and the duty to continue treatment of potentially dangerous patients—balancing duties to patients and the public. *Pace Law Rev.* 2000;231–262.

36. Gerber PC. Abandonment and the nonpaying patient. *Physicians Manage.* 1984;86–83,96.

37. Gutheil TG, Simon RI. Abandonment of patients in split treatment. *Harv Rev Psychiatry.* 2003;175–179.

38. Hongsathavij v. Queen of Angels/Hollywood Presbyterian Med. Ctr. (1998). 695[62 Cal. App. 4th 1123, 1138, 73 Cal. Rptr. 2d 695, 704]. 1998.

39. *Black's Law Dictionary.* In: 1990;1311.

40. Jorgenson LM, Sutherland PK, Bisbing SB. Transference of liability: employer liability for sexual misconduct by therapists. *Brooklyn Law Rev.* 1995;1421–1481.

41. Schouten R. Legal aspects of consultation. In: Cassem NH, Stern TA, Rosenbaum JF, Jellinek MS, eds. *Massachusetts General Hospital Handbook of General Hospital Psychiatry.* St. Louis, MO: Mosby-Year Book, 1997;415–436.

42. Fox BC, Siegel ML, Weinstein RA. "Curbside" consultation and informal communication in medical practice: a medicolegal perspective 435. *Clin Infect Dis.* 1996;616–622.

43. Sederer L, Ellison J, Keyes C. Guidelines for prescribing psychiatrists in consultative, collaborative, and supervisory relationships. *Psychiatric Services.* 1998;1197–1202.

44. Cohen MH. Malpractice and vicarious liability for providers of complementary & alternative medicine. *Benders Health Care Law Mon.* 1996;3–13.

45. Josefek K. Alternative medicine's roadmap to mainstream. *Am J of Law and Med.* 2000; 295.

46. Cohen MH. *Beyond Complementary Medicine: Legal and Ethical Perspectives on Health Care and Human Evolution.* Ann Arbor, MI: University of Michigan Press; 2000.

47. Eisenberg DM, Cohen MH, Hrbek A, Grayzel J, van Rompay MI, Cooper RA. Credentialing complementary and alternative medical providers. *Ann Intern Med.* 2002;965–973.

48. Ryan M. Medical malpractice: a review of issues for providers. *Hematol Oncol Clin North Am.* 2002;106:1331–1350.

49. Torres A, Proper S. Medicolegal developments and the dermatologist. *Adv Dermatol.* 1997;299–322.

50. Health Insurance Portability and Accountability Act of 1996. Public Law 104–191. 1996.

51. Office of the Secretary DoHaHS. Standards for privacy of individually identifiable health information. 67:53182–53273. Federal Register 2002.

52. Brendel RW, Bryan E. HIPAA for Psychiatrists. *Harv RevPsychiatry.* 2004.

53. Stone J. Ethical issues in complementary and alternative medicine. *Complement Ther Med*. 2000;207–213.

54. Beck JC. Legal and ethical duties of the clinician treating a patient who is liable to be impulsively violent. *Behavioral Sciences and the Law*. 1998;375–389.

55. Kennedy I. Duty to warn third parties: Bradshaw v. Daniel. *Med Law Rev*. 1994;237–239.

56. McAbee FB. Physician's duty to warn third parties about the risk of genetic diseases. *Pediatrics*. 1998;140–142.

57. Schloendorff v. Society of New York Hospital. 92[105]. 1914. Northeast Reporter.

58. Schouten R. Informed consent: resistance and reappraisal. *Critical Care Med*. 2004; 1359–1361.

59. Monaco GP, Smith G. Informed consent in complementary and alternative medicine: current status and future needs. *Semins Oncol*. 2002;1:601–608.

60. Ubel PA. "What should I do, Doc?": some psychologic benefits of physician recommendations. *Arch of Intern Med*. 2002;977–980.

61. English DC. Valid informed consent: a process, not a signature 72. *Am Surgeon*. 2002; 45–48.

62. *Precourt v. Frederick*. [481], 1144. 1985. Northeast Reporter 2d, Massachusetts Supreme Judicial Court.

63. Appelbaum PS, Lidz CW, Meisel A. *Informed Consent: Legal Theory and Clinical Practice*. New York, NY: Oxford University Press, 1987.

64. *Harnish v. Children's Hospital Medical Center*. [439], 240. 1982. Northeast 2d, Massachusetts Supreme Judicial Court.

65. *Moore v. Baker*, 98 F.2d 1129 (11th Circuit 1993). 1129[98]. 1993. F.2d, 11th Circuit.

66. Schouten RDKS. Medical-legal and ethical issues in the pharmacological treatment of children. In: Werry JSAMG, ed. *Practitioner's Guide to Psychoactive Drugs in Children and Adolescents*. New York, NY: Plenum Publishing; 1993:161–178.

67. Grisso T, Appelbaum PS. *Assessing Competence to Consent to Treatment: A Guide for Physicians and Other Health Professionals*. New York, NY: Oxford Univesity Press; 1998.

68. Brock DW, Wartman SA. When competent patients make irrational choices. *N Engl J of Med*. 1990;1595–1599.

69. Kerridge I, Lowe M, Mitchell K. Competent patients, incompetent decisions. *Ann Intern Med*. 1995;878–881.

70. Moskop JC. Informed consent in the emergency department. *Emerg Med Clin North Am* 1999;22:327–329.

71. Nora LM, Benvenuti RJ, III. Medicolegal aspects of informed consent. *Neurol Clin*. 1998;26:207–216.

72. Sprung CL, Winick BJ. Informed consent in theory and practice: legal and medical perspectives on the informed consent doctrine and a proposed reconceptualization. *Crit Care Med*. 1989;43:1346–1354.

73. *Shine v. Vega*. [709], 58. 1999. Northeastern Reporter 2d, Massachusetts Supreme Judcicial Court.

74. Roth LH, Meisel A, Lidz CW. Tests of competency to consent to treatment. *Am J Psychiatry*. 1977;279–284.

75. President's Commission for the Study of Ethical Problems in Medicine and Biomedical and Behavioral Research. Making Health Care Decisions: A Report on the Ethical and Legal Implications of Informed Consent in the Patient-Practitioner Relationship. 1982. Washington, DC: U.S. Government Printing Office.

76. *Rogers v. Commissioner of Department of Mental Health*. Mass Rep Mass Supreme Judic Court. 1983;489–513.

77. *Canterbury v. Spence.* 772[464]. 1972. F.2d, D.C. Cir. *cert. denied,* 409 U.S. 1064.
78. Dickerson DA. A doctor's duty to disclose life expectancy information to terminally ill patients. *Cleveland State Law Rev.* 1995;319–350.
79. Beck JM, Azari ED. FDA, off-label use, and informed consent: debunking myths and misconceptions. *Food Drug Law J.* 1998;71–104.
80. Choonara I, Conroy S. Unlicensed and off-label drug use in children: implications for safety. *Drug Saf.* 2002;1–5.
81. Smith JJ, Berlin L. Off-label use of interventional medical devices. *AJR Am J Roentgenol.* 1999;539–542.
82. Federation of State Medical Boards. Model guidelines for the use of complementary and alternative therapies in medical practice. Federation of State Medical Boards. 2002.
83. Council on Ethical and Judicial Affairs. Sexual misconduct in the practice of medicine. American Medical Association. *JAMA* 1991;2741–2745.
84. ACOG Committee. Sexual misconduct in the practice of obstetrics and gynecology: ethical considerations. Opinion No. 144. *ACOG Comm Opin.* 1994;3.
85. Schouten R. Maintaining boundaries in the doctor-patient relationship. In: Stern TA, Herman JB, Slavin PL, eds. *The MGH Guide to Psychiatry in Primary Care.* New York: McGraw Hill, 1998:655–659.
86. Simon R. Therapist-patient sex: from boundary violations to sexual misconduct. *Psychiatr Clin North Am.* 1999;31–47.
87. Bisbing SB, Jorgenson LM, Sutherland PK. Causes of action. In: Jorgenson LM, Sutherland PK, eds. *Sexual Abuse by Professionals: A Legal Guide.* Charlottesville, NC: The Michie Company, 1995:121–154.
88. Bemmann KC, Goodwin J. New laws about sexual misconduct by therapists: knowledge and attitudes among Wisconsin psychiatrists. *Wis Med J.* 1989;11–16.
89. Young JL, Griffith EE. Developments in clergy malpractice: the case of Sanders v. Casa View Baptist Church. *J Am Acad Psychiatry Law.* 1999;143–147.
90. Gutheil T, Jorgenson L, Sutherland P. Prohibiting lawyer-client sex. *Bull Am Acad Psychiatry Law.* 1992;365–382.
91. Cohen MH. *Future Medicine: Ethical Dilemmas, Regulatory Challenges, and Therapeutic Pathways to Health and Healing in Human Transformation.* Ann Arbor, MI: University of Michigan Press, 2003.
92. Snyderman R, Weil AT. Integrative medicine: bringing medicine back to its roots. *Arch Intern Med.* 2002;1:395–397.
93. Charles SC. Coping with a medical malpractice suit. *West J Med.* 2001;271:55–58.
94. Ryan M. Medical malpractice: a review of issues for providers. *Hematol Oncol Clin North Am.* 2002;106:1331–1350.
95. Localio AR, Lawthers AG, Brennan TA, et al. Relation between malpractice claims and adverse events due to negligence. Results of the Harvard Medical Practice Study III. *N Engl J Med.* 1991;245–251.
96. Brennan TA, Hebert LE, Laird NM, et al. Hospital characteristics associated with adverse events and substandard care. *JAMA.* 1991;3265–3269.
97. Gutheil TG, Appelbaum PS. Malpractice and other forms of liability. In: Appelbaum PS, ed. *Clinical Handbook of Psychiatry and the Law.* Philadelphia, PA: Lippincott Williams & Wilkins, 2000:135–214.
98. Localio AR. *Medical malpratice American style: Lies, damned lies, and statistics.* Center for Clinical Epidemiology and Biostatistics, University of Pennsylvania. 4 A.D. 5–15–2003, unpublished manuscript.
99. Adamson TE, Tschann JM, Gullion DS, Oppenberg AA. Physician communication skills and malpractice claims. A complex relationship. *West J Med.* 1989;769:356–360.

100. Moore PJ, Adler NE, Robertson PA. Medical malpractice: the effect of doctor-patient relations on medical patient perceptions and malpractice intentions. *West J Med.* 2000;282:244–250.

101. Charles SC, Gibbons RD, Frisch PR, Pyskoty CE, Hedeker D, Singha NK. Predicting risk for medical malpractice claims using quality-of-care characteristics. *West J Med.* 1992;10:433–439.

102. Levinson W. Physician-patient communication: The relationship with malpractice claims among primary care physicians and surgeons. *JAMA.* 1997;553–559.

103. Gutheil T, Bursztajn H, Brodsky A. Malpractice prevention through the sharing of uncertainty. *N Engl J of Med.* 1984;49–51.

104. Kellett AJ. Healing angry wounds: the roles of apology and mediation in disputes between physicians and patients. *Spec Law Dig Health Care (Mon.)* 1989;7–27.

105. Finkelstein D, Wu AW, Holtzman NA, Smith MK. When a physician harms a patient by a medical error: ethical, legal, and risk-management considerations. *J Clin Ethics.* 1997;330–335.

106. Blackston JW, Bouldin MJ, Brown CA, Duddleston DN, Hicks GS, Holman HE. Malpractice risk prevention for primary care physicians. *Am J Med Sci.* 2002;117:212–219.

107. Frank-Stromborg M, Bailey LJ. Cancer screening and early detection: managing malpractice risk. *Cancer Pract.* 1998;206–216.

108. Ernst E. Second thoughts about safety of St John's wort. *Lancet.* 1999;2014–2016.

109. Fugh-Berman A. Herb-drug interactions. *Lancet.* 2000;134–138.

110. Piscitelli SC, Burstein AH, Chaitt D, Alfaro RM, Falloon J. Indinavir concentrations and St John's wort. *Lancet.* 2000;547–548.

111. Alford DM. The clinical record: recognizing its value in litigation. *Geriatr Nurs.* 2003;228–230.

112. Weintraub MI. Documentation and informed consent. *Neurol Clin.* 1999;371–381.

113. *Schneider v. Revici* . 987[817]. 1987. Federal Reporter 2d, Second Circuit.

114. *Charell v. Gonzales.* 665[660]. 1997. New York Supplement 2d], S.Ct., N.Y. County. Affirmed and modified to vacate punitive damages award, 673 New York Supplement 2d 685 (App Div., 1st Dept., 1998), reargument denied, appeal denied, 1998 New York Appellate Division LEXIS 10711 (App. Div., 1st Dept., 1998), appeal denied, 706 Northeastern Reporter 2d 1211 (1998).

115. *Tunkl v. Regents of the Univ. of California.* 441[383]. 1963. Pacific Reporter 2d, California Supreme Court.

116. Sade RM. Autonomy and beneficence in an information age. *Health Care Anal.* 2001;247–254.

117. Ethics Committee, Society for Academic Emergency Medicine. An ethical foundation for health care: an emergency medicine perspective. *Ann Emerg Med.* 1992;1381–1387.

118. American College of Obstetrics and Gynecology. Ethical decision-making in obstetrics and gynecology. *ACOG Tech Bull.* 1989;1–7.

119. Blustein J. Doing what the patient orders: maintaining integrity in the doctor-patient relationship. *Bioethics.* 1993;290–314.

120. Ernst E, Cohen MH. Informed consent in complementary and alternative medicine. *Arch Intern Med.* 2001;2288–2292.

121. Ernst E. The risk-benefit profile of commonly used herbal therapies: ginkgo, st. john's wort, ginseng, echinacea, saw palmetto, and kava. *Ann Intern Med.* 2002;42–53.

122. Ernst E. Complementary medicine: where is the evidence? *J Fam Pract.* 2003;630–634.

123. Thompson Coon JS, Ernst E. Herbs for serum cholesterol reduction: a systematic view. *J Fam Pract.* 2003;468–478.

124. Ende J, Kazis L, Ash A, Moskowitz MA. Measuring patients' desire for autonomy: decision making and information-seeking preferences among medical patients. *J Gen Intern Med.* 1989;23–30.
125. Adams KE, Cohen MH, Jonsen AR, Eisenberg DM. Ethical considerations of complementary and alternative medical therapies in conventional medical settings. *Ann Intern Med.* 2002;660–664.
126. Sugarman J, Burk L. Physicians' ethical obligations regarding alternative medicine. *JAMA.* 1998;1623–1625.
127. Cohen M, Ruggie M, Micozzi M. *The Practice of Integrative Medicine: A Legal and Operational Guide.* New York: NY: Springer Publishing; 2007.

Index